Cognitive-Communication
Disorders of Dementia

Cognitive-Communication Disorders of Dementia

Kathryn A. Bayles, Ph.D., CCC-SLP
Cheryl K. Tomoeda, M.S., CCC-SLP

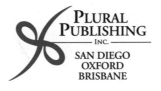

PLURAL
PUBLISHING
INC.

SAN DIEGO
OXFORD
BRISBANE

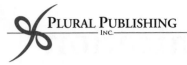

5521 Ruffin Road
San Diego, CA 92123

e-mail: info@pluralpublishing.com
Web site: http://www.pluralpublishing.com
49 Bath Street

Abingdon, Oxfordshire OX14 1EA
United Kingdom

Typeset in 10½/13 Palatino by Flanagan's Publishing Services, Inc.
Printed in the United States of America by McNaughton and Gunn

Library of Congress Cataloging-in-Publication Data:

Bayles, Kathryn.
    Cognitive-communication disorders of dementia / Kathryn Bayles and Cheryl Tomoeda.
        p. ; cm.
    Includes bibliographical references.
    ISBN-13: 978-1-59756-111-2 (hardcover : alk. paper)
    ISBN-10: 1-59756-111-8 (hardcover : alk. paper)
  1. Dementia—Complications. 2. Cognition disorders in old age. 3. Communicative
disorders in old age.   I. Tomoeda, Cheryl K. II. Title.
    [DNLM: 1. Dementia—complications. 2. Cognition Disorders—diagnosis. 3. Cognition
Disorders—etiology. 4. Cognition Disorders—therapy. 5. Communication Disorders—
diagnosis. 6. Communication Disorders—etiology. 7. Communication Disorders—therapy.
WM 220 B358c 2007]
    RC521.B393 2007
    616.8'3—dc22

                                                                        2007007594

Contents

Preface

This book is designed to provide students and practicing professionals the knowledge needed to diagnose and treat dementia-associated communication disorders. Whereas only meager information about the behavioral sequelae of dementing diseases was available 40 years ago, a voluminous literature exists today. And, whereas information on dementia was almost never included in speech, language, and hearing science program curricula, even 20 years ago, the American Speech-Language-Hearing Association now requires it for program accreditation. To become certified, graduate students must provide documentation of coursework on the cognitive-communicative disorders associated with dementing diseases. This knowledge requirement is highly appropriate because dementia is the premier challenge facing health care providers in the 21st century. Whereas the prevalence of individuals with dementia rose steadily in the last half of the 20th century, it will explode in the 21st century with the graying of the baby boomers and elderly population worldwide. Communicative function is inevitably affected when an individual has memory and other intellectual deficits sufficient to meet the diagnostic criteria for dementia. In short, individuals with the cognitive-communicative disorders of dementia are the profession's fastest growing clinical population.

Organization of Text

The text can be divided conceptually into four topic areas:

1. Cognition and communication
2. Dementing diseases and their effects on cognition and communication
3. Assessment of cognitive-communicative function
4. Treatment of cognitive-communication disorders

Cognition and Communication— Chapters 1 to 3

Chapter 1 is a short chapter in which the syndrome of dementia is defined and the primary dementing diseases specified. Throughout the book are references to neuroanatomic structures and **Chapter 2** by Sarah Orjada provides a review of neuroanatomy and the neural bases of cognition and language. Chapter 2 also contains a discussion of aphasia types and neuroimaging procedures. The topic of **Chapter 3** is communication and cognition. Its purpose is to provide the reader an understanding of cognition and the relation of cognition to communication. Because cognition is affected by normal aging, the chapter contains an overview of aging and cognitive-communicative functioning to assist clinicians in differentiating individuals with mild dementia from healthy elders.

Dementing Diseases— Chapters 4 to 10

Each dementing disease has unique pathology, the distribution of which accounts for a characteristic cognitive-communication disorder. **Chapters 4** through **10** are devoted to explaining the primary dementia producing diseases likely to be seen by the speech-language pathologist: Alzheimer's, Down syndrome, vascular, Parkinson's, Lewy body, Huntington's, and frontotemporal degeneration. These chapters follow a similar topical format: diagnostic criteria, neuropathology, risk factors, effects on cognitive and communicative functioning, and a summary of key points.

Assessment—Chapter 11

Assessment of cognitive-communicative disorders of dementia is the focus of **Chapter 11**. It begins with a discussion of the process of assessment followed by a discussion of tests appropriate for screening and comprehensive evaluation of cognitive-communicative functioning. The third segment of the chapter contains information about differentiating Alzheimer's dementia, the most common form, from normal aging, delirium, depression, the behavioral and language variants of frontotemporal dementia, vascular dementia, and Lewy body dementia.

Treatment—Chapters 12 to 14

Chapters **12**, **13**, and **14** are devoted to the treatment of cognitive-communication disorders of dementia and care planning. In **Chapter 12** the focus is on empirically based, *direct* interventions that are carried out by the clinician with the patient. Readers will learn many techniques for facilitating information processing (learning and retrieval) and the communicative functioning of individuals with dementia. Also included are guidelines for planning treatment. *Indirect* interventions, or those recommended by clinicians but carried out by other caregivers, are the focus of **Chapter 13**. Indirect interventions are subcategorized as linguistic

manipulations that improve language comprehension and production and environmental manipulations that support function. In **Chapter 14** the reader is familiarized with the laws governing the provision of services to residents of long-term care facilities, the use of test performance data to develop treatment plans, and the importance of documentation. Sample treatment plans for a mild and moderate Alzheimer's dementia patient are included. Good clinical practice requires consideration of the caregiver as well as the patient with dementia. Thus, this chapter also contains a section on caregiving and the importance of caregiver counseling.

Appendix: Culture and Dementia

Ours is a culturally diverse society and consideration of culture is crucial to management of individuals with dementia and their caregivers. The Appendix contains a listing of the ASHA specified knowledge needed for achieving cultural competence. The foundation for cultural competence is understanding one's own cultural identity and Appendix A contains an exercise to help readers gain insight to their cultural orientation. Many, if not most readers will be American, thus a summary of the values held by the majority of Americans is included. The characteristics of the major cultural groups in the United States follow with suggestions for providing culturally sensitive care. The Appendix concludes with guidelines for using interpreters and resources for learning more about cultural diversity and intercultural skill building.

Use of the Text

The authors have tried to provide a comprehensive and up-to-date account of the cognitive-communication disorders associated with dementia-producing diseases. Understanding the diseases and how they affect communicative functioning requires knowledge of the brain and cognition. Thus the first unit of the book is a primer on the brain, cognition, and the neural bases of cognition and communication. Memory systems are well described because of the profound effects of dementing diseases on memory and the fact that patient function can often be improved by using spared memory systems to compensate for those impaired. Whereas all readers may not need the information in Chapter 2, on the neural bases of cognition and language, the information in Chapter 3, on cognition and communication, is essential to the rest of the book. If the topic of dementia is one of many in a course, and time is limited, the instructor can focus on certain of the dementing diseases. Because Alzheimer's disease is the most common cause of dementia and more is published about it than other dementing diseases, we recommend including Chapter 4 in a unit on dementia. The information in Chapter 12 on strategies for improving information processing is relevant to therapy planning for all types of language disorders whereas the information in Chapter 13 is more specific to the management of individuals with dementia, as is the information in Chapter 14.

Throughout the text, less familiar terms are defined and important information is highlighted in boxes. Also, the headings in text provide a guide to the logic of the chapters for both instructors and students. At the end of each chapter is a summary of important points. Their review will provide instructors, students, and practicing professionals a good overview of the chapter's content. In sum, our goal in writing the book is to improve the knowledge of students and practicing professionals for the benefit of the millions of individuals with dementing diseases.

Acknowledgments

Writing a technical book is an awesome enterprise, and many individuals helped make it a reality. First, we thank Sarah Orjada for the chapter on the neural bases of cognition and communication. Katie Leake, Alyssa Glanzman, and Michelle Gutmann provided assistance with literature searches, proofreading, formatting, and obtaining permissions. We also thank the National Institute on Aging (NIH-NIA), the National Institute on Mental Health (NIMH), the AARP— Andrus Foundation, the Robert Wood Johnson Foundation, and the University of Arizona Vice President for Research Office that funded our research studies, the data from which form the foundation of this book. Without the commitment to research of many individuals with dementia and their caregivers, our research would not have been possible. We are indebted to these selfless individuals.

Words alone are inadequate to express our thanks to family members for their support while we burned the proverbial midnight oil to write this book. Bob, Zachary, Jackson, and Sandy, your support was invaluable. In closing, we dedicate this book to friends and members who have modeled how to age gracefully and cope with dementia. You are our inspiration.

Kathryn Bayles, Ph.D.
Cheryl Tomoeda, M.S.

Contributor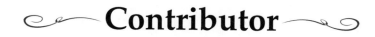

Sarah A. Orjada, M.A., CCC-SLP
Doctoral Candidate
University of Arizona
Department of Speech, Language, and Hearing Sciences
Tuscon, Arizona
Chapter 2

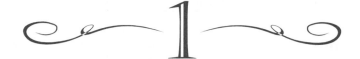

Introduction to Dementia

Dementia Is a Syndrome

Dementia is a syndrome. In medical terms, a syndrome is a constellation of signs and symptoms associated with a morbid process. The word "dementia" comes from the Latin phrase *de* (out of) *mens* (mind) and over the centuries has been associated with various mental abnormalities. Today the term is used to refer to a characteristic pattern of mental and behavioral impairment defined by the American Psychiatric Association's DSM-IV-TR (American Psychiatric Association, 2000). According to the DSM-IV-TR criteria, the clinical features necessary for the diagnosis of dementia are *multiple* deficits manifested by memory impairment and one or more of the following cognitive disturbances: aphasia, apraxia, agnosia, or disturbance in executive functioning. These cognitive impairments must be sufficient to interfere with social and occupational functioning and occur in the absence of delirium. Because many diseases and conditions are associated with the dementia syndrome (Table 1–1), there are additional disease specific criteria in the DSM-IV-TR that are provided in the book chapters on the primary dementia-producing diseases.

Table 1–1. Primary Causes of Dementia

Irreversible Causes	Reversible Causes
Alzheimer's disease	Infection
Pick's disease	Drug toxicity
Frontotemporal degeneration	Vitamin deficiency
Creutzfeldt-Jakob's disease	Tumor
Huntington's disease	Depression
Multiple infarctions	Normal pressure hydrocephalus
Vascular disease	Renal failure
Wilson's disease	Congestive heart failure
Parkinson's disease	Thyroid disease
Lewy body disease	Hypoglycemia
Binswanger's disease	Syphilis

Causes of Dementia

The most common cause of dementia is Alzheimer's disease (AD), accounting for half the cases. Other common causes are vascular disease (VaD), Lewy body disease (LBD), and Parkinson's disease (PD). Although VaD is widely regarded as the second most common cause, recent evidence suggests that pure vascular dementia is uncommon (Nolan, Lino, Seligman, & Blass, 1998). Many experts now consider "mixed" dementia, in which vascular disease and Alzheimer's disease co-occur, as the second most common cause (Bowler, Munoz, Merskey, & Hackinski, 1998; Snowdon, 1997). Epidemiologists also believe LBD to be considerably more common than previously recognized and may challenge vascular disease as the second most common cause of dementia. Like VaD, LBD can co-occur with AD. Gearing, Schneider, Rebeck, Hyman, and Mirra (1995) reported the presence of Lewy bodies in as many as 20% of AD cases coming to autopsy.

Individuals with PD can develop dementia though not all do. Determining the frequency of dementia in individuals with PD and an individual's risk for dementia have been the goals of many epidemiologic investigations. Both age and duration of disease appear important in the calculation of risk. Older age at onset and longer duration are associated with increased risk. Aarsland, Anderson, Larsen, Lolk, and Kragh-Sorensen (2003) conducted a prospective study of the prevalence of dementia in a community-based population after four and eight years of follow-up. At baseline testing, 26% of the 224 individuals with PD were judged to have dementia, after four years, 52%, and after eight years, 78%. Mayeux and colleagues (1990) reported a cumulative risk of dementia in persons with PD of 65% by age 85. Estimates from these two studies are higher than the 38% reported by Hughes and colleagues (2000) who studied individuals who came to a health clinic over a 10-year period. These quite variable results are likely due to differences in the definitions of dementia used by the investigators and the age and duration of disease in subjects studied.

Prevalence of Dementia Increasing

Because dementia is associated with many age-related diseases, its prevalence has steadily risen with the growth in the elderly segment of the population. And, as the "baby boom" generation reaches 65, the number of individuals with dementia will rise dramatically. Health care planners estimate that the number of new cases of AD alone will double annually, and by the year 2050, 14 million elderly Americans will carry the diagnosis of Alzheimer's dementia (Figure 1–1).

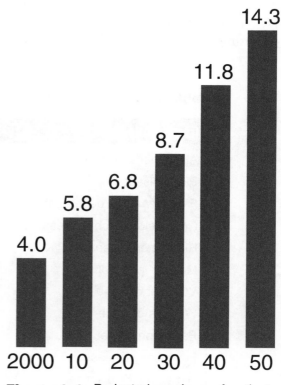

Figure 1–1. Projected numbers of patients with Alzheimer's disease in the U.S., in millions.

Many dementia patients live for more than a decade after diagnosis and the current cost of caring for them is staggering, $100 billion annually (National Institute on Aging, 2003). In the early stages of dementia, the cost comes from the loss of the affected individual's productivity in the workforce and often that of family caregivers. In the late stages, the cost comes mainly from the expense of institutionalization. This dramatic rise in the prevalence of dementia is the major challenge facing health care professionals in the United States and, indeed, worldwide.

Role of the Speech-Language Pathologist

Thirty years ago, most Americans, including speech-language pathologists (SLPs), were unfamiliar with dementia. Few clinicians had training in the provision of care for individuals with dementia. However, as the number of people with dementia increased, demand for services increased. Legislators, health care professionals, and researchers responded. Today a vast literature on dementia exists and many more resources are available to persons with dementia and their families.

Beginning in the mid-1970s, SLPs were increasingly called on to evaluate the cognitive-communicative and swallowing disorders associated with dementing diseases. The first formal recognition of the role of SLPs in treating individuals with cognitive impairments, among them those associated with dementia, came in 1987 when the American Speech-Language-Hearing Association (ASHA) published a technical report on the habilitation and rehabilitation of cognitively impaired individuals (ASHA, 1987). This document made explicit the inextricable relation between cognition and language, "The interrelationship between cognition and language serves as the basis for effective communication. A cognitive impairment can result in a communication breakdown, requiring speech-language intervention to improve functional ability" (p. 53). Between 1975 and 2005, ASHA produced several documents elaborating the role of SLPs with individuals with cognitive-communicative impairments (see Bayles et al., 2005 for a review). Most recently, ASHA (2005) published a technical report entitled, "The Roles of Speech-Language Pathologists Working with Individuals with Dementia-Based Communication Disorders," in which SLPs were stated to have a primary role in screening, assessment, and treatment as well as a role in caregiver training and counseling. The purpose of this book is to provide clinicians and practicing professionals the information needed to carry out these roles.

Summary of Important Points

- Dementia is a syndrome, not a disease.
- The key feature that defines dementia is the presence of multiple cognitive deficits sufficient to interfere with social and occupational functioning.
- Many diseases produce dementia, the most common of which is Alzheimer's disease.
- Some causes of dementia are reversible, most are not.
- With the advent of pharmacologic treatments, it is important to diagnose dementia early so affected individuals can receive treatment.
- The prevalence of dementia is increasing because of the disproportionate growth of the elderly population.
- The cost of caring for individuals with dementia is extremely high and challenges health care professionals worldwide.
- Speech-language pathologists have a role in screening for dementia, assessing its

effect on cognition, communication, and swallowing, and facilitating function.

- The American Speech-Language-Hearing Association has published documents specifying the role of SLPs with individuals with dementia and a listing of the knowledge and skills needed to be clinically proficient with this population.

References

Aarsland, D., Anderson, K., Larsen, J. P., Lolk, A., & Kragh-Sorensen, P. (2003). Prevalence and characteristics of dementia in Parkinson's disease: An 8-year prospective study. *Archives of Neurology, 60*, 387–392.

American Psychiatric Association. (2000). *Diagnostic and statistical manual of mental disorders DSM-IV-TR.* Washington, DC: Author.

American Speech-Language-Hearing Association. (1987). Role of speech-language pathologists in the habilitation and rehabilitation of cognitively impaired individuals. *Asha, 29*, 53–55.

American Speech-Language-Hearing Association. (2005). *The roles of speech-language pathologists working with individuals with dementia-based communication disorders: Position statement.* Rockville, MD: Author.

Bayles, K., Kim, E., Azuma, T., Chapman, S., Cleary, S., Hopper, T., et al. (2005). Developing evidence-based practice guidelines for speech-language pathologists serving individuals with Alzheimer's dementia. *Journal of Medical Speech-Language Pathology, 13*, xiii–xxv.

Bowler, J.V., Munoz, D.G., Merskey, H., & Hachinski, V. (1998) Fallacies in the pathological confirmation of the diagnosis of Alzheimer's disease. *Journal of Neurology, Neurosurgery, and Psychiatry, 64*, 18–24.

Gearing, M., Schneider, J. A., Rebeck, G. W., Hyman, B. T., & Mirra, S. S. (1995). Alzheimer's disease with and without coexisting Parkinson's disease changes: Apolipoprotein E genotype and neuropathologic correlates. *Neurology, 45*, 1985–1990.

Hughes, T. A., Ross, H. F., Musa, S., Bhattacherjee, S., Nathan, R. N., Mindham, R. H., et al. (2000). A 10-year study of the incidence of and factors predicting dementia in Parkinson's disease. *Neurology, 54*, 1596–1602.

Mayeux, R., Chen, J., Mirabello, E., Marder, K., Bell, K., Dooneief, G., et al. (1990). An estimate of the incidence of dementia in idiopathic Parkinson's disease. *Neurology, 40*, 1513–1517.

National Institutes of Health (2003). *2001–2002 Alzheimer's disease progress report.* NIH publication number 03-5333. Washington, DC: Author.

Nolan, K. A., Lino, M. M., Seligman, A.W., & Blass, J. P. (1998). Absence of vascular dementia in an autopsy series from a dementia clinic. *Journal of the American Geriatric Society, 46*, 597–604.

Snowdon, D.A., Greiner, L.H., Mortimer, J.A., Riley, K.P., Greiner, P.A., & Markesbery, W.R. (1997). Brain infarction and the clinical expression of Alzheimer disease. The Nun study, *JAMA, 227*, 813–817.

The Neural Bases of Cognition and Language

Sarah A. Orjada

This introductory neuroanatomy chapter provides information about the neural bases of cognition and language that will be useful in understanding the chapters that follow. Because the focus of this book is cognitive-communication disorders related to dementia, neuroanatomic regions and connections most directly related to language and memory are covered in the greatest detail. The first section is an overview of the nervous system in which key structures, their locations, and general functions are discussed. It is meant to be a reference for information about structures mentioned throughout the book. The second section describes the types of neuroimaging procedures routinely used by researchers and physicians for identifying areas of brain function and damage. Third, emphasis is given to the neural architecture of language and the types of aphasia associated with damage to the left hemisphere of the brain. Finally, a disorder called *agnosia* is briefly discussed, as well as terminologic issues related to cognitive-communication disorders.

Structures of the Nervous System and Their Function

The nervous system consists of a number of different components, each of which performs unique functions. These components are connected by pathways, resulting in a great deal of interaction among parts of the nervous system. For example, the executive system (which is involved in analyzing information, making decisions, and planning actions) and other parts of the brain share extensive connections. This interconnectivity enables us to use information from the environment to guide behavior. In addition, areas of the nervous system important for emotion are highly interconnected, allowing emotion to be associated with sensation, and for that information to be sent to structures associated with the executive system. Major structures and pathways within the nervous system are discussed below, beginning with the most basic unit, the neuron.

The Cells of the Nervous System

The neuron, or nerve cell, is the cell the nervous system uses to process and transmit information. Estimates of the number of neurons in the human brain reach 100 billion, with possibly 10 times more supporting, or glial, cells (Nolte, 2002).

Although some neurons look vastly different from others, most have common identifiable features (Figure 2–1).

The soma, or cell body, contains organelles necessary for the metabolic demands of the neuron. Branching from the soma are dendrites, which collect signals from other neurons and transmit that information *to* the cell body. Neurons differ in the number of extensions, varying from only one or two (unipolar and bipolar neurons, respectively) to an unlimited number of extensions, (multipolar neurons). One type of multipolar neuron that possesses a very complex dendritic tree is the Purkinje cell of the cerebellum (Figure 2–2).

Typically, each neuron has one long process called an axon. The purpose of the axon is to transmit information *away* from the cell body. The axon can divide into a number of terminal branches that "connect" to other neurons over a synapse.

A synapse consists of a space (synaptic cleft) between neurons where information is transmitted from one neuron (presynaptic element) to another (postsynaptic element). The presynaptic element contains synaptic vesicles, which contain chemicals called *neurotransmitters* that are used by the nervous system to convey information. If the presynaptic neuron receives the correct trigger, it will cause the release of neurotransmitters into the synaptic cleft. The neurotransmitters bind with receptors on the postsynaptic end, causing electrical activity to occur in the postsynaptic neuron.

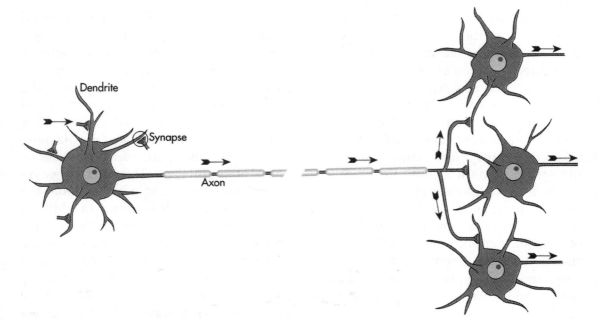

Figure 2–1. Schematic of a typical neuron and its connections to other neurons. Arrows indicate the direction of signal propagation. Reprinted with permission from *The Human Brain: An Introduction to Its Functional Anatomy*, J. Nolte, p. 3. Copyright 2002, Elsevier.

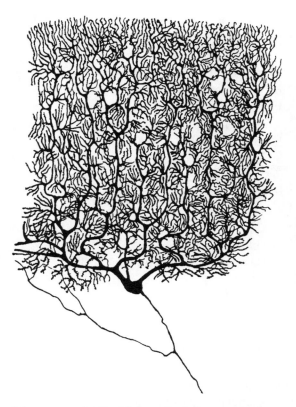

Figure 2–2. Purkinje cell of the cerebellum, demonstrating the complexity of the dendritic tree of one type of multipolar neuron. Reprinted with permission from *The Human Brain: An Introduction to Its Functional Anatomy*, J. Nolte, p. 4. Copyright 2002 Elsevier.

The nervous system utilizes a number of neurotransmitters to facilitate different cognitive functions, four of which are important for this book. The first neurotransmitter to be discovered, called acetylcholine, is most important for learning, memory, and attention. Dopamine is implicated in memory, attention, and executive functioning (such as problem-solving), and dopaminergic neurons terminate mostly in the frontal lobes and limbic (emotional) areas of the brain. Norepinephrine is also involved in attentional abilities and is widely used throughout the brain. Serotonin is important for regulating behaviors such as sleep and appetite, and neurons that use serotonin terminate in many parts of the brain.

Particular types of glial cells assist in the transmission of signals from neuron to neuron, and act as an insulator for the axon. The type of glial cell used to provide insulation differs according to whether the neuron is in the peripheral nervous system (PNS) or central nervous system (CNS). Schwann cells are the glial cells of the PNS that form myelin by wrapping around a segment of one axon, whereas oligodendrocytes, the glial cells of the CNS, form myelin by wrapping around segments of multiple axons (Figure 2–3).

Neurons with a myelin sheath are considered myelinated and those without, unmyelinated. There are gaps in the myelinated axons called *nodes of Ranvier* that are necessary for the axon to have some communication with extracellular space so that ions can diffuse across the membrane. In this way, the neuron can continue propagating (i.e., transmitting) the electrical signal. Myelin and the glial cells comprising it have numerous functions, the best understood of which is speeding propagation of the electrical signal. Myelinated axons in the CNS are called "white matter" because myelin is a fatty substance white in color. Gray matter, which can go by a number of different names such as cortex, nucleus, or ganglion, is made up of neuronal cell bodies that process information.

The great number of cells in the nervous system and the even greater number of synaptic connections between those cells make it possible for the nervous system to support complex cognitive functions. Vast networks of neurons and their connections must be engaged to produce high-level activities such as language and memory. An important principle is that connections between neurons can strengthen with use; thus, changes in the strength of neural connections may provide a mechanism for memory at the cellular level (discussed later in the chapter).

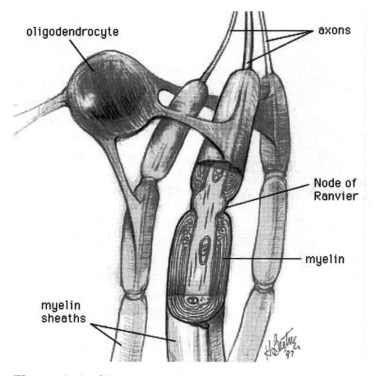

Figure 2–3. Oligodendrocyte forming myelin around numerous axons. Photo courtesy of the National Institutes of Health Office of Science Education, Free Resources for Science Teachers (http://science-education.nih.gov).

Major Components of the Central and Peripheral Nervous Systems

The nervous system consists of central and peripheral divisions. The CNS is made up of the cerebrum, brainstem, cerebellum, and spinal cord. Major components of the PNS are spinal and cranial nerves (Figure 2–4).

Central Nervous System

In the CNS, the cerebrum consists of the cerebral hemispheres and diencephalon (thalamus and hypothalamus). The right and left cerebral hemispheres each contain subcortical structures that lie deep inside the brain, such as the hippocampus, amygdala, thalamus, and the basal ganglia, as well as white matter pathways and an outer layer of cerebral cortex. Cerebral cortex is topographically divided into lobes: frontal, parietal, occipital, temporal, and limbic. The limbic lobe (also called the cingulate gyrus) is on the medial surface of the cerebral hemispheres, wrapping around the corpus callosum, the largest band of white matter that connects the hemispheres. The cerebellum sits at the back of the brain, behind the brainstem (midbrain, pons, and medulla). The spinal cord is a continuation of the pathways that travel through the brainstem.

Peripheral Nervous System

The major components of the PNS are spinal and cranial nerves. Spinal nerves either proj-

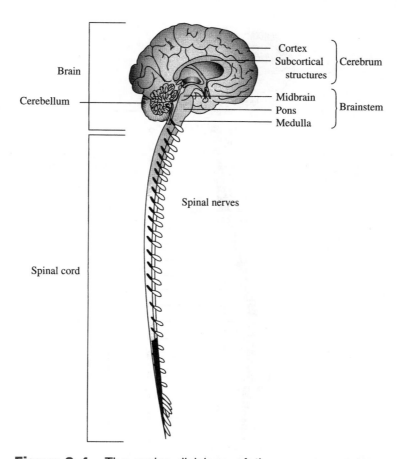

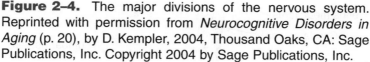

Figure 2–4. The major divisions of the nervous system. Reprinted with permission from *Neurocognitive Disorders in Aging* (p. 20), by D. Kempler, 2004, Thousand Oaks, CA: Sage Publications, Inc. Copyright 2004 by Sage Publications, Inc.

ect from the anterior horn of the spinal cord to ultimately innervate muscles, or they gather sensory information for the body below the neck and converge on the posterior horn of the spinal cord. There are 31 pairs of spinal nerves distributed along the five segments of the spinal cord: cervical (8), thoracic (12), lumbar (5), sacral (5), and coccygeal (1) (Figure 2–5).

Cranial nerves control motor and sensory information for the head and neck. There are 12 pairs of cranial nerves (see Table 2–1), most of which arise from the brainstem. Generally they are numbered

such that the first cranial nerve is the most superior (highest) on the brainstem and the twelfth cranial nerves is most inferior (lowest) (Figure 2–6).

Anatomic Orientation

Anatomic Directions

Parts of the CNS are often discussed in terms of anatomic directions and/or planes. Because of the bend that occurs between the brain and spinal cord (cephalic flexure), anatomic

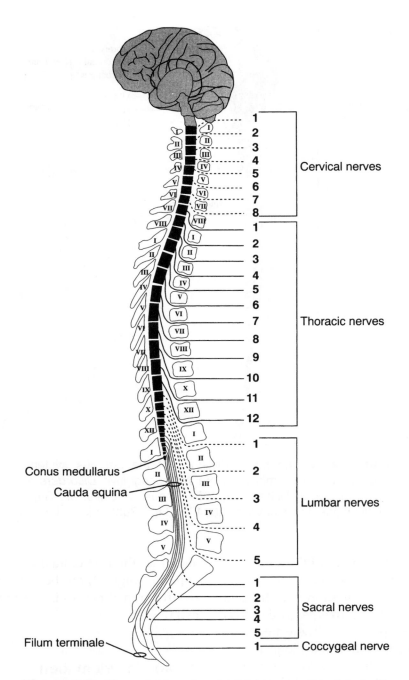

Figure 2–5. The spinal cord and spinal nerves. Reprinted with permission from *Neuroscience for the Study of Communicative Disorders*, by S. Bhatnagar and O. Andy, p. 195, Copyright 1995 by Williams & Wilkins.

Table 2–1. The Cranial Nerves and Their Function

Number	Cranial Nerve	General Function	Specific Function and/or Structures Innervated
CN I	Olfactory	Sensory	Smell, Taste
CN II	Optic	Sensory	Vision
CN III	Oculomotor	Motor	Innervation of most muscles that move the eye, pupil, and upper eyelid
CN IV	Trochlear	Motor	Innervation of the superior oblique muscle of the eye
CN V	Trigeminal	Sensory and Motor	Mastication and sensation to the face, innervation of the palate and pharynx
CN VI	Abducens	Motor	Abducts the eye
CN VII	Facial	Sensory and Motor	Movement of facial muscles, innervates taste receptors and salivary glands
CN VIII	Auditory/Vestibular	Sensory	Hearing and equilibrium
CN IX	Glossopharyngeal	Sensory and Motor	Taste, elevation of palate, pharynx, and larynx, salivary glands
CN X	Vagus	Sensory and Motor	General sensation of soft palate and upper larynx; motor innervation to muscles of soft palate and pharynx
CN XI	Spinal Accessory	Motor	Controls trapezius and sternocleidomastoid, controls swallowing movements
CN XII	Hypoglossal	Motor	Controls tongue movement

directions may change depending on the part of the CNS being described; however, they are important to discuss as they are often used. An example of how anatomic directional terms can be problematic is the dichotomy of dorsal (toward the back) versus ventral (toward the belly); this refers to different directions when discussing the brain or spinal cord (Figure 2–7). Another set of problematic terms is rostral (toward the head) versus caudal (toward the tail). This is self-explanatory when describing the spinal cord but loses its descriptive power when discussing the brain.

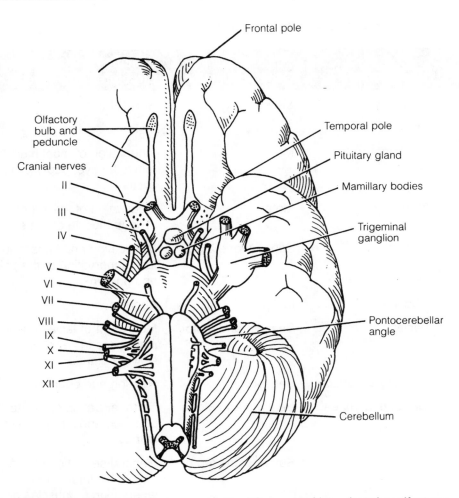

Figure 2–6. The brainstem and cranial nerves. Note that the olfactory nerve is CN I. The frontal and temporal poles are the most anterior portions of the frontal and temporal lobes, respectively. The enlarged trigeminal ganglion reflects the complexity of the trigeminal nerve. From *Correlative Neuroanatomy* (20th ed.), by J. deGroot and J. G. Chusid, p. 144. Copyright 1988 by Appleton and Lange. Reproduced with permission from the McGraw-Hill Companies.

When discussing the brain, other terms for anatomic directions are preferable. Anterior is used to mean "in front of," whereas posterior means "behind." Superior means "above," and "inferior" means "below." Medial refers to "toward the middle," and "lateral" refers to "toward the outside." Some examples of use of this terminology include, (a) the midbrain is superior to the pons, (b) the amygdala is anterior to the hippocampus, and (c) the third ventricle is medial to the thalamus.

Anatomic Planes

Anatomic planes are useful in discussing sections of the brain, and are often used when

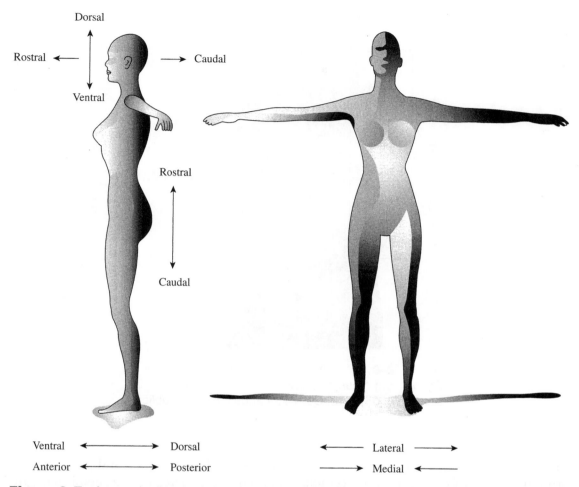

Figure 2–7. Anatomic directions for the head and body. Reprinted with permission from *Neurocognitive Disorders in Aging*, by D. Kempler, 2005, p. 18. Copyright 2005 by Sage Publications, Inc.

examining radiologic scans (Figure 2–8). The sagittal plane divides the hemispheres of the brain, leaving two equal halves. Parasagittal planes are any that are parallel to the sagittal plane. Coronal (frontal) planes are perpendicular to the sagittal plane. Transverse (axial) planes are horizontal in orientation.

Major Structures of the Brain

The major anatomic structures of the brain that are integral to the later discussion of communication and memory are outlined here in terms of their basic function, location, and structure.

Cerebral Hemispheres: Lateral and Medial Views

Within the cerebral hemispheres are five lobes, each specialized for a different type of information processing. In general, (a) the frontal lobes are important for executive functioning and motor planning/control; (b) the parietal lobes mediate somatic sensation and

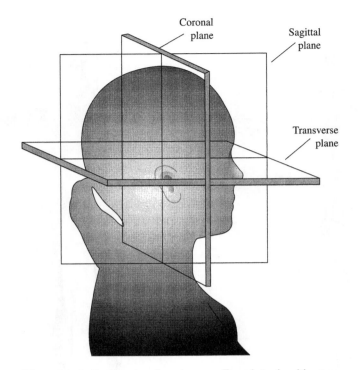

Figure 2–8. Anatomic planes. Reprinted with permission from *Neurocognitive Disorders in Aging,* by D. Kempler, 2005, p. 19. Copyright 2005 by Sage Publications, Inc.

spatial awareness; (c) the occipital lobes are primarily responsible for visual processing; (d) the temporal lobes process auditory information and contain structures important for particular types of memory; and (e) the limbic lobes (cingulate gyri) are responsible for processing emotions, and are integrally involved in numerous complex cognitive functions.

The outer covering of the cerebral hemispheres, or cortex, folds in on itself during nervous system development, thereby creating a larger cortical surface area. A large cortical surface with greater numbers of neurons enables humans to perform complex mental activities. The areas of cortex that are folded in are called *sulci* (or fissures). Certain sulci are used as landmarks (Figure 2–9); the central sulcus divides the frontal and parietal lobes of each hemisphere and the lateral sulci provide a boundary between the frontal and temporal lobes. A cortical area that partially contributes to language production is the insula, which lies inside the lateral fissure. It can be seen by separating or cutting away the frontal, temporal, and parietal opercula (Latin for *lid*) that cover it. The insula also contains gustatory (taste) and autonomic areas, which control body functions such as heart rate. There is no prominent sulcus dividing the parietal from the occipital lobe on the lateral surface of the brain, but on the medial surface of the hemispheres, the parieto-occipital sulcus provides a boundary. The cingulate sulcus divides the cingulate gyrus from the frontal lobe medially.

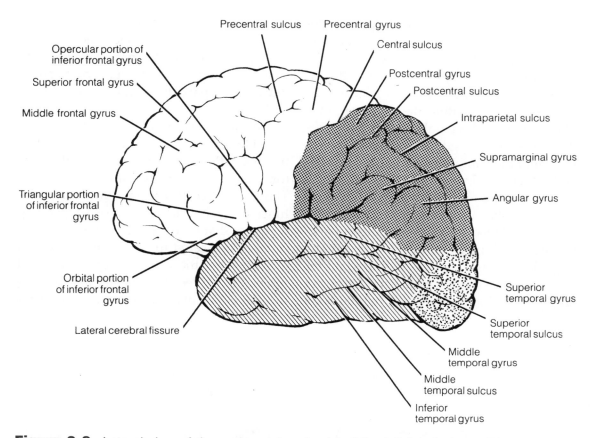

Figure 2–9. Lateral view of the major gyri and sulci of the left hemisphere. Reprinted from *Correlative Neuroanatomy* (20th ed.), by J. deGroot and J. G. Chusid, p. 194. Copyright 1988 by Appleton and Lange, reproduced with permission from the McGraw-Hill Companies.

The outfolded parts of cerebral cortex are called *gyri*. Some prominent gyri on the lateral surface of the cerebral hemispheres are the precentral gyri (anterior to the central sulcus, within the frontal lobe), which are important for motor function. The postcentral gyri (posterior to the central sulcus) play a large role in processing sensory information. Together, the precentral and postcentral gyri form the sensorimotor cortex in each cerebral hemisphere. The frontal lobes are divided into superior, middle, and inferior gyri, divided by superior and inferior frontal sulci. The inferior frontal gyri are further subdivided into orbital, triangular, and oper-cular parts. Gyrus rectus is the only named portion of the inferior surface of the frontal lobe, and is part of the orbitofrontal cortex. The parietal lobes contain the superior parietal lobule and the supramarginal and angular gyri, both of which are involved in language functioning, particularly those in the left hemisphere. Homologous areas in the right hemisphere are generally specialized for spatial awareness. The temporal lobes are divided into superior, middle, and inferior temporal gyri by superior and inferior temporal sulci. Heschl's gyri, or primary auditory cortex, lie in the lateral sulcus on the surface of the temporal lobes.

Medially (Figure 2–10), the parahippocampal gyrus runs from the inferior portion of the temporal lobe posteriorly toward the inferior surface of the occipital lobe. It is so named because it overlies the hippocampus, a structure deep within the temporal lobe. The portion of the parahippocampal gyrus that covers the amygdala is called the uncus. Lateral to the parahippocampal gyrus is the occipitotemporal, or fusiform, gyrus, a portion of which is implicated in facial recognition, particularly in the right hemisphere. In the occipital lobe, the calcarine sulcus marks the area of primary visual processing. The lingual gyrus and cuneus are important for higher level visual processing and are found on the medial surface of the occipital lobe.

The precuneus is a landmark on the medial surface of the parietal lobe. The fornix, a C-shaped white matter pathway that connects the hippocampi to subcortical structures, can be partially seen in a medial view of the brain.

Although specific areas of cortex are dedicated to sensory, motor, and other cognitive functions, there is some degree of plasticity (or ability to change), even in adult brains. The areas of cortex devoted to a particular function can increase or decrease depending on use of that tissue. For example, the cortical area dedicated to hand movement will increase when the hands are repeatedly used for highly skilled movements like playing the piano. The plasticity of neural tissue has

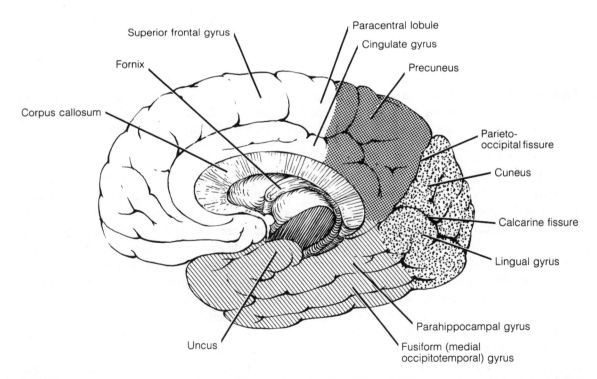

Figure 2–10. Medial view of the major gyri and sulci of the right hemisphere. Reprinted from *Correlative Neuroanatomy* (20th ed.), by J. deGroot and J. G. Chusid, p. 195. Copyright 1988 by Appleton and Lange, reproduced with permission from the McGraw-Hill Companies.

important implications for learning and memory (see Cooke & Bliss, 2006 for more information on neural plasticity and its role in learning and memory).

The Thalamus(i)

The thalami (one in each hemisphere) are collections of nuclei near the middle of the brain that relay incoming sensory information to the cortex and route information within the brain. In fact, nearly all information that reaches the cortex synapses in the thalamus first. Functionally, the thalamus needs to be organized such that it can reliably send information to particular areas of cortex. Thus, it is composed of a number of nuclei that are responsible for different types of information.

Thalamic nuclei are of different types, two of which are important for this chapter: *relay* and *association*. Relay nuclei receive specific sensory information and pass it on to cortical areas. Relay nuclei include the (a) anterior nucleus, which relays information from subcortical areas of the limbic system to the cingulate gyrus; (b) ventral anterior and (c) ventral lateral nuclei, which receive motor information from the basal ganglia and cerebellum and send it to motor cortex; and (d) ventral posterior nucleus, which receives somatosensory information and projects to primary sensory cortex. Association nuclei receive information from and project to association cortices. Association nuclei include the (a) dorsomedial nucleus, which has connections with prefrontal association cortices and as such deals with information related to frontal lobe and cingulate gyrus functions; and (b) the pulvinar, which has connections with parieto-temporal-occipital association cortices, and mostly processes visual and somatosensory information.

The thalamus, by virtue of its location and vast connections, plays a major role in communication and cognition. Damage to various nuclei of the thalamus and/or its connections with the basal ganglia (described below), areas of the limbic system, and cortex can cause impairments in regulation of emotion, executive functioning, speech motor control, and comprehension. Language impairments that occur after damage to the thalamus are discussed later in the chapter.

The Basal Ganglia

The basal ganglia comprise a group of subcortical structures commonly associated with the production and modulation of movement. Damage to structures of the basal ganglia can result in movement disorders, such as Parkinson disease and Huntington's disease. In Parkinson disease, there is a general reduction in movement, whereas Huntington's disease is expressed as excessive motor movements; this dichotomy results because different areas of the basal ganglia are involved in these two diseases.

The core structures of the basal ganglia are the caudate nucleus, putamen, globus pallidus, and substantia nigra (Figure 2–11). Often the caudate nucleus and the putamen are referred to as the *striatum* because of the narrow, parallel (striated) fibers that connect them, whereas the putamen and globus pallidus are called the *lenticular nucleus* because of their slightly curved shape (*lenticular* means "lens-like"). The basal ganglia have complex interconnections both within its own structures, and with the thalamus and cortex.

Although the basal ganglia are most commonly associated with motor function, there is evidence that components of the basal ganglia are important in higher cognitive function. The caudate nucleus, in particular, is implicated in cognitive rather than motor

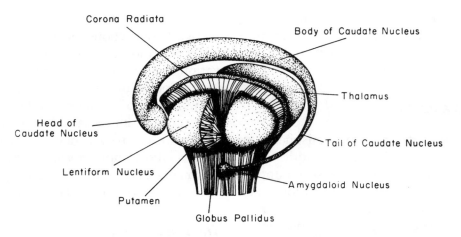

Figure 2–11. Major components of the basal ganglia. Reprinted with permission from *Neurology for the Speech-Language Pathologist*, (2nd ed.), by R. J. Love and W. G. Webb, p. 96. Copyright 1992 Elsevier.

function (Nolte, 2002). Damage to frontal-subcortical circuits (Figure 2–12) involving the caudate nucleus can cause cognitive dysfunction, such as difficulty with executive functioning and initiation, in particular. Impaired functioning of the caudate nucleus and its circuitry with prefrontal cortex also has been found to result in obsessive-compulsive disorder (OCD) (Friedlander & Desrocher, 2006).

The Hippocampus(i)

The hippocampi (one in each cerebral hemisphere) are major structures of the limbic system that support consolidation of new memories. The hippocampi lie deep within the temporal lobes, underneath the parahippocampal gyri. They have a number of components: the dentate gyrus, the hippocampus proper (also called *Ammon's horn*), and the subiculum. Information leaving the hippocampus travels through a white matter pathway called the fornix, which projects to other subcortical areas, eventually resulting in the storage of memories in various regions of the brain. Damage to the hippocampi—or

progressive loss of hippocampal cells, as in Alzheimer's disease—can cause anterograde amnesia, wherein the individual is unable to create new memories for facts and events even though memories created before the damage remain intact.

The Amygdala(e)

The amygdalae are core structures of the limbic system and are important in emotional response and learning. They lie in the medial temporal lobe, just anterior to the hippocampi. Considered to be one structure, each amygdala is composed of a number of nuclei that are highly interconnected with one another. The amygdalae also receive projections from and project to many brain regions. The extensive connections of the amygdalae illustrate the central role emotion plays in memory and learning. The amygdalae are most commonly associated with a fear response. Hence, damage to the amygdalae can impair the ability to learn an appropriate response to dangerous stimuli. In general, the amygdalae are important in forming memories that have emotional components.

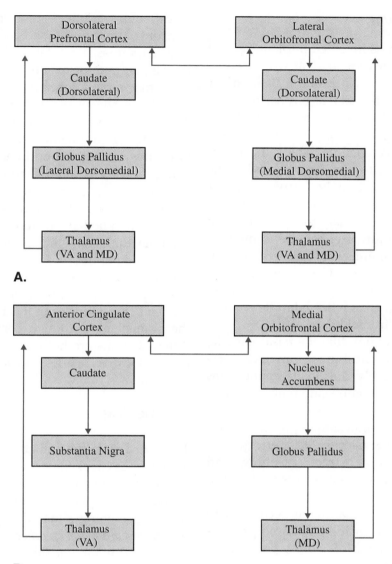

Figure 2–12. A. Prefrontal and orbitofrontal subcortical circuits (*VA* ventral anterior nucleus of the thalamus; *MD*, mediodorsal nucleus of the thalamus). **B.** Anterior cingulate and orbitofrontal subcortical circuits. The substantia nigra is an area in the brainstem, part of which produces the neurotransmitter dopamine. The nucleus accumbens is an important limbic system structure. Reprinted with permission from "Frontal-subcortical Neuronal Circuits and Clinical Neuropsychiatry: An Update," by S. Tekin and J. L. Cummings, pp. 648–649, *Journal of Psychosomatic Research, 53.* Copyright 2002 Elsevier.

The Cerebellum

The cerebellum is involved in planning and coordinating movement. The word *cerebellum* literally means "little brain." It is similar to the cerebrum in that it also consists of two hemispheres that are divided into lobes (anterior and posterior). The vermis is the center of the cerebellum where the hemispheres connect to one another, and is the structure believed to be responsible for movement of the trunk and adjustments of posture. The intermediate zone, which is just lateral to the vermis on either side, is involved in limb movement. The cerebellar hemispheres (lateral to the intermediate zone) are involved in planning of learned, skilled movement, which is reflected in its connections with the frontal lobes.

The cerebellum, like the basal ganglia, also appears to contribute to various aspects of cognition, likely due to its connections with frontal, association, and limbic cortices. Cerebellar damage has been implicated in impairments of emotional processes and behavior (Riva & Giorgi, 2000), error monitoring, planning, abstract reasoning, and working memory (Fiez, Peterson, Cheney, & Raichle, 1992; Schmahmann & Sherman, 1998). Language impairments secondary to cerebellar lesions include impaired processing and production of words, particularly verb generation (Fiez et al., 1998) and impaired verbal fluency and grammatical construction (Riva & Giorgi, 2000; Schmahmann & Sherman, 1998).

White Matter

As mentioned earlier, white matter consists of myelinated axons. These axons carry information to cerebral cortex (generally from the thalamus), or from the cortex to other structures. White matter pathways are of different varieties—projection, association, or commissural—and go by a dizzying array of names (tract, fasciculus, funiculus, lemniscus, peduncle). Projection fibers are those that carry information from the brain to the brainstem and spinal cord or vice versa. Association fibers connect different parts of the same cerebral hemisphere (e.g., arcuate fasciculus). Commissural fibers connect the hemispheres (e.g., anterior commissure, corpus callosum, posterior commissure).

Occasionally, the same collections of axons are called by different names. For example, the same white matter is called the corona radiata (if it is above the level of the corpus callosum), the internal capsule (if it is between the structures of the striatum), or the cerebral peduncles (if it is funneling into the brainstem). Although confusing, these different terms are helpful in communicating the location of a lesion such as a stroke.

The Meninges

The word meninx, which is singular for meninges, is Greek for *membrane*. The meninges form a membrane around the CNS to protect and support the brain and spinal cord. The meninges include the dura mater (Latin for *hard mother*), arachnoid (Greek for *spider*), and pia mater (Latin for *soft mother*) (Figure 2–13). The dura is attached to the inside of the skull so that there is essentially no space between them (unless trauma occurs, causing blood to accumulate between the dura and the skull, resulting in an *epidural hematoma*). The dura is tightly connected on its inferior surface to the arachnoid layer, again so that there is essentially no space between them (trauma can cause bleeding and the accumulation of blood under the dura, or a *subdural hematoma*). The arachnoid layer has a series of arachnoid tra-

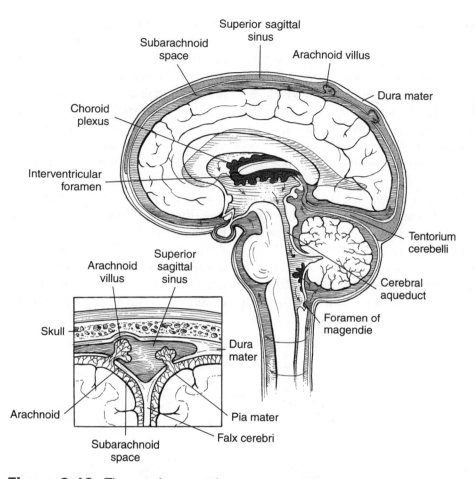

Figure 2–13. The meninges and components of the ventricular system. Reprinted with permission from *Introduction to Neurogenic Communication Disorders* (6th ed.), by R. Brookshire, p, 8. Copyright 2003 by Mosby, Inc.

beculae (strands of supportive connective tissue) that look like filaments that connect the arachnoid to the pia mater. There is subarachnoid space between the arachnoid and pia mater where blood vessels and cerebrospinal fluid travel. The subarachnoid space is also where small protrusions of the arachnoid layer, called arachnoid villi, take in cerebrospinal fluid and mix it with the outgoing venous blood; this process primarily takes place in areas called sinuses (cavities), such as the superior sagittal sinus. The pia mater closely adheres to the surface of the brain, covering all the gyri and sulci.

The meninges also project inward in particular areas, such as between the cerebral hemispheres, where it is called the *falx cerebri* and between the cerebellum and the cerebral hemispheres, where it is called the *tentorium cerebelli*. The same layers of the meninges (dura, arachnoid, and pia) travel down the spinal cord, as well, but in the spinal cord real epidural space exists between the dura and the vertebrae.

The Ventricles

The consistency of the brain is similar to gelatin. Thus, when the brain is taken out of the skull and placed on a tray, it quickly loses its shape under the force of gravity. When in the skull, however, the brain floats in cerebrospinal fluid (CSF), which enables it to keep its shape and also reduces the impact of external forces. CSF is secreted by the choroid plexus (Figure 2–13), which is a special type of secretory tissue located in the ventricles.

There are two C-shaped lateral ventricles filled with CSF, one in each cerebral hemisphere (Figure 2–14). They are connected to a third ventricle by the interventricular foramen, which is a narrow structure through which CSF flows from one ventricle to the next. The third ventricle is located between the thalamus of each hemisphere, and in most people the interthalamic adhesion connects the thalami within the third ventricle. The third ventricle is then connected to a fourth ventricle by the cerebral aqueduct, a structure similar to the interventricular foramen. CSF flows out of the fourth ventricle through the median and lateral apertures, into large cisterns (areas that hold liquid). The fluid then flows up around the cerebral hemispheres and into the superior sagittal sinus, an indentation between the cerebral hemispheres, where it is absorbed by arachnoid villi. Some of the CSF moves from the cisterns and down into the spinal cord.

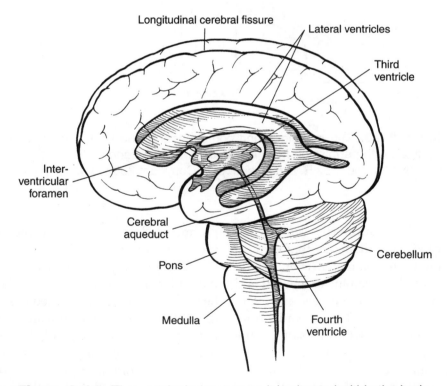

Figure 2–14. The ventricular system as it is situated within the brain. Reprinted with permission from *Introduction to Neurogenic Communication Disorders* (6th ed.), by R. Brookshire, p. 14. Copyright 2003 by Mosby, Inc.

Cerebral Blood Supply

The primary blood supply of the brain comes from the internal carotid arteries and the vertebral arteries (Figure 2–15). The internal carotid arteries supply a majority of the brain with blood, particularly the anterior, lateral, and medial aspects. The middle cerebral artery (MCA) is a continuation of the internal carotid artery. It travels laterally, supplying the insula and lateral regions of the right and left cerebral hemispheres. The

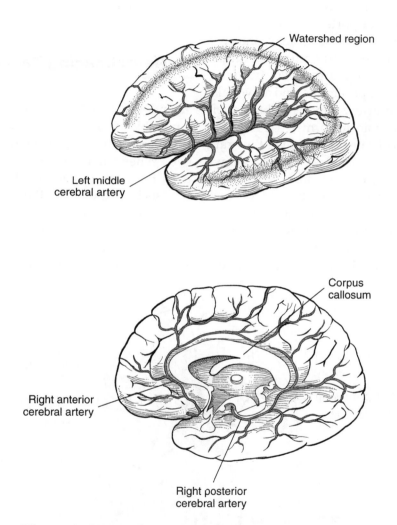

Figure 2–15. The cerebral arteries. The watershed region is that which is supplied by the edges of the cerebral arteries. A lack of oxygen to the brain (anoxia) often affects the watershed regions most severely because the available oxygen cannot reach the outermost parts of the arteries. Reprinted with permission from *Introduction to Neurogenic Communication Disorders* (6th ed.), by R. Brookshire, p. 26. Copyright 2003 by Mosby, Inc.

left MCA supplies areas of the brain critical for language functioning. The anterior cerebral arteries (ACA) supply the medial surface of the anterior part of the brain. The vertebral arteries travel along the cervical vertebrae and join to form the basilar artery as they ascend. The posterior cerebral arteries (PCA) branch from the basilar artery to supply the medial and inferior portions of the posterior part of the brain. Collateral, or small, branches of major arteries feed structures deep in the brain, such as the basal ganglia, thalamus, hypothalamus, hippocampus, and amygdala.

The basilar artery and the right and left carotid arteries join to form what is called the circle of Willis near the base of the brain (Figure 2–16). The circle of Willis allows blood to continue to reach areas of the brain that would otherwise be without blood supply, were that part of the vasculature to become compromised, as in blockage of the internal carotid artery. The internal carotids, ACA, and PCA are the major arteries of the circle of Willis. Two smaller arteries, the anterior communicating (AcomA) and posterior communicating (PcomA) arteries, connect the anterior and posterior portions of the circle of Willis, respectively. The AcomA connects the ACAs in most people. The PcomA connect the PCA with the internal carotid arteries.

Neuroimaging Techniques

Techniques have been developed that make it possible to view structures within the body that cannot be visualized with the naked eye. When such imaging techniques are used for viewing parts of the nervous system such as the brain, they are called *neuroimaging*. The neuroimaging techniques described below are of two types: anatomic (or structural) and functional. Anatomic scans (such as CT and MRI) provide detailed

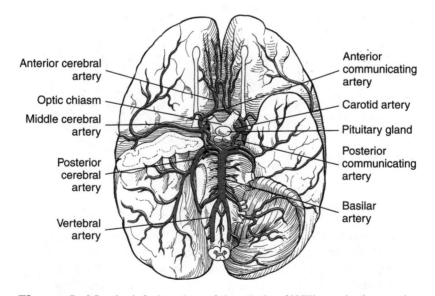

Figure 2–16. An inferior view of the circle of Willis and other major structures. Reprinted with permission from *Introduction to Neurogenic Communication Disorders* (6th ed.), by R. Brookshire, p. 26. Copyright 2003 by Mosby, Inc.

images of structures, whereas functional scans provide information about brain activity. In the case of anatomic scans, neuroimaging can provide useful information regarding what structures have been compromised due to trauma, stroke, or disease. Functional neuroimaging (such as PET, SPECT, and fMRI) can provide information about cognitive processes by revealing areas of brain activity related to particular tasks, or reduced activation in the case of damage to the brain. Images, particularly from functional scans, often can be used for differential diagnosis in the case of disorders that are difficult to distinguish based upon clinical signs and symptoms alone.

Computerized Tomography (CT)

CT refers to the fact that computers are used to construct pictures of a structure using slices, or two-dimensional images ("tomos" is Greek for *slice*). CT scans have been used medically since the 1970s. They can be used to scan various parts of the body, but head CT is the focus here. In a head CT, the patient lies quietly on a table while the scanner moves around the head. One side of the scanner emits x-rays, while the other side collects data from the x-ray signal. The information gathered is sent to a computer, where a three-dimensional reconstruction of the patient's head is created. That image can be "sliced" in a number of different anatomic planes so that structures of interest can be visualized from *a number of* different angles. Sometimes a contrast agent will be delivered to the patient via an intravenous (IV) injection so that particular structures or the blood can be visualized more clearly.

The major advantages of CT scans are that they are relatively inexpensive compared to other neuroimaging techniques, they can be used to diagnose a number of

medical problems, they can detect a cerebral hemorrhage (bleeding in the brain) early in its course, and individuals with implanted metal devices can receive the scan. Limitations include varying levels of exposure to radiation that depend on the length of the procedure, potential allergic reactions to the contrast agent or even kidney failure (most likely when there is a pre-existing kidney condition), and difficulty in discovering an ischemic lesion (caused by a decrease in blood supply) early in its course.

Magnetic Resonance Imaging (MRI)

Like CT, MRI is used to visualize structures within the body, such as the brain. However, MRI is better at visualizing soft tissue than is CT. In MRI, the patient lies flat on a table and is positioned within a hole in the scanner, called the bore. The MRI scanner uses a strong magnetic field and radio signals to obtain information about structures within the patient's brain.

MRI has several advantages over CT. No x-rays are used in MRI, which reduces the risk associated with x-ray exposure. MRI is particularly useful in early detection of ischemic stroke, identifying the lesion hours before a CT scan. MRI also has greater contrast resolution than CT, which allows one to distinguish between similar structures. Improvements in technology have resulted in MRI being used to diagnose an increasing number of medical conditions, such as diseases in which myelin is attacked (demyelinating diseases). In addition, techniques associated with MRI, such as voxel-based morphometry, have improved the ability to detect and quantify brain atrophy (i.e., tissue loss).

Many of the risks associated with MRI are related to the strong magnetic field used by the scanner. For example, patients with pacemakers are often unable to have an MRI, as the magnetic field may interfere with the functioning of the device. Other metallic objects, such as hair pins, can become dangerous projectiles. Small metallic flakes embedded in the skin or eyes of individuals who were metal workers can heat up during a MRI and potentially burn the patient. Some patients have metallic plates, pins, or screws in various parts of their bodies, and even if they are made of nonferrous metal that is not dangerous in the scanner, they might cause artifacts or changes in the image quality around that object. MRIs can also be uncomfortable and frightening in that patients are exposed to loud noises from the scanner, and some patients may experience claustrophobia because of the relatively small size of the bore. MRI is also expensive in terms of equipment costs and upkeep.

Positron Emission Tomography (PET)

Unlike CT and MRI, PET is not used to visualize particular anatomic structures. Rather, the function of the brain is indirectly measured through blood flow and brain metabolism. In PET, the patient is first injected with a radioactive tracer isotope (typically ^{11}C, ^{13}N, ^{15}O, or ^{18}F) with a short half-life, meaning it decays very quickly to half its injected value. The tracer undergoes changes within the body that allow the scanner to determine where the tracer has become concentrated. PET is used medically in diagnosis of cancerous tumors, as the tracer gathers in higher concentrations in cancerous cells. PET is also used to diagnose Alzheimer's disease or to differentiate it from other types of dementia, as Alzheimer's disease is linked with reduced brain metabolism. Researchers use PET to aid in the identification of brain areas that are associated with certain functions.

Although it has utility in diagnosis of particular structural abnormalities and dis-

eases, PET has a number of limitations, including exposure to small amounts of the radioactive tracer, high equipment cost related to creation of the isotopes (a machine called a *cyclotron* is required), slow speed of image acquisition, and low spatial and temporal resolution. Poor spatial resolution results in a reduced ability to distinguish structures of interest from nearby structures, and poor temporal resolution results in difficulty determining the time sequence of changes in brain activity.

Single Photon Emission Computed Tomography (SPECT)

SPECT, like PET, measures brain metabolism indirectly through a tracer that is injected into the patient, although the tracer typically used in SPECT (^{99m}Tc-HMPAO) is different and does not require the same high-cost equipment as used in PET. The signal emitted by the tracer is picked up by a special sensor, called a gamma camera, and the image is reconstructed on a computer. SPECT is often used in scanning the brain and in diagnosis of tumor. This neuroimaging technique has proven to be increasingly accurate in diagnosing Alzheimer's disease and in differentiating it from vascular dementia and frontotemporal dementia, surpassing clinical assessments in sensitivity in some research studies (see Dougall, Bruggink, & Ebmeier, 2004). SPECT can differentiate between the more global reduced brain metabolism seen in Alzheimer's disease versus the more scattered reduced metabolism seen in vascular dementia.

SPECT is less expensive and more widely available than PET. A limitation of SPECT is that it has poorer image resolution than PET, which makes it more difficult to distinguish between neighboring structures. SPECT also involves exposure to small amounts of radiation because of the injected tracer.

Functional Magnetic Resonance Imaging (fMRI)

fMRI is a relatively new neuroimaging technique in which brain activity is measured, as in PET and SPECT. fMRI uses a magnetic field to measure the blood oxygenation level dependent (BOLD), which is a signal from the blood that indirectly indicates brain activity. Because of the use of magnets rather than x-rays, there are no risks associated with radiation. Risks associated with the magnet, however, must be carefully considered.

Limitations of fMRI include poor temporal resolution, which makes it difficult to determine the time sequence in which certain activities in the brain occur. Scanning sessions may be long, depending on the tasks in which patients are engaged. Patients must lie still throughout the scan, thus some patients are not considered good candidates for fMRI, such as small children or individuals with AD. The interested reader is referred to a text by Huettel, Song, and McCarthy (2004) for more information on fMRI.

Language—What It Is and Where It Is

Language is a symbol system used to communicate. It is not a unitary phenomenon; rather, language is composed of a number of different types of knowledge—phonologic, semantic, syntactic, morphologic, and pragmatic. The components of language are differentially represented in the cerebral hemispheres, with phonology, morphology, and syntax strongly lateralized to the left hemisphere. Semantic knowledge is distributed throughout both cerebral hemispheres. Pragmatics is generally considered to be the purview of the right hemisphere, as damage to the right hemisphere often impairs social interaction.

Different areas of language can be impaired depending on the site of damage. Typically, language impairments are the result of damage to areas surrounding the left lateral sulcus (Sylvian fissure) (Figure 2–17) because most components of language are

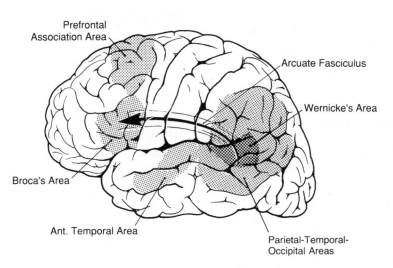

Figure 2–17. Primary language areas and association areas of the left hemisphere. Reprinted with permission from *Neurology for the Speech-Language Pathologist*, (2nd ed.), by R. J. Love and W. G. Webb, p. 20. Copyright 1992 Elsevier.

mediated by the left cerebral hemisphere in the great majority of the population. Nearly all right-handed individuals have language-dominant left hemispheres (approximately 99%), as do most left-handed individuals (approximately 70%) (Helm-Estabrooks & Albert, 1991).

Aphasia

Damage to the language-dominant hemisphere (left hemisphere, henceforth) due to stroke, trauma, or disease typically results in disordered language. The person who has sustained damage to the language areas of the brain is said to have aphasia, or an acquired impairment of language. Individuals who have damage to the right hemisphere of the brain are not said to have aphasia (unless they are right hemisphere-dominant for language). Because no particular right hemisphere syndromes have been identified, they are generally described in terms of their particular impairments (i.e., pragmatic impairment, impairment in comprehending multiple meanings, impaired prosody, etc.). There are a number of aphasia syndromes, however, that differ by location of left hemisphere damage. One shared characteristic of all aphasia types is an impaired naming ability called *anomia*.

Aphasia Classification

Aphasia classification is based on behavior rather than lesion location and is a useful tool for communicating relative areas of impaired and preserved language functions. It can be used to succinctly describe an individual's language status and to track change over time, as aphasia type may change as the individual improves in particular areas of language.

Four parameters are used to differentiate aphasia types: naming, fluency, auditory comprehension, and repetition. In the clinical evaluation of aphasia, four considerations are important. The first consideration is whether the individual has a naming impairment; if not, the individual does not have aphasia. The next consideration is the degree of speech fluency, which takes into account a number of language factors: the number of words in a phrase, ratio of content (nouns) and function (grammatical) words, syntactic structures used, and the existence of *paraphasias* (errors in word use) (Helm-Estabrooks & Albert, 1991). Individuals with aphasia can be classified as fluent or nonfluent. Next, auditory comprehension is assessed, ranging from asking basic biographical questions to following complex instructions. Repetition is then considered and is assessed by asking the individual to imitate a series of words, phrases, and sentences of increasing complexity. Together, these four parameters (naming, fluency, auditory comprehension, and repetition) enable clinicians to classify individuals with the different types of aphasia (Figure 2–18) that are discussed in the following section.

Aphasia Types

Broca's, Wernicke's, conduction, anomic, transcortical motor, transcortical sensory, and global aphasias are typically considered to be cortical aphasias. However, lesions resulting in aphasia may extend to subcortical structures, such as the thalamus or basal ganglia. Aphasia can result from damage to subcortical structures alone.

Broca's Aphasia. Broca's area (see Figure 2–17) is best known for its role in formulating the motor plans for spoken language, although evidence exists that it may also support working memory related to syntactic processing (Fiebach, Schlesewsky, Lohmann, von Cramon, & Friederici, 2005; Fiebach,

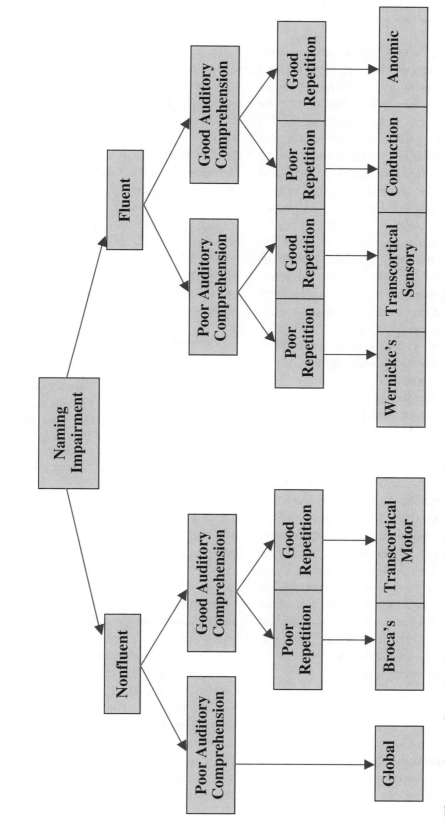

Figure 2–18. Classification of cortical aphasias (after Helm-Estabrooks & Albert, 1991).

Vos, & Friederici, 2004). Broca's area is composed of the triangular and opercular parts of the inferior frontal gyrus. Its name comes from Paul Broca, who was considered to be the first to discover the function of this region of cortex, although attributing this discovery to him is not without controversy. Broca was a French physician whose 1861 paper included a discussion of the famous patient M. Leborgne, who was nicknamed "Tan" for his repetitive use of that word. Damage to Broca's area alone is not sufficient to produce Broca's aphasia; rather, the lesion must also include subcortical white matter and adjacent cortex. Individuals with Broca's aphasia are anomic, nonfluent, have good auditory comprehension, and poor repetition. They typically speak in short, agrammatic utterances with more content words than functors.

Language samples can be obtained from picture descriptions. The picnic scene from the Western Aphasia Battery (WAB; Kertesz, 1982) was used for the examples in this chapter. In the picture, a man and a woman are sitting on a picnic blanket with a picnic basket between them and a radio next to the woman. The man is reading a book, and the woman is pouring a drink. Other items in the picture include a tree, a house with a car in the garage, a flag on a pole, a man flying a kite with a dog next to him, someone fishing off of a pier, two people sailing in a lake, and a boy kneeling in the lake with a bucket. A language sample from an individual with Broca's aphasia who has been asked to describe this picture follows.

"Sailing a boat. Or ship. Fishing outside. Lunch. Reading a book. Going fishing. Guy and a girl. A dog. A kite. Sailing."

Wernicke's Aphasia. Wernicke's area (see Figure 2–17) is located on the posterior part of the superior temporal gyrus, near the primary auditory cortex (Heschl's gyrus). Wernicke's area is part of the auditory association area, and thus is important for comprehension of spoken language. It is named after Karl Wernicke, a German neuropsychiatrist, who was the first to publish a description of the function of this area of cortex in 1874. Individuals with Wernicke's aphasia are anomic, fluent, and have impaired auditory comprehension and poor repetition. Their spoken language is characterized by a number of paraphasias and *neologisms* (nonsense words) as can be seen in the language sample that follows. A language sample of an individual with Wernicke's aphasia describing the same picture follows.

"I'm assuming these are three people right here. Two boys and a girl. You'll be the outside your children. Not too big either, not too small. Look happy, very happy. Family tree. White people, that's important in my job. Well, knowing who they are. Having a very good time. It's a nice day, probably shillin' the summer. Could be a . . . I'm poniting about where I'm trying to say the words."

Conduction Aphasia. White matter association pathways, such as the arcuate fasciculus (see Figure 2–17), also play a role in language. The arcuate fasciculus enables us to repeat what we hear because it connects the language comprehension area (Wernicke's area) to the language production area (Broca's area). Conduction aphasia results from damage to the arcuate fasciculus or the cortex that overlies it because information that is comprehended cannot be "conducted" to the language production area. Thus, a distinctive feature of conduction aphasia is the inability to repeat words and sentences. Individuals with conduction aphasia are anomic, fluent, have good auditory comprehension, and poor repetition.

Anomic Aphasia. As previously mentioned, anomia is the hallmark feature of all aphasias. Individuals with anomic aphasia are impaired only in their ability to retrieve the correct name, and so are fluent and have good auditory comprehension and repetition ability. Anomia can occur after damage to numerous areas of the language regions of the left hemisphere, and as such is of little use in terms of localization. Although the ability to name is disrupted in anomic aphasia it is generally not the case that semantic representations are destroyed, but rather that the anomia is the result of an impaired ability to retrieve the correct name. Widespread (rather than focal) damage is needed to cause a loss of conceptual knowledge.

The following is a language sample from an individual with anomic aphasia who is describing the same picture as the patients with Broca's and Wernicke's aphasia.

"Well we have a . . . a mother. Well . . . yes, it is a, a mother and father and, uh, looks like, uh, the woman is, uh, putting a drink in a glass and the father is, uh, looking with the book. There's a nice, uh, tree. And then there's a . . . I guess it's a, there's a woman . . . not a woman but a man . . . is a . . . I know what that's doing . . . but I can't put the name on that. There's a child and then I can't remember what you call this . . . but there's a person that's fishing. There are two people here . . . oh, the, uh . . . boat. It's not called a boat . . . and there's uh . . . I know what that is . . . I know it's a person there."

Transcortical Motor Aphasia. Areas of the motor cortex responsible for speech, such as Broca's area, require input from motor planning areas, such as premotor and supplementary motor cortices. When Broca's area is disconnected from other motor cortical areas, a transcortical motor aphasia can result. Individuals with transcortical motor aphasia are anomic, nonfluent, have good auditory comprehension, and good repetition. The hallmark feature, though, is reduced initiation of speech, which results in reduced output.

Transcortical Sensory Aphasia. Similar to transcortical motor aphasia, transcortical sensory aphasia results from a disconnection of perisylvian and extrasylvian regions, in this case those important for auditory comprehension. Individuals with transcortical sensory aphasia are anomic, fluent, have poor auditory comprehension, and good repetition. Because of their pattern of spared and impaired language abilities, they tend to repeat what others say even without a cue to do so.

Global Aphasia. Large perisylvian lesions are typically required to result in global aphasia. As the label implies, individuals with global aphasia are impaired in all areas of language represented in the aphasia classification system. They are anomic, nonfluent, have poor auditory comprehension, and poor repetition. The communication of those with global aphasia may be restricted to repetitive utterances, gestures, or drawing.

Subcortical Aphasias. Damage to the anterior limb of the white matter fibers that are situated between structures of the striatum (called the internal capsule), can result in impaired language production. After a lesion in this location, individuals typically speak in short phrases with moderately impaired syntax. Conversely, a lesion in the posterior limb of the internal capsule can cause impaired language comprehension, poor repetition, and relatively fluent language output. A lesion that affects both the anterior and posterior limbs of the internal capsule can cause global aphasia. Finally, lesions of the thalamus can cause a type of aphasia in which repetition is spared, but fluency and auditory comprehension are variably impaired.

Agnosia

The word *agnosia* refers to a lack of knowledge (*a* = without; *gnosis* = knowledge). Agnosias can occur in a number of sensory domains, and typically come about because of a lesion in the sensory association cortex subserving a particular sensation. In agnosia, primary sensory cortex is intact and thus perception of sensory information is normal; however, recognizing the meaning of what has been perceived is impaired. For example, auditory agnosia is a lack of knowledge of sound, which can manifest as an inability to recognize and attach meaning to sounds (such as the ring of a telephone). The individual with auditory agnosia can perceive sound, but they are unable to recognize or process its meaning. Other types of sensory agnosias include visual and tactile agnosia. Additionally, *anosognosia* (literally, "without disease knowledge") is typically seen after right hemisphere damage. Individuals with anosognosia deny that they are impaired or fail to recognize the significance of their impairment.

Communication Disorders of Dementia

Individuals who have dementia also have communication disorders. These disorders are referred to as cognitive-communication disorders, in order to designate that the communication impairment co-occurs with other cognitive impairments. The term *aphasia* is typically reserved for those individuals who have acquired language impairments without other cognitive impairments. Chapter 3 contains a comprehensive overview of cognitive-communication impairments.

Summary

The focus of this chapter has been on the major structures of nervous system, with particular attention to neuroanatomic substrates and impairments of language. Having knowledge of the neural basis of cognition and language enables clinicians to understand the behavioral sequelae of the various dementing diseases.

References

Bhatnagar, S., & Andy, O. (1995). *Neuroscience for the study of communicative disorders*. Baltimore: Williams & Wilkins.

Brookshire, R.H. (2003). *Introduction to neurogenic communication disorders* (6th ed.). St. Louis, MO: Mosby.

Cooke, S. F., & T.V. P. Bliss (2006). Plasticity in the human central nervous system. *Brain*, *129*, 1659–1673.

deGroot, J., & Chusid, J. G. (1988). *Correlative neuroanatomy* (20th ed.). East Norwalk, CT: Appleton & Lange.

Dougall, N. J., Bruggink, S., & Ebmeier, K. P. (2004). Systematic review of the diagnostic accuracy of 99mTc-HMPAO-SPECT in dementia. *American Journal of Geriatric Psychiatry*, *12*(6), 554–570.

Eichenbaum, H. (2002). *The cognitive neuroscience of memory: An introduction*. New York: Oxford University Press.

Fiebach, C. J., Schlesewsky, M., Lohmann, G., von Cramon, D. Y., & Friederici, A.D. (2005). Revisiting the role of Broca's area in sentence processing: Syntactic integration versus syntactic working memory. *Human Brain Mapping*, *24*, 79–91.

Fiebach, C. J., Vos, S. H., & Friederici, A. D. (2004). Neural correlates of syntactic ambiguity in sentence comprehension for low and high span readers. *Journal of Cognitive Neuroscience*, *16*(9), 1562–1575.

Fiez, J. A., Peterson, S. E., Cheney, M. K., & Raichle, M. E. (1992). Impaired non-motor learning and error detection associated with cerebellar damage. *Brain, 115,* 155–178.

Friedlander, L., & Desrocher, M. (2006). Neuroimaging studies of obsessive-compulsive disorder in adults and children. *Clinical Psychology Review, 26,* 32–49.

Helm-Estabrooks, N., & Albert, M.L. (1991). *Manual of aphasia therapy.* Austin, TX: Pro-Ed.

Huettel, S. A., Song, A .W., & McCarthy, G. (2004). *Functional magnetic resonance imaging.* Sunderland, MA: Sinauer Associates.

Kempler, D. (2005). *Neurocognitive disorders in aging.* Thousand Oaks, CA: Sage.

Love, R. J., & Webb, W. G. (1992). *Neurology for the speech-language pathologist* (2nd ed.). Boston: Butterworth-Heinemann.

Nolte, J. (2002). *The human brain: An introduction to its functional anatomy* (5th ed.). St. Louis, MO: Mosby.

Riva, D., & Giorgi, C. (2000). The cerebellum contributes to higher functions during development: Evidence from a series of children surgically treated for posterior fossa tumours. *Brain, 123,* 1051–1061.

Schmahmann, J. D., & Sherman, J. C. (1998). The cerebellar cognitive affect syndrome. *Brain, 121,* 561–579.

Tekin, S., & Cummings, J. L. (2002). Frontal-subcortical neuronal circuits and clinical neuropsychiatry: An update. *Journal of Psychosomatic Research, 53,* 647–654.

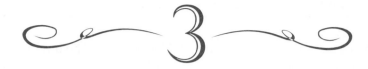

Cognition and Communication

Among the most fascinating of questions are how humans communicate, the relation of language and thought, and brain function in linguistic communication. These questions intrigue scientists and lay persons alike because communication is among the most complex of human behaviors and probably the most important.

From the moment of birth, infants are busy analyzing language. Within just a year's time, they learn the sounds of their language and the meaning of many words. Preschool children love language play and delight in rhyming words, reciting tongue twisters, and creating make-believe dialogues. Parents are fascinated by a child's developing language for through it they witness cognitive and emotional development.

Most lay individuals take for granted their ability to express ideas linguistically until exposed to the tragedy of language loss. It is only when a child fails to develop language normally, or a parent becomes aphasic after having a stroke, that they grasp how incredibly important communication is to life. Increasingly, it is dementing disease that reveals the importance of communication because individuals with dementia inevitably develop communication impairment.

Communication Defined

Communication can be defined as the sharing of information by means of a symbol system. It is linguistic when words are used and nonlinguistic when other symbol systems, such as mathematical notation, are used. To communicate, either linguistically or nonlinguistically, an individual must have an idea to share and a symbol system through which to express the idea. For example, the symphony conductor communicates ideas about tempo, loudness, and style by waving the baton in prescribed ways understood by members of the orchestra. The coach of a baseball team communicates plays by hand signals known to the players. These are examples of nonlinguistic communication, and although nonlinguistic communication can be impaired as a consequence of dementing illness, the focus of this book is linguistic impairment and its relation to cognition.

A clarification that needs to be made is that when the term "communication" is used, the authors mean "intentional" communication. Persons with dementia, like other people, can unintentionally communicate by many means: posture, facial expressions, and eye contact. It is intentional communication that is disordered, but to continue to use the term "intentional" would be burdensome; therefore, it will henceforth be assumed that the reader understands that it is implied.

Other distinctions critical to proper characterization of the effects of dementing illness are the differences between the terms "speech," "language," and "linguistic communication." For our purposes, "speech" refers to the motor production of sounds rather than an acoustic representation of language. "Language" refers to the symbol system by which sound is paired with meaning for a particular purpose. "Linguistic communication" is the cognitive process of sharing ideas through language. In some dementing illnesses, like Alzheimer's disease, the ability to communicate is affected more than speech and language.

Meaningful communication requires the production and comprehension of ideas. The act of speaking, in and of itself, does not constitute communication because that which is spoken may be structurally and semantically meaningless. Nor does knowing the grammar of a language ensure the ability to communicate. One can know the rules for combining sounds into words, and words with each other, without being able to intentionally communicate. Communication occurs only when sounds and words have been structured in such a way that the idea of the speaker is derived by the listener.

Communication Is a Manifestation of Cognition

Consider just the simple act of naming an object, for example, a parsnip. First you must perceive the features of the parsnip. They must be matched to those in long-term memory for recognition to occur. Thereafter, you must form an intention to say the object's name. The linguistic representations for objects are part of long-term lexical memory and must be retrieved and brought to consciousness. Perhaps you are uncertain about what a parsnip looks like and therefore are unsure whether you are perceiving a parsnip, turnip, or rutabaga. If so, you have to make a decision as to whether you should indicate your uncertainty. To articulate uncertainty of the object's name or to simply state the name, a motor plan must be formed. Thus, the simple act of object naming requires perception, access to long-term memory, association, recognition, lexical retrieval, decision-making, motor planning, and self-monitoring.

Because individuals with dementia have multiple cognitive deficits, including memory impairment, communicative function is always affected. The profiles of cognitive-communicative deficits of individuals with dementia reflect the distribution of neuropathology associated with their disease. In later chapters, the distribution of pathology of the primary dementing diseases and their effects on cognition and communicative function are specified. The purpose of this chapter is to provide an overview of communication and cognition and how they are related. This knowledge is fundamental to assessment, developing effective therapies, and caregiver counseling.

Cognition Defined

Cognition is a general term that refers to both *stored knowledge* and the *processes for making and manipulating knowledge*. The human brain is a pattern recognition system, and memories are stored patterns. The ability to access memory stores enables us to interpret our ever changing environments and modify our behavior to ensure survival and achieve lesser objectives.

The "Company of Cognition"

A helpful analogy for conceptualizing cognition is to think of it as a large company whose mission is to analyze sensation, detect and remember regularities in incoming sensory information, and use experience to guide behavior. The "company of cognition" has numerous departments whose personnel perform unique functions but nonetheless work in parallel with personnel in other departments. Each department is responsible for analyzing a certain kind of sensory input (auditory, visual, tactile, gustatory, and olfactory). For example, there is a department for processing auditory sensations and one for processing visual stimuli, and so on. Ultimately, all departments report to an executive division that analyzes information, makes decisions, and plans action.

Each department in the "company of cognition" has unique neural architecture. The department that processes auditory sensations is the province of the temporal lobes. Processing visual sensations is the province of the occipital lobes, and somatic sensations are processed by the parietal lobes. The frontal lobes make decisions and carry out executive functions. All departments share information by virtue of fiber tracts connecting them and all send their output via fiber tracts to the frontal lobes. In similar fashion, the lobes of the brain are connected to the limbic system which is responsible for linking emotion with sensation; the limbic system, in turn, is linked to the frontal executive system.

Thinking of cognition as a company, with many departments working together to process information, is similar to how Alexander Luria (1973), the late renowned Soviet psychologist, described cognitive functioning. In Luria's three-unit model, one neural unit governs arousal and tone, another unit processes sensory information, and a third makes decisions and initiates action. The integrity of all three units is essential to normal cognitive functioning. If the level of arousal is poor, then information processing by other units is compromised. If a sensory processing system is damaged, individuals can develop agnosias and/or other processing deficits. When the executive unit is dysfunctional, judgment, attention and decision-making are compromised.

Memory Defined

Memory is not a unitary phenomenon (Eichenbaum & Cohen, 2001; Schacter, Wagner, & Buckner, 2000; Squire, Stark, & Clark, 2004) nor does it serve a single psychological function. Consider that you have memory for facts, faces, sensations, various procedures, music, symbol systems, words, and contexts. In fact, many memory systems exist (Cohen & Squire, 1980; Gaffan, 1974; Hirsch 1974; Nadel & O'Keefe, 1974; Schacter, 1985). A popular and clinically useful schema (after Squire, 2004) for characterizing the types of memory is shown in Figure 3–1. These different memory systems rely on distinct neurologic substrates, process different kinds of information, and have different rules of operation. Of great importance to clinicians is that these systems can be separately impaired by neurologic disease and injury. Thus, clinicians need an understanding of the different memory systems, their operational principles, and neural architecture to understand why an individual with a particular type and distribution of neuropathology has certain symptomatology.

Sensory Memory

At the earliest stage of information processing is the registration of sensation. Sensations are received by our peripheral receptor

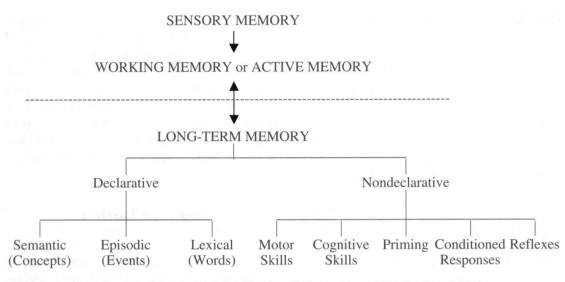

Figure 3–1. A model of memory (after Bayles & Tomoeda, 1997; Squire, 2004).

organs (e.g., eyes, ears, chemical receptors) and interpreted in sensory cortices. A helpful way to think about sensory memory is as a playback system in which incoming sensory information is sustained long enough that it can be reviewed for further processing (Emery, 2003). The auditory playback system is known as *echoic memory*. The visual playback system is called *iconic memory*.

Sensory Memory Is a Preattentive System

The term sensory memory applies to sensations that occur at the level of the peripheral receptor organs before they are consciously realized. Higher order attentional processes bring some sensations to consciousness, though not all. As you might suspect, information in sensory memory rapidly decays to make way for the representation of new incoming sensations. The duration of sensory memory is estimated to range from a third of a second to as long as two seconds (Dick, 1974; Harrell, Parente, Bellingrath, & Lisicia, 1992).

When an individual has a deficit in a peripheral receptor organ, sensation is altered and the quality of information coming from the environment is degraded. To facilitate sensory memory, clinicians must ensure that clients with sensory impairments, such as impaired vision or hearing, wear their glasses and hearing aids.

Working Memory

When sensations are consciously realized, they are in what is widely known as "*working memory*." Alan Baddeley (1986) introduced the term "working memory" to refer to information in conscious awareness *and* the processes active in the conscious awake person. The term is popular because it implies that much work is going on in consciousness, and indeed, there is. One activity is the focusing of attention that enables individuals to bring certain sensations to consciousness. But attention is only one of many processes referred to by the term working memory. Consider that when sensation is brought to consciousness, it must be interpreted. Multiple working memory subsystems enable us to review newly received information. Two that are of particular relevance to SLPs are the *articulatory/phonological loop* and the *visuospatial sketchpad*. The articulatory/phonological loop makes possible the subvocal rehearsal of that which we have just heard and the visuospatial sketchpad enables us to recirculate, in our "mind's eye," that which we have just seen.

To interpret new information, we rely on previous experience. Thus, working memory must activate past experience and bring that knowledge to consciousness. Generally, decisions must be made about the new information the organism is receiving. Baddeley called the decision-making component of working memory the *central executive*. The central executive system focuses attention, encodes information, retrieves information from long-term stores, plans action, and solves problems.

When information in working memory is encoded in long-term memory, it is linked with other similar memories. For example, new concepts are linked with those previously learned, new procedures are linked with other procedures, and new words with other words. The two-way arrows in Figure 3–1 signify that information is transferred from working memory to long-term memory and is retrieved from long-term memory when needed. Encoding and retrieval are carried out by the working memory system.

Active Memory

A synonym for working memory is active memory. It is whatever is on your mind. Said another way, it is what you are thinking about. Working memory can be conceptualized as containing buffers that store incoming sensory information but the buffers have a limited capacity. In a classic experiment in 1956, Miller demonstrated that the buffer span capacity of working memory is, on average, seven plus or minus two units of unrelated information. When the amount of information exceeds buffer capacity, some falls from consciousness. The terms used to refer to the buffer span capacity of an individual's working memory are "*short-term memory*," "*primary memory*," or "*memory span*." Encoded information that has fallen from consciousness, regardless of whether it was a few seconds or years ago, is long-term memory. Many people mistakenly refer to information that fell from consciousness a short time ago as short-term memory. However, short-term memory only refers to the amount of information that can be *held* in consciousness. Long-term memory refers to information that has fallen from consciousness even if it was a short time ago.

Neural Substrates of Working Memory

As you may have surmised, the frontal lobes are essential to working memory, particularly prefrontal regions which are extensively connected with the sensory processing systems of the brain and structures that underlie emotion. Eichenbaum (2002) notes that prefrontal cortex (PFC) has the capacity to hold items in consciousness for manipulation and the encoding of stimuli and events. Its subdivisions are "highly connected with one another and with posterior areas of the cortex to operate as a complex and widespread network for conscious control over memory and other intellectual functions" (p. 336). Dorsolateral prefrontal cortex bilaterally comprises the CEO of the "company of cognition" (Smith & Jonides, 1999).

The articulatory/phonological loop is subserved by Broca's area and surrounding cortex as well as inferior parietal and inferior temporal cortex. The visuospatial sketchpad is supported by occipitoparietal cortex which mediates the visual and spatial components, respectively (Baddeley, 2003). Individuals with dementia typically have damage to the frontal lobes and structures that input to the frontal lobes. As a consequence, the functioning of working memory is compromised in dementia.

Long-Term Memory

Long-term memory is commonly dichotomized as *declarative* knowledge and *nondeclarative* knowledge (Squire, 2004). Declarative knowledge is factual information that can be declared. A synonym for declarative memory is explicit memory because fact knowledge can be made explicit. Nondeclarative memory is a broader term referring to movement or motor memory, certain cognitive skills, priming, conditioned responses, and reflexes.

Declarative Memory

Declarative knowledge, or fact memory, can be subdivided into three related systems: semantic memory (SM), episodic memory (EM), and lexical memory (LM).

Semantic memory (SM). Semantic memory (SM) is that domain in the nervous system in which conceptual knowledge is represented. The term SM was introduced by Quillian (1966) who proposed a theory of information processing that included a long-term store of conceptual knowledge (Cohen, 1983; Tulving, 1972; Wickelgren, 1979). Concepts are constructs we form about the world based on our experiences. As Smith and Medin (1981) wrote in their book about categories and concepts, "Without concepts, mental life would be chaotic. If we perceived each entity as unique, we would be overwhelmed by the sheer diversity of what

we experience and unable to remember more than a minute fraction of what we encounter" (p. 1).

The word "semantic" in the term "semantic memory" may make some readers think that the contents of SM are words. However, the elemental unit of SM is theorized to be the concept, not the word. If you find the previous sentence hard to accept, consider that humans can conceptualize things for which they have no words. For example, you can conceptualize the following for which no word exists: an amorphous mass of gelatinous material about the size of a basketball seeming to have a self-contained propulsion system that enables it to continually change shape.

Other evidence that the units of SM are not in one-to-one correspondence with words is that many concepts can be referred to by a single word, for example "net." "Net" is associated with the concept of a tennis court barrier, a fisherman's tool, what is left after expenses, and a material used to make prom formals, just to name a few of its referents. Conversely, one concept can be associated with many words. For example, the concept "religion" is associated with Taoism, Protestantism, Catholicism, Judaism, Buddhism, Islam, and so forth.

Concepts can be activated by words, but conceptual activation can occur nonlinguistically as well, from objects and pictures, for example. A picture of a parallelogram may activate the spatial concepts of parallel lines and opposing lines of equal length but not the word parallelogram. Every day, individuals obtain new information by nonlinguistic means, and unless the need arises, much of this knowledge is never given linguistic representation. Consider that individuals who are profoundly deaf develop concepts without forming a linguistic representation for them. When a child who is deaf touches a hot stove, the concept of hot is encoded; however, without language training, the child will never develop the word "hot." Also, consider that an individual can lose the word for a concept without losing the concept, namely, individuals with anomic aphasia.

Words certainly help us conceptualize and indeed are so helpful that much thinking is done in words. However, when information is stored, the words that conveyed the information are generally forgotten; instead, we remember the concepts expressed by the words.

SM is a hierarchically organized network of associations such that related concepts are linked. Thus, when a concept such as "ice" is activated, the related concepts of "cold," "hard," and "water" are also activated. Although the concept is the elemental structural unit of SM, it is not the only unit. Propositions and schemata, that are combinations of concepts, also have representation.

Proposition. A proposition can be defined as a relational expression. It is grammatically analogous to a clause and contains a relational term, such as a verb, and one or more nouns or noun phrases that function as subjects and objects of the relation. For example, the following are propositions:

The hurricane, Katrina, devastated New Orleans.

Children dress up in costumes on Halloween.

Fall is the season after summer.

These propositions have been given linguistic representation, though not all propositions are translated into words.

Considerable evidence exists for the psychological reality of propositions. For example, regardless of the grammatical form of a sentence, it is reducible to the same constituent propositions; that is, it makes no difference whether the propositions are couched in a complex syntactic frame, a compound construction, or a simple construction (Franks & Bransford, 1974; Wang, 1977). People can recognize when two sentences or clauses are equivalent paraphrases because they perceive the relational expression, or proposition contained in them. The following two sentences, which are equivalent paraphrases, illustrate this fact:

1. A strong desire of Tyler's is to purchase an acre of land with a panoramic view of Tucson.
2. Tyler really wants to buy an acre-sized lot with a valley-wide view of the "Old Pueblo."

Sachs (1967) demonstrated that people remember the propositions (or conceptual meaning) and ultimately forget the grammatical form in which they were expressed. Some investigators have demonstrated that it is the number of propositions, rather than the number of words, that affects the memorability of the meaning of a sentence (Kintsch & Glass, 1974; Rochon, Waters, & Caplan, 1994).

Schemata. A schema is an attentional set formed by the simultaneous activation of a group of related concepts (Figure 3–2). Schemata are another structural unit of SM. People have schemta for a multitude of activities, for example, packing a carry-on bag for an airplane, being a member of a wedding party, using a cell phone, making an appointment with a doctor.

The process of building new schemata involves learning the associations between a particular set of concepts and propositions. For example, individuals exposed to the game of golf learn a host of propositions, for example, that certain clothes and shoes are worn when playing golf, that the angle of

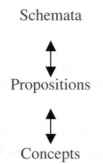

Figure 3–2. Semantic memory: A hierarchically organized representational system.

the club face influences the trajectory of the golf ball, that different clubs are used for different kinds of shots, that the person who had the fewest strokes on the previous hole hits first on the new hole, and that it is rude to talk when someone is hitting the ball. By playing golf, the schema is strengthened until the conventions of golf become second nature. Schemata help us know what to expect and guide our behavior.

Episodic Memory (EM). Episodic memory (EM) is the system that "receives and stores information about temporally dated episodes or events, and temporal-spatial relations among them" (Tulving, 1984, p. 223). One way to think about episodic memory is that it is semantic memory plus a context. An example may make this point clearer. Consider that "golf" is a concept represented in SM. Now, let's assume that you played golf last Sunday morning. That was an event, an episode. If you can remember the event of having played golf last Sunday morning, that is EM. Notice that a context, "last Sunday morning," was added to the conceptual base of golf as a game in the EM example. SM is what you *know*, you know golf is a game; EM is an event you can *remember*, namely, playing golf last Sunday. Likely you do not remember the context in which you

learned that golf is a game, it is just something you know, like knowing that an apple is a fruit. But, being able to remember the last time you played golf or ate an apple is EM.

A Synonym for EM Is Chronologic Memory. EM enables us to travel back in time to recall past events. It is more fragile than SM. In fact, we forget most of the events of our lives. Likely you cannot remember what you ate for dinner on the 25th of last month, or the color of the car parked next to yours in the parking lot last Friday, or how the napkins were arranged at the last dinner party you attended. Insignificant events are forgotten.

Lexical Memory (LM). Lexical memory (LM) is memory for words, their referents and meaning, spelling, and pronunciation. Some cognitive scientists argue that LM is a subsystem of semantic memory (Butters, Granholm, Salmon, Grant, & Wolfe, 1987). Certainly concepts and their linguistic representations are intimately connected; however, it is well recognized that we have concepts that have no lexical representation and lexical information can be impaired without impairment of conceptual knowledge. Individuals with aphasia typically have preserved conceptual knowledge but struggle with linguistic representations.

Neural Substrates of Declarative Memory. The declarative memory system is supported by three primary components: the cortex, parahippocampal region, and the hippocampus. Together, these brain regions enable us to acquire factual knowledge and remember events. Recall that the cortex is the endpoint for incoming sensory information. Within each sensory modality (or lobe) sensations are analyzed by a hierarchy of cells that perform increasingly complex analyses. The results of the analyses are sent to association areas of the cortex that have the capacity to form multimodal representations of information. These multimodal association areas have extensive inputs to the medial temporal lobes and parahippocampal regions. The parahippocampal region is able to sustain this input for short periods of time thereby enabling the hippocampus to "process comparisons among the various current stimuli and events and between current stimuli and representations of previous stimuli and events" (Eichenbaum, 2002, p. 235). It is the hippocampus that makes it possible to add new cortical representations of information or restructure existing cortical representations. Cells in the hippocampi have the capacity for long-term potentiation meaning they can stay active for extended periods of time enabling them to replay information recently received. The replay of information during sleep provides the cortex the opportunity to repeatedly strengthen the link between new, recently experienced sensations and previously existing representations of knowledge. Because the hippocampi function like an index to link new, incoming information with previously learned information, individuals with hippocampal damage have a deficit in EM.

Just anterior to the hippocampi lie the amygdalae which are important in the processing of emotion (Cahill, Babinsky, Markowitsch, & McGaugh, 1999; Hyman, 1998; Iversen, Kupfermann, & Kandel, 2000). There is strong evidence that the amygdalae modulate declarative memory on the basis of emotion (Cahill, Babinsky, Markowitsch, & McGaugh, 1995; Cahill et al., 1996). Emery (2003) theorizes that autobiographical memory developed phylogenetically from emotional memory, a theory that has considerable appeal because the emotional significance of an event greatly influences its memorability. Emery's research, from a life themes study, indicates that episodic memory may be coded in both pictures (visual code) and words (verbal code) (Emery, 2003).

Factual knowledge, is said to be "distributed" throughout the brain. That is, it is not stored in a single area. Take, for example, your fact knowledge of your maternal grandmother. You have knowledge of what she looks like, how her voice sounds, what she smells like, how she feels when you hug her, as well as event knowledge about times you have spent with her. This diverse knowledge is not represented in one cell or cell assembly. Rather, it is theorized that your knowledge of how grandmother looks has representation in visual association cortex and how her voice sounds in auditory association cortex and so on. Multimodal association cortex, where information from the various sensory processing systems converges contains a more complex representation of grandmother. This explanation is very simplistic but makes the point that conceptual knowledge is distributed across cortical sensory association areas. For a more in-depth account of the brain system that supports declarative memory, the reader is referred to *The Cognitive Neuroscience of Memory* by Eichenbaum (2002).

Although word knowledge is represented in both cerebral hemispheres, it is cortical regions of the left temporal lobe that are key in the process of naming. Individuals with left temporal lobe damage have difficulty naming visually presented words or objects (Farah & Wallace, 1992; McCarthy & Warrington, 1988). By studying the naming errors of people with brain damage and the brain activation patterns of neurologically normal adults during picture naming, Damasio, Grabowski, Tranel, Hichwa, and Damasio (1996) identified three brain regions of particular importance to word knowledge: the anterior inferior temporal pole; the middle part of the inferior temporal gyrus; and the posterior region of the temporal lobe. Several investigators report that the left inferior prefrontal cortex also subserves word knowledge because this area has been shown to be active during object naming (Martin, Haxby, Lalonde, Wiggs, & Ungerleider, 1995) and when adults make semantic decisions about words (Demb et al., 1995; Gabrieli, Desmond, Demb, & Wagner, 1996).

Nondeclarative Memory

As previously mentioned, nondeclarative memory is a general term referring to several kinds of memory: motor skills, cognitive skills, priming, conditioned responses, and reflexes (nonassociative learning). A characteristic of these different types of nondeclarative memory is that they are strengthened by repetition and practice.

Motor Skill Memory. Motor skill memory refers to motor procedures that are learned and the processes that support them. Examples of motor skill memory are riding a bicycle, driving a car, typing, and articulating (Figure 3–3). Unlike declarative memory which comprises factual knowledge that can be stated, motor procedural memory refers to the *performance* of an action. One can think about the mechanics of driving a car but that is not procedural memory. Motor procedural memory is exhibited in the act of driving the car. One has knowledge about how to ski or play tennis, but motor procedural memory is evident only when one actually skis or hits the tennis ball.

Neural Substrate of Motor Skill Memory. Motor skill memory (also known as motor procedural memory) is supported by the corticostriatal system including premotor and motor cortex, basal ganglia, and cerebellum (Mishkin, Malamut, & Bachevalier, 1984; Mishkin, Siegler, Saunders, & Malamut, 1982; Zola-Morgan, Squire, & Mishkin, 1982).

Cognitive Skill Memory. The term cognitive skill memory is an umbrella term for various cognitive procedures that occur without conscious awareness. Examples are mirror-reversed reading and recognizing holographic images nested in pictures (Figure 3–4). The

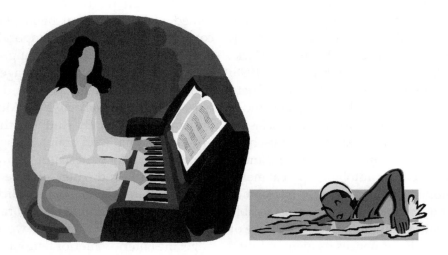

Figure 3–3. Examples of motor skill memory include playing a piano and swimming.

Figure 3–4. Cognitive skill memory is used to see the image within this stereogram.

neural substrates for various cognitive skills differ making it impossible to specify a single neural architecture.

Priming. Priming is the facilitation of performance as a consequence of previous experience with a stimulus and is typically measured in terms of accuracy of judgment or latency of response. Priming can be conceptual or perceptual. Conceptual priming is the spreading of activation between related concepts. An example of conceptual priming is the activation of the concepts "cold," "hard," and "water" when we hear the word "ice."

In perceptual priming the prior exposure to perceptual features of the stimulus facilitates the response. For example, the word "cake" may be activated by having previously seen the word "cake" or a word similar in appearance.

Neural Substrates of Priming. Priming occurs in the neocortex but certain subcortical structures may facilitate priming, notably the basal ganglia. The areas of cortex involved depend on the nature of the stimu-

lus, that is, whether it is a concept or a set of perceptual features. When the stimulus is visual, areas of the occipital lobe and/or inferior temporal lobe are involved. When the stimulus is auditory, both the left and right auditory cortices are involved. The left auditory cortex processes cues related to phonologic information; the right auditory cortex processes cues related to the speaker's voice.

Habits and Conditioned Behaviors. Habits are chains of behavioral events. The events in the chain are associated with each other such that the execution of one behavior triggers the next behavior. Most of us have a chain of behaviors we follow upon awakening and before we go to bed. We can carry out this routine while thinking about something else. Humans can develop habits because of the brain's capacity to form associations between repeated events. Conditioned behaviors are behaviors that are automatically produced in response to a particular stimulus or set of stimuli. The behavior is associated with the stimulus and reinforced by the events subsequent to the behavior or the eradication of an unpleasant antecedent event. An example is feeling afraid when approached by a growling dog.

Neural Substrates of Habit Memory and Conditioned Behaviors. The corticostriatal system, in particular the striatum, underlie the formation of habits (Knowlton, Mangels, & Squire, 1996). Eichenbaum (2002) explains that the striatum receives cortical sensory input and has direct motor outputs that make possible the association of stimuli with behavioral outputs. The striatum also has pathways for reward signals that enhance the association of stimuli and responses. Individuals with damage to the striatum are impaired in developing stimulus-response sequences.

The cerebellum is important in motor conditioning (Squire, 2004). It has complex connections with the brainstem and receives vestibular, visual, and auditory inputs. Also, its circuitry enables it to make a topographic representation of the entire body surface (Eichenbaum, 2002). Individuals with damage to the cerebellum are impaired in the acquisition of classically conditioned responses.

Relation of Cognition and Memory to Communication

Production of Linguistic Information

Ideation begins the process of producing meaningful linguistic output. The ideas that people communicate can be reduced to concepts represented in their SM. Once an idea or idea sequence has been formulated, it must be translated into a linguistic symbol system for communication to occur. A point to be underscored is that a translation process occurs; that is, ideation and thinking may be done in a different language than what is seen on the written page or heard in a lecture. The brain appears to have a language of its own, a machine language, as Fodor (1975) says, a language of thought, the output of which is translatable into human natural language. To utter or write an idea, we have to rely on complex motor skills (articulation or writing) that are forms of nondeclarative procedural memory. To ensure that what we say is what we intended to say, we have to monitor our utterances and make judgments about them. Thus, the production of linguistically expressed information uses semantic memory, lexical memory, working memory, motor procedural memory, and the central executive system. Although this is an oversimplification of what occurs in producing language, it makes the point that the cognitive-memorial systems make communicating an idea possible.

Comprehension of Linguistic Information

Linguistic comprehension ultimately involves deriving the right concepts and propositions. It is the product of sequential and parallel processes that involve many parts of the nervous system. For example, the perception of a spoken concept or proposition can be traced from its detection by the auditory system in which feature, segmental, and word analyses occur to the level of semantic memory and consciousness. During its journey through the nervous system, linguistic stimuli undergo lexical, structural, and logical analyses, the output of which is a conceptual set, a propositional set, or both.

The context of a communicative event biases the interpretation of information exchanged. Context can be defined as the physical setting, the emotional climate, the social organization between participants, and the purpose underlying the communicative event. Tracking these variables is a complex constructive process, and participants in a communicative exchange need to be attentive to phonetic and paraverbal features such as pitch, intonation, gestures, facial expressions, and emotional loading of words. It is our cognitive ability to analyze context that enables us to develop appropriate expectations about linguistic information that is forthcoming.

The process of forming expectations results from the intellectual process of relating past experience to immediate experience. It involves being able to identify commonalities between a particular context and a past event so that a reasonable prediction can be made about what propositions will follow. Our stored representations of the world guide us in interpreting new information and influence the way in which new information is processed. When miscommunication occurs, people find themselves systematically reviewing the context of the communicative event in terms of their expectations to discover where the breakdown occurred.

The ability to infer is fundamental to comprehension. An inference is a conclusion derived from an analysis of facts and premises. During listening and reading, a selection process is occurring; that is, not everything that is heard or read is stored. Most likely to be stored is the moral or point of the discourse. Making inferences, analyzing context, and building expectancies require conscious processing, in other words, working memory.

Why Communication Is Affected in Dementia

The production and comprehension of language cannot be separated from cognition. Rather, communication is a manifestation of cognition. Persons with dementia have trouble producing linguistic information because they have trouble thinking and generating and ordering ideas, in part because

information-processing capabilities of declarative and working memory systems are disturbed, in part because of degradation of knowledge. These same individuals have difficulty comprehending language because of deficits in the cognitive processes of perception, recognition, attention, inferencing, memory, and degradation of knowledge.

With an understanding of the types of memory and their neural architecture, and the relation of communication to cognition, clinicians can make reasonably valid predictions about the cognitive-communicative disorders associated with damage to different brain areas. For example, individuals with AD have early damage to the hippocampi that causes impairment of EM. Impaired EM causes individuals to forget what they just heard, read, or thought. As a result they produce many sentence fragments, and comprehension suffers. Also, they have difficulty acquiring new factual knowledge.

The different dementia producing diseases have signature patterns of neuropathology and as a result, signature cognitive-communicative disorders. In later chapters you will learn about the type and distribution of neuropathology of the primary dementing diseases and their effects on cognition and communication. First, however, it is important to understand how cognition and communicative functioning are affected in normal aging. Dementing diseases primarily affect people later in life; thus, clinicians must be able to discriminate between the effects of normal aging on cognition and the effects of pathologic processes associated with age-related dementing diseases.

Aging and Memory

People frequently blame their memory failures on aging; indeed, it is generally known that memory suffers with age. However, not all memory systems are equally affected. Effects are most pronounced on working memory and the episodic subsystem of declarative memory.

Working Memory

Executive functions (attention, inhibition, planning, monitoring, and encoding) are particularly vulnerable (Morris, Gick, & Craik, 1988; West, 1996) because they depend on dorsal prefrontal cortex, a brain region known to be particularly susceptible to the effects of aging (Fuster, 1989; Good et al., 2001; Raz, Briggs, Marks, & Acker, 1999). Nonetheless, the span capacity of working memory holds well. Most elders can repeat a telephone number (7 digits) as well as young adults. However, when the information to be recalled exceeds the average of seven units of unrelated information, the effect of age is apparent.

Declarative Memory

Of the subtypes of declarative memory, EM is affected most by aging, more than SM or LM (Nilsson et al., 1997). From middle age on, individuals experience gradual deterioration in the ability to recall names, faces, and events, particularly recent events (Nyberg et al., 2003). Typically, *recall* of information is affected more than the ability to *recognize* previously seen or heard information.

Whereas consensus exists about age effects on EM, the literature is conflicted about age effects on SM. What some investigators interpret as an SM deficit, others interpret as a deficit in the cognitive processes required by the neuropsychologic tests used to evaluate SM. Some investigators have used verbal fluency tests (generative naming of items in a category) to study

integrity of SM and reported an age effect (Rönnlund, Nyberg, Backman, & Nilsson, 2005). But the question arises as to whether the decline in performance on verbal fluency tests reflects a true degradation of conceptual knowledge or impairment in the process of accessing exemplars. Furthermore, some investigators suggest that SM increases from middle-age to young old-age (Nyberg et al., 2003).

Nondeclarative Memory

Motor procedural knowledge is well preserved in aging as is the ability to learn new motor skills (Smith, 1996; Woodruff-Pak, 1997). Although individuals may be slower in performing skills like hitting the golf ball, or playing tennis, they do not lose their ability to execute the movement. Many people who enjoy golf have been humbled by the experience of playing with individuals in their 70s whose scores approximate their age. Habits and conditioned responses persist into old age and new habits can be learned. Considerable research has been done on the cognitive procedure known as priming with mixed results. When an age effect is reported, it typically is small.

Four Summary Statements About Aging and Memory

The voluminous literature on aging and cognition is beyond the scope of this book to review, but four summary statements can be made that are clinically useful in differentiating early dementia from normal aging.

First, with increasing age, humans slow down physically and psychologically (Salthouse, 1996). Slowing is thought to result from cellular and structural changes in the brain (Raz, 2000), decreases in white matter due to demyelination of neurons (Kemper, 1994), and a decrease in the number of dopamine receptors (Backman et al., 2000). The volume of frontal cortex decreases from mid-life on. As a result, individuals 65 and older are slower in perceiving, processing, and reacting especially when the situation requires rapid processing of complex information (Birren, Woods, & Williams, 1980; Salthouse, 1985; Schaie, 1989). Clinicians can mistake age-related slowness for early dementia.

Second, aging affects the processing and retrieval of information more than the fund of knowledge. Aging does not diminish our knowledge. We continue to learn from experience throughout life. However, aging makes us less facile at processing and retrieving information.

Third, not all types of memory are equally vulnerable to the effects of normal aging. Most affected by normal aging is episodic memory. From middle-age on, people recognize that they have more trouble remembering things like who starred in a particular movie, or the name of someone they met recently at a party. Because EM deficit is a hallmark feature of early Alzheimer's, clinicians must know how to differentiate the changes in EM of normal elders from those associated with early AD. In the chapter on assessment is a table showing the typical performance of normal elders on episodic memory tasks and how it differs from that of individuals with dementia from Alzheimer's disease and Parkinson's disease. Note how rapidly the individuals with dementia forget recent information after a short delay.

Fourth, great variability exists in the psychological and physical status of individuals over age 65. Elders with a long history of good health, exercise, and cognitively stimulating jobs typically perform significantly better on cognitive-communicative and other neuropsychological tests than elders with a his-

tory of health problems, no exercise, and little cognitive stimulation (Emery, 1985; Hickman, Howieson, Dame, Sexton, & Kaye, 2000; Schaie & Willis, 1991; Snowdon, 2001). Clinicians must discard stereotypic notions about elders. An individual who is 65 and destined to be a centenarian, by virtue of lifestyle and heritage, is likely to perform quite differently on neuropsychological tests than an individual who is 65 and homebound with poor health. Table 3–1 shows documented risk factors for functional decline and disability (Fried & Guralnik, 1997; Stuck et al., 1999).

Table 3–1. Risk Factors for Decline in Functional Abilities of Community-Dwelling Elderly (Stuck et al., 1999)

Increasing age
Fewer years of schooling
Lower socioeconomic status
Low frequency of social contacts
Poor self-rated health
Smoking
Abstinence from alcohol or heavy alcohol consumption
Lower extremity limitation
Falls
High or low body mass index
Weight loss
Little physical activity
Visual impairment
Depression
Cognitive impairment
Number of chronic conditions
Use of multiple medications

Aging and Communication

Age effects have been demonstrated on confrontation-naming (Goodglass, 1980; Nicholas, Barth, Obler, Au, & Albert, 1997) and generative-naming tests (Coppens & Frisinger, 2005; Kempler, Teng, Dick, Taussig, & Davis, 1998), but in a functional sense, elders are not impaired in their ability to communicate. Elders continue to learn new words and concepts throughout life although they may be less efficient learners. There are some reports in the literature of reduction in syntactic complexity in the language of elders (Kemper, Kynette, Rash, O'Brien, & Sprott, 1989) but these may reflect memory impairments rather than loss of syntactic knowledge. The same is true for language comprehension that is influenced by the type and amount of information to be comprehended (Kahn & Cordon, 1993; Obler, Nicholas, Albert, & Woodward, 1985). When the information to be comprehended is complex, and presented rapidly, age effects are most apparent.

In summary, knowledge of vocabulary and grammar are preserved in aging. Elders retain their ability to acquire new vocabulary and understand words. They form grammatical sentences and can distinguish grammatical from ungrammatical constructions. The reported effects of aging on language are primarily the consequence of decrements in sensory processing and psychomotor slowing rather than loss of linguistic knowledge.

Summary of Important Points

- Communication is the sharing of information by means of a symbol system.
- Communication is a manifestation of cognition.
- Persons with dementia have trouble with intentional communication because by definition, they have multiple cognitive deficits.
- The effects of dementing diseases on cognitive-communicative functioning reflect the nature and distribution of neuropathology.
- Cognition is stored knowledge and the processes for making and manipulating knowledge.
- Cognition can be likened to a large company whose mission is to analyze sensation, detect and remember regularities in incoming sensory information, and use experience to guide behavior.
- Memory is stored knowledge and the processes for making and manipulating it.
- Humans have many memory systems each with distinct neural architecture that can be separately impaired by trauma or disease.
- Sensory memory is the brief registration of sensation at the level of the peripheral receptor organ. It is preattentive and sensations rapidly fade making way for new sensations.
- Working memory is information in conscious awareness and the processes active in the reception, encoding, and retrieving of information.
- Much work goes on in working memory that is directed by a central executive that enables us to make decisions and plan action.
- Long-term memory can be dichotomized as declarative knowledge and nondeclarative knowledge.
- Declarative memory is fact memory and can be subdivided into semantic, episodic, and lexical memory.
- Semantic memory comprises our conceptual knowledge, it is what we know. The elemental unit is the concept.
- Episodic memory enables us to remember the events of our life. It is our autobiographical memory and the most fragile of the memory systems.

- Lexical memory is our memory for words, their referents and meaning, spelling, and pronunciation.
- Nondeclarative memory is a general term that refers to several kinds of memory: skills (motor and cognitive), habits, priming, conditioned responses, and reflexes.
- Motor skill memory is often referred to as procedural memory. It is realized in the doing of a skill such as driving a car or hitting a tennis ball.
- Cognitive skill memory refers to myriad cognitive operations that occur without conscious awareness, one of which is mirror-reversed reading.
- Priming is the facilitation of performance as a consequence of previous experience with a stimulus or its associates. Priming can be conceptual or perceptual.
- Habits are chains of behavioral events in which the execution of one behavior triggers the next behavior.
- The production and comprehension of linguistic information cannot be separated from cognition but rather reflect cognition.
- Persons with dementia have difficulty producing linguistic information because they have trouble thinking, generating, and ordering ideas. They have difficulty comprehending language because of deficits in the cognitive processes and degradation and loss of knowledge.
- With an understanding of the types of memory and their neural substrates, clinicians can reasonably predict the cognitive-communicative disorders associated with damage to different brain areas.
- Aging affects the functioning of working memory, particularly executive functions.
- Of the declarative memory systems, episodic memory is most affected by age. From mid-life on, individuals experience gradual deterioration in their ability to recall names, faces, and events.

- Motor procedural memory holds well with age although individuals may be slower in performing motor skills.
- Differentiating the early dementia patient from the healthy elder can be challenging because normal aging causes deterioration in episodic memory.
- In normal aging, individuals slow down physically and psychologically. Aging affects the processing and retrieval of information more than the fund of knowledge.
- Great variability exists in the psychological and physical status of individuals over age 65.
- Knowledge of vocabulary and grammar are preserved in aging and reported effects of aging on language are primarily the consequence of decrements in sensory processing and psychomotor slowing rather than loss of linguistic knowledge.

References

Backman, L., Ginovart, N., Dixon, R. A., Wahlin, R. R., Wahlin, A., Halldin, C., et al. (2000). Age-related cognitive deficits mediated by changes in the striatal dopamine system. *American Journal of Psychiatry, 157,* 635–637.

Baddeley, A.D. (1986). *Working memory.* Oxford: Clarendon Press.

Baddeley, A. D. (2003). Working memory: Looking back and looking forward. *Nature Reviews Neuroscience, 4,* 829–839.

Bayles, K. A., & Tomoeda, C. K. (1997). *Improving function in dementia and other cognitive-linguistic disorders.* Austin, TX: Pro-Ed.

Birren, J. E., Woods, A., & Williams, M. V. (1980). Behavioral slowing with age: Causes, organization, and consequences. In L. Poon (Ed.), *Aging in the 1980s* (pp. 293–308). Washington, DC: American Psychological Association.

Butters, N., Granholm, E. L., Salmon, D. P., Grant, I., & Wolfe, J. (1987). Episodic and semantic memory: A comparison of amnesic and demented patients. *Journal of Clinical and Experimental Neuropsychology, 9,* 479–497.

Cahill, L., Babinsky, R., Markowitsch, H. J., & McGaugh, J. L. (1995). The amygdala and emotional memory. *Nature, 377,* 295–296.

Cahill, L., Haier, R. J., Fallon, J., Alkire, M. T., Tang, C., Keator, D., et al. (1996). Amygdala activity at encoding correlated with long-term, free recall of emotional information. *Proceedings of National Academy of Science USA, 93,* 8016–8021.

Canli, T., Zhao, A., Desmond, J. E., Kang, E., Gross, J., & Gabrieli, J. D. (1999). fMRI identified a network of structures correlated with retention of positive and negative emotional memory. *Psychobiology, 27,* 441–452.

Cohen, G. (1983). *The psychology of cognition* (2nd ed.). New York: Academic Press.

Cohen, J. N., & Squire, L. (1980). Preserved learning and retention of pattern-analyzing skill in amnesia: Dissociation of "knowing how" and "knowing that." *Science, 210,* 207–209.

Coppens, P., & Frisinger, D. (2005). Category-specific naming effect in non-brain-damaged individuals. *Brain and Language, 94,* 61–71.

Damasio, H., Grabowski, T. J., Tranel, D., Hichwa, R. D., & Damasio, A. R. (1996). A neural basis for lexical retrieval. *Nature, 380,* 499–505.

Demb, J. B., Desmond, J. E., Wagner, A. D., Vaidya, C. J., Glover, G. H., & Gabrieli, J. D. (1995). Semantic encoding and retrieval in the left inferior prefrontal cortex: A functional MRI study of task difficulty and process specificity. *Journal of Neuroscience, 15,* 5870–5878.

Dick, A. O. (1974). Iconic memory and its relation to perceptual processes and other memory mechanisms. *Perception and Psychophysics, 16,* 575–596.

Eichenbaum H. (2002). *The cognitive neuroscience of memory.* Cambridge: Oxford University Press.

Eichenbaum, H., & Cohen, N. J. (2001). *From conditioning to conscious recollection: Memory systems of the brain.* New York: Oxford University Press.

Emery, V. O. B. (1985). Language and aging. *Experimental Aging Research Monographs II,* 71–89.

Emery, V. O. B. (2003). "Retrophylogenesis" of memory in dementia of the Alzheimer type. In V. O. B. Emery & T. E. Oxman (Eds.), *Dementia: Presentation, differential diagnosis, and nosology* (pp. 177–236). Baltimore: The John Hopkins University Press.

Farah, M. J., & Wallace, M. A. (1992). Semantically-bounded anomia: Implications for the neural implementation of naming. *Neuropsychologia, 30,* 609–621.

Fodor, J. A. (1975). *The language of thought.* New York: Thomas Y. Crowell.

Franks, J. J., & Bransford, J. D. (1974). Memory for syntactic form as a function of semantic context. *Journal of Experimental Psychology, 103,* 1037–1039.

Fried, L. P., & Guralnik, J. M. (1997). Disability in older adults: Evidence regarding significance, etiology and risk. *Journal of the American Geriatric Society, 45,* 92–100.

Fuster, J. M. (1989). *The prefrontal cortex* (2nd ed). New York: Raven Press.

Gabrieli, J. D. E., Desmond, J. E., Demb, J. B., & Wagner, A. D. (1996). Functional magnetic resonance imaging of semantic processes in the frontal lobes. *Psychological Science, 7,* 278–283.

Gaffan, D. (1974). Recognition impaired and association intact in the memory of monkeys after transection of the fornix. *Journal of Comparative and Physiological Psychology, 86,* 1100–1109.

Good, C. D., Johnsrude, I. S., Ashburner, J., Henson, R. N. A., Friston, K. J., & Frackowiak, R. S. J. (2001). A voxel-based morphometric study of ageing in 465 normal adult brains. *NeuroImage, 14,* 1–16.

Goodglass, H. (1980). Naming disorders in aphasia and aging. In L. Obler & M. Albert (Eds.), *Language and communication in the elderly* (pp. 37–45). Lexington, MA: DC Heath.

Harrell, M., Parente, F., Bellingrath, E. G., & Lisicia, K. A. (1992). *Cognitive rehabilitation of memory: A practical guide.* Gaithersburg, MD: Aspen.

Hickman, S. E., Howieson, D. B., Dame, A., Sexton, G., & Kaye, J. (2000). Longitudinal analysis of the effects of the aging process and neuropsychological test performance in the healthy young-old and older-old. *Developmental Neuropsychology, 17,* 323–337.

Hirsh, R. (1974). The hippocampus and contextual retrieval from memory: A theory. *Behavioral Biology 12,* 421–444.

Hyman, S. E. (1998). A new image of fear and emotion. *Nature, 393,* 417–418.

Iversen, S., Kupfermann, I., & Kandel, E. R. (2000). Emotional states and feelings. In E. R. Kandel, J. Schwartz, & T. M. Jessell (Eds.), *Principles of neural science* (pp. 982–997). New York: McGraw-Hill.

Kahn, H. J., & Cordon, D. (1993). Qualitative differences in working memory and discourse comprehension in normal aging. In H. H. Brownell & Y. Joanette (Eds.), *Narrative discourse in neurological impaired and normally aging adults* (pp. 103–114). San Diego, CA: Singular.

Kemper, S., Kynette, D., Rash, S., O'Brien, K., & Sprott, R. (1989). Life-span changes to adults' language: Effects of memory and genre. *Applied Psycholinguistics, 10,* 49–66.

Kemper, T. L. (1994). Neuroanatomical and neuropathological changes during aging and in dementia. In M. L. Albert & E. J. E. Knoepfel (Eds.), *Clinical neurology of aging* (2nd ed., pp. 3–67). New York: Oxford University Press.

Kempler, D., Teng, E. L, Dick, M., Taussig, I. M., & Davis, D. S. (1998). The effects of age, education, and ethnicity on verbal fluency. *Journal of the International Neuropsychological Society, 4,* 531–538.

Kintsch W., & Glass G. (1974). Effects of propositional structure upon sentence recall. In W. Kintsch (Ed.), *The representation of meaning in memory* (pp. 140–151). Hillsdale, NJ: Lawrence Erlbaum Associates.

Knowlton, B. J., Mangels, J. A., & Squire, L. R. (1996). A neostriatal habit learning system in humans. *Science, 273,* 1399–1402.

Luria, A. (1973). *The working brain.* New York: Basic Books.

Martin, A., Haxby, J. V., Lalonde, F. M., Wiggs, C. L., & Ungerleider, L. G. (1995). Discrete cortical regions associated with knowledge of color and knowledge of action. *Science, 270,* 102–105.

McCarthy, R. A. & Warrington, E. K. (1988). Evidence for modality-specific meaning systems in the brain. *Nature, 334,* 428–430.

Miller, G. A. (1956). The magical number seven, plus or minus two: Some limits on our capacity for processing information. *Psychological Review, 63,* 81–97.

Mishkin, M., Malamut, B., & Bachevalier, J. (1984). Memories and habits: Two neural systems. In G. Lynch, J. McGaugh, & N. Weinberger (Eds.), *Neurobiology of learning and memory* (pp. 65–77). New York: Guilford Press.

Mishkin, M., Siegler, B., Saunders, R. C., & Malamut, B. J. (1982). An animal model of global amnesia. In S. Corkin, K. L. Davis, J. H. Growdon, E. Usdin, & R. J. Wurtman (Eds.), *Toward a treatment of Alzheimer's disease* (pp. 235–247). New York: Raven Press.

Morris, R. G., Gick, M. L., & Craik, F. I. M. (1988). Processing resources and age differences in working memory. *Memory and Cognition, 16,* 362–366.

Nadel, L., & O'Keefe, J. (1974). The hippocampus in pieces and patches: An essay on modes of explanation in physiological psychology. In R. Bellairs & E. G. Gray (Eds.), *Essays on the nervous system. A festschrift for JZ Young.* Oxford: The Clarendon Press.

Nicholas, M., Barth, C., Obler, L. K, Au, R., & Albert, M. L. (1997). Naming in normal aging and dementia of the Alzheimer's type. In H. Goodglass & A. Wingfield (Eds.), *Anomia: Neuroanatomical and cognitive correlates* (pp. 166–188). San Diego, CA: Academic Press.

Nilsson, L. G., Backman, L., Nyberg, L., Erngrund, K., Adolfsson, R., Bucht, G., et al. (1997). The Betula prospective cohort study: Memory, health, and aging. *Aging, Neuropsychology, and Cognition, 4,* 1–32.

Nyberg, L., Maitland, S. B., Rönnlund, M., Backman, L., Dixon, R. A., Wahlin, A., et al. (2003). Selective adult age differences in an age-invariant multi-factor model of declarative memory. *Psychology and Aging, 18,* 149–160.

Obler, L. K., Nicholas, M., Albert, M. L., & Woodward, S. (1985). On comprehension across the adult lifespan. *Cortex, 21,* 273–280.

Quillian, M. R. (1966). *Semantic memory.* Unpublished doctoral dissertation. Carnegie Institute of Technology. Reprinted in part in M. Minsky (Ed.), (1968). *Semantic information processing.* Cambridge, MA: MIT Press.

Raz, N. (2000). Aging of the brain and its impact on cognitive performance: integration of structural and functional findings. In F. I. M. Craik & T. A. Salthouse (Eds.), *The handbook of aging and cognition* (2nd ed., pp. 1–90). Mahwah, NJ: Lawrence Erlbaum Associates.

Raz, N., Briggs, S. D., Marks, W., & Acker, J. D. (1999). Age-related deficits in generation and manipulation of mental images: II The role of the dorsolateral prefrontal cortex. *Psychology and Aging, 14*, 436–444.

Rochon, E., Waters, G. S, & Caplan, D. (1994). Sentence comprehension in patients with Alzheimer's disease. *Brain and Language, 46*, 329–349.

Rönnlund, M., Nyberg, L., Backman, L., Nilsson, L-G. (2005). Stability, growth, and decline in adult life span development of declarative memory: Cross-sectional and longitudinal data from a population-based study. *Psychology and Aging, 20*, 3–18.

Sachs, J. S. (1967). Recognition memory for syntactic and semantic aspects of connected discourse. *Perception and Psychophysics, 2*, 437–444.

Salthouse, T. A. (1985). Speed of behavior and its implications for cognition. In J. E. Birren & T. A. Salthouse (Eds.), *Handbook of the psychology of aging* (2nd ed., pp. 400–426). San Diego, CA: Academic Press.

Salthouse, T. A. (1996). The processing-speed theory of adult age differences in cognition. *Psychological Review, 103*, 403–428.

Schacter, D. L. (1985). Multiple forms of memory in humans and animals. In N. Weingerger, J. McGaugh, & G. Lynch (Eds.), *Memory systems of the brain: Animal and human cognitive processes* (pp. 351–379). New York: Guilford Press.

Schacter D. L., Wagner A.D., & Buckner, R. L. (2000). Memory systems of 1999. In E. Tulving & F. I. M. Craik (Eds.), *Oxford handbook of memory* (pp. 627–643). New York: Oxford University Press.

Schaie, K. W. (1989). Perceptual speed in adulthood: Cross-sectional and longitudinal analyses. *Psychology and Aging, 4*, 443–453.

Schaie, K. W., & Willis, S. (1991). *Adult development and aging*. New York: HarperCollins.

Smith, A. D. (1996). Memory. In J. E. Birren & K.W. Schaie (Eds.), *Handbook of the psychology of aging* (pp. 236–250). San Diego, CA: Academic Press.

Smith, E. E., & Jonides, J. (1999). Storage and executive processes in the frontal lobes. *Science, 283*, 1657–1661.

Smith, E. E., & Medin, D. L. (1981). *Categories and concepts*. Cambridge, MA: Harvard University Press.

Snowdon, D. (2001). *Aging with grace*. New York: Bantam Books.

Squire, L. R. (2004). Memory systems of the brain: A brief history and current perspective. *Neurobiology of Learning and Memory, 82*, 171–177.

Squire, L. R., Stark, C. E. L., & Clark, R. E. (2004). The medial temporal lobe. *Annual Review of Neuroscience, 27*, 279–306.

Stuck, A. E., Walthert, J. M., Nikolaus, T., Bula, C. J., Hohmann, C., & Beck, J. C. (1999). Risk factors for functional status decline in community-living elderly people: A systematic literature review. *Social Science and Medicine, 48*, 445–469.

Tulving, E. (1972). Episodic and semantic memory. In E. Tulving & W. Donaldson (Eds.), *Organization of memory* (pp. 381–403). New York: Academic Press.

Tulving, E. (1984). Elements of episodic memory (precis). *Behavioral and Brain Sciences, 7*, 223–268.

Wang, M. D. (1977). Frequency effects in the abstraction of linguistic ideas. *Bulletin of the Psychonomic Society, 9*, 303–306.

West, R. L. (1996). An application of prefrontal cortex function theory to cognitive aging. *Psychological Bulletin, 120*, 272–292.

Wickelgren, W. A. (1979). *Cognitive psychology*. Englewood Cliffs, NJ: Prentice-Hall.

Woodruff-Pak, D. S. (1997). *The neuropsychology of aging*. Cambridge, MA: Blackwell.

Zola-Morgan, S., Squire, L., & Mishkin, M. (1982). The neuroanatomy of amnesia: Amygdala-hippocampus versus temporal stem. *Science, 218*, 1337–1339.

4

Alzheimer's Dementia

Alzheimer's disease (AD) is the most common cause of dementia. An age-associated disease, it rarely affects individuals younger than 65 years of age. Diagnosis is challenging and historically has been made by excluding other conditions that can produce changes in mental status and intellectual functioning. Computer tomography and magnetic resonance imaging are generally used to rule out tumor, cerebrovascular disease, and normal pressure hydrocephalus and to look for disease-associated atrophy in the medial temporal lobe and amygdalohippocampal system (Knopman et al., 2001).

Diagnostic Criteria for AD

The diagnostic criteria for dementia of the Alzheimer type (American Psychiatric Association, 1994) build on the basic criteria for dementia (multiple intellectual deficits sufficient to interfere with social and occupational functioning) and are as follows:

A. Gradual onset and progressive cognitive deterioration.
B. Cognitive deficits are not due to:
    1. other central nervous system etiologies
    2. systemic conditions

3. substance-induced conditions.
C. Cognitive deficits are not due to an Axis I disorder (e.g., schizophrenia or major depressive disorder).

Because the diagnosis of AD is still presumptive until autopsy or brain biopsy, criteria have been established for designating the degree of confidence that can be placed in the diagnosis.

Criteria for "Possible" AD

The term "possible" AD is applied if there is uncertainty about the diagnosis. The criteria for the designation of "possible" AD (McKhann et al., 1984) include:

1. Dementia in the absence of other dementia-producing etiologies, but with atypical onset, presentation, or course.
2. Dementia presenting concurrently with another systemic or brain disorder sufficient to produce dementia, but which is not considered to be *the cause* of the dementia.
3. Severe progressive decline of a single cognitive function in the absence of another specific cause.

Criteria for "Probable" AD

Patients are described as having "probable" AD if the following criteria (McKhann et al., 1984) are met:

1. Dementia is established by clinical examination documented by mental status examinations and confirmed by neuropsychological tests.
2. Deficits exist in two or more areas of cognition.
3. Progressive worsening of memory and other cognitive functions has occurred.
4. No disturbance of consciousness.
5. Onset was between the ages of 40 and 90, most often after age 65.
6. Absence of systemic disorders or other brain diseases that, in and of themselves, could account for the progressive deficits in memory and cognition.

Further support for the diagnosis of "probable" AD is evidence of progressive difficulties with activities of daily living, a family history of dementia, laboratory results (e.g., computerized tomography [CT] or magnetic resonance imaging [MRI] scan data) and other clinical features consistent with the onset and course of AD.

Neuropathology of AD

Alzheimer's disease (AD) begins in perirhinal cortex (Figure 4–1), the hippocampal complex in the temporal lobes, and the basal forebrain, areas important to episodic memory (Braak, Braak, & Bohl, 1993; Van Hoesen, 1997). As the disease worsens, and structural changes occur in the frontal lobes, working memory is affected. When neuropathology extends to temporal and parietal cortices, semantic memory is affected. Most spared are motor and visual cortices (Farkas et al., 1982; Haxby, Grady, Duara, et al., 1986; Haxby, Grady, Koss, et al., 1990). Because of the sparing of motor cortex, speech is spared.

Motor symptoms can develop late in the disease, among them change in muscle tone, cogwheel phenomenon, postural instability, and difficulty walking. Collectively, these motor changes are referred to as "extrapyramidal signs" (Wilson et al., 2000) and their presence is associated with greater dementia severity (Mayeux, Stern, & Spanton, 1985; Soininen, Laulumaa, Helkala, Hartikainen, & Riekkinen, 1992; Stern, Mayeux, Sano, & Hauser, 1987; Stern, Albert, et al., 1994).

When tissue from the brain of an AD patient is examined microscopically, changes are apparent in the form of neuritic plaques, neurofibrillary tangles, atrophy, and areas of granulovacuolar degeneration. Deposits of amyloid within blood vessels may also be seen.

Neuritic plaques (Figure 4–2), called senile plaques in the older literature, are bits and pieces of degenerating neurons that clump together and have a beta-amyloid core. Beta-amyloid is a protein fragment that has been separated from a larger protein called amyloid precursor protein. The disjoined beta-amyloid fragments aggregate and mix with other molecules, neurons, and nonnerve cells. Neuritic plaques are most prevalent in the outer half of the cortex where the number of neuronal connections is largest.

Neurofibrillary tangles (Figure 4–3) are disintegrating microtubules (microtubules are part of the internal support structure of healthy neurons). They break down because of changes in the protein, tau. As they disintegrate, they become tangled and are a signature morphologic change that the pathologist looks for to confirm the presence of AD.

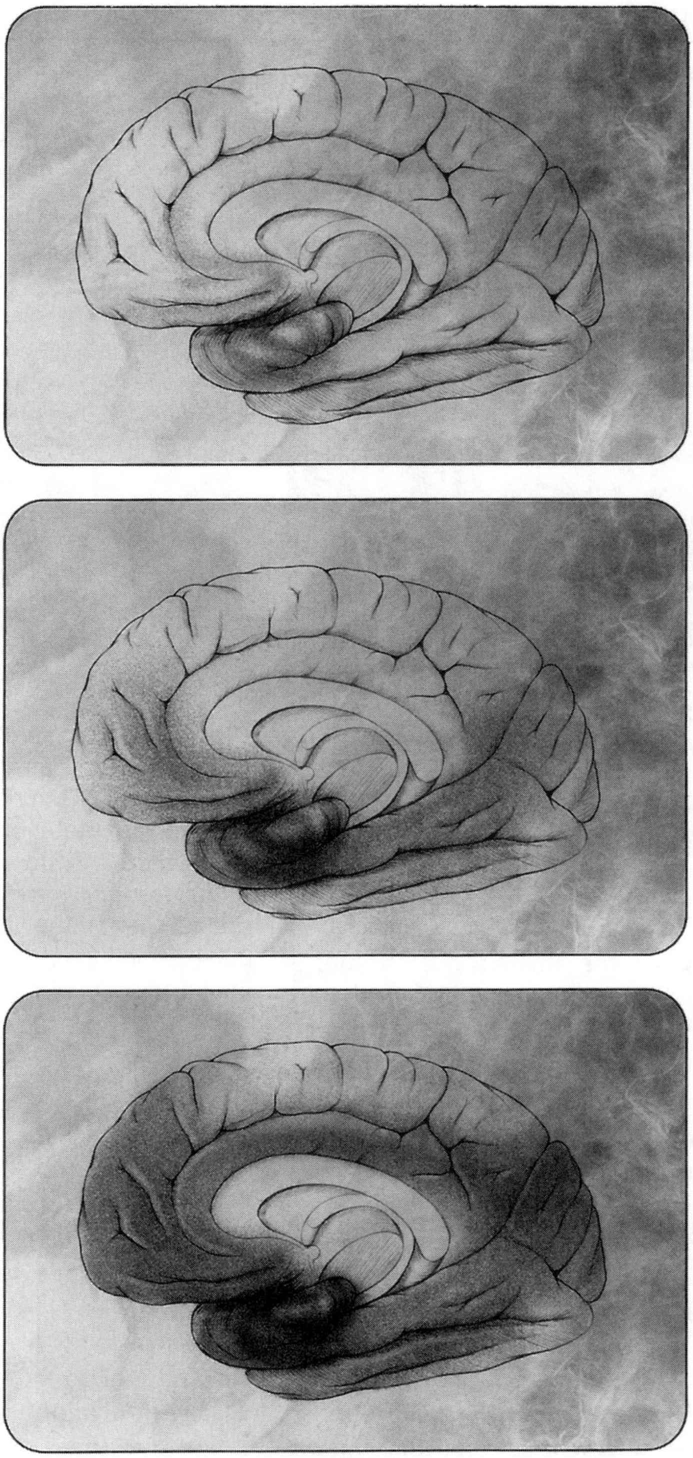

Figure 4–1. Brain areas affected by Alzheimer's disease over the course of the condition. Darker shades indicate areas affected at the various stages of AD. From National Institute on Aging (2002). *Alzheimer's Disease: Unraveling the Mystery*. Silver Spring, MD: Alzheimer's Disease Education and Referral (ADEAR) Center. NIH Publication 02-3782.

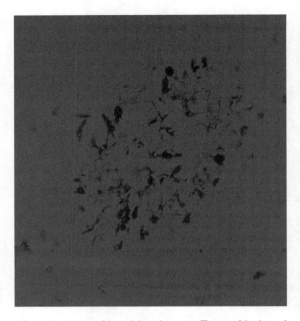

Figure 4–2. Neuritic plaque. From: National Institute on Aging (2002). *Alzheimer's Disease: Unraveling the Mystery*. Silver Spring, MD: Alzheimer's Disease Education and Referral (ADEAR) Center. NIH Publication 02-3782.

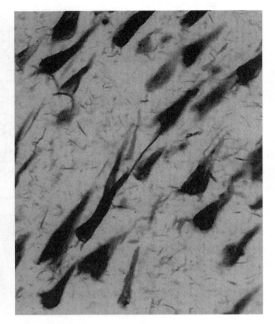

Figure 4–3. Neurofibrillary tangle from the hippocampus of an AD case. From Hof, P. R., Bussière, T., & Morrison, J. H. (2004). Neuropathology of the Ageing Brain. In M. M. Esiri, V. M.-Y. Lee, & J. Q. Trojanowski (Eds.), *The Neuropathology of Dementia* (pp. 113–127). Cambridge: Cambridge University Press. Copyright 2004 Cambridge University Press. Reprinted with the permission of Cambridge University Press.

Atrophy, or the shrinking of tissue, is common in AD (Figures 4–4, 4–5, and 4–6), though it may not be visible on a CT scan if the patient is in the early stage of the disease. Positron emission tomography (PET) scans show prominent changes in the temporal and parietal lobes and inconsistent changes in frontal lobes. Magnetic resonance imaging shows substantial atrophy in entorhinal cortex (Krasuski et al., 1998; Pearlson et al., 1992) and the hippocampal complex (Jack, Petersen, O'Brien, & Tangalos, 1992; Johnson, Saykin, Flashman, & Riordan, 1998).

Granulovacuolar degeneration refers to fluid-filled spaces within cells that contain granular debris. Together these changes (neuritic placques, neurofibrillary tangles, and granulovacuolar degeneration) in brain cells interrupt intercellular communication and thus information processing.

Risk Factors for AD

Evidence has accumulated that the following factors may place an individual at increased risk for developing AD:

- Age
- Family history
- Less education
- Head trauma
- Gender
- Age of mother
- Having two copies of the type 4 allele of apolipoprotein E
- Having minimal cognitive impairment

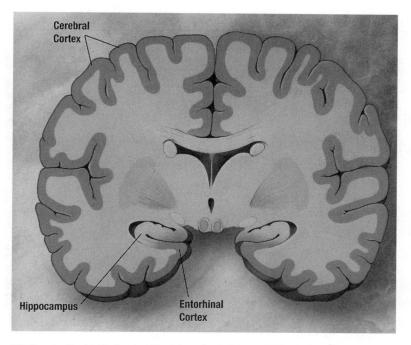

Figure 4–4. Schematic showing brain regions affected in the preclinical stage of AD. From National Institute on Aging (2002). *Alzheimer's Disease: Unraveling the Mystery*. Silver Spring, MD: Alzheimer's Disease Education and Referral (ADEAR) Center. NIH Publication 02-3782.

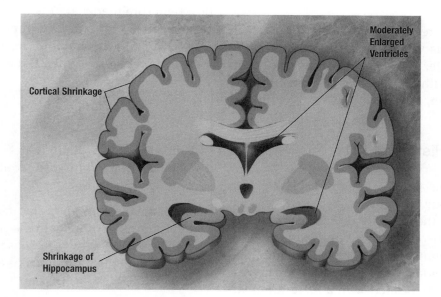

Figure 4–5. Schematic showing brain regions affected in mild AD. From National Institute on Aging (2002). *Alzheimer's Disease: Unraveling the Mystery*. Silver Spring, MD: Alzheimer's Disease Education and Referral (ADEAR) Center. NIH Publication 02-3782.

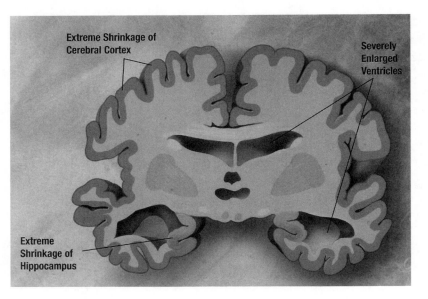

Extreme Shrinkage of
Cerebral Cortex

Severely
Enlarged
Ventricles

Extreme
Shrinkage of
Hippocampus

Figure 4–6. Schematic showing brain regions affected in severe AD. From National Institute on Aging (2002). *Alzheimer's Disease: Unraveling the Mystery.* Silver Spring, MD: Alzheimer's Disease Education and Referral (ADEAR) Center. NIH Publication 02-3782.

Age

Clinically recognizable AD is unusual in individuals younger than 60 but for every decade after the sixth, the number of individuals with AD doubles (Khachaturian & Radebaugh, 1998).

Family History of AD

Individuals with a first-order relative with AD are four times more likely to develop it. However, the majority of AD cases are sporadic with only 5% having familial/autosomal dominant inheritance. Familial AD often develops when individuals are in their 40s and is associated with a more fulminating course (Jacobs, Sano, Marder, & Bell, 1994; Lovestone, 1999; Selkoe, 2000). Results of twin studies indicate that when one twin develops AD, in only 35 to 50% of the cases

will it develop in the other genetically identical twin (Breitner et al., 1993).

Scientists have linked three genes to early onset AD: the amyloid precursor protein gene on chromosome 21, the presenilin

Definitions

Familial—occurring in more members of a family than would be expected by chance.

Autosomal—the gene is located on a chromosome other than the sex chromosome, so the disease is not sex-linked; males and females are equally likely to be affected.

Dominant—the defective gene dominates its normal partner gene from the unaffected parent.

gene 1 on chromosome 14, and the presenilin gene 2 on chromosome 1. Note that the amyloid precursor protein gene is located on the same chromosome that is affected in Down syndrome, chromosome 21. The presenilin gene 1 on chromosome 14 is suspected of being responsible for the majority of early onset cases.

Less Education

Individuals with less education have been reported to be more likely to develop AD (Kawas & Katzman, 1999). Uneducated individuals, who are older than 75, have almost twice the risk of dementia compared to elders with eight or more years of education. A popular explanation for this finding is that educated individuals have a richer network of interneuronal connections (and therefore greater cognitive reserve) that developed from the stimulation provided by more education.

History of Head Trauma

Individuals with prior head injury may be at higher risk for AD (Kawas & Katzman, 1999). Although the specific mechanism underlying the association of AD and head injury is not well understood, scientists theorize that head injury can alter the brain's protective system. Recently, researchers found head injury to be a risk factor only for those individuals with the ApoE4 allele (Mayeux et al., 1995).

Gender

Women have a higher age-specific prevalence (Hebert et al., 1995; Schoenberg, Anderson, & Haeren, 1985) and incidence (Kokmen, Chandra, & Schoenberg, 1988; McGonigal et al., 1993) of AD than men. The reason for the gender effect remains to be explained, though some attribute it to the greater longevity of women (Jagger, Clarke, & Stone, 1995).

Maternal Age

Your mother's age at the time of your birth may influence your risk of developing AD. Both advanced (Cohen, Eisdorfer, & Leverenz, 1982) and early (van Duijn, Hoffman, & Kay, 1991) maternal age have been reported as influential. The pathogenetic mechanism underlying the association of advanced or early maternal age and AD remains open for speculation.

Apolipoprotein E4 Allele

A type of cholesterol carrying protein has been found to be a major risk factor for late-onset AD, namely, the type 4 allele of apolipoprotein E (ApoE). ApoE in the body varies in composition across individuals. The specific composition of ApoE is influenced by the presence or absence of three major variants of the gene which are called E2, E3, and E4. An individual inherits one gene that codes for the ApoE protein from each parent. The most common type is ApoE3 and most people inherit one or two copies. People who develop AD more commonly have the ApoE4 allele, and those with two copies of the ApoE4 gene have eight times greater risk of developing late onset AD than individuals with no copies of ApoE4 (Corder et al., 1993). However, almost half the individuals with AD do not have the ApoE4 genotype, and the presence of an E4 allele accounts for a relatively small percentage of the cases of AD (Evans et al., 1997; Myers et al., 1996).

Minimal Cognitive Impairment

The term minimal cognitive impairment (MCI) is widely used to describe a population of individuals who report memory problems and changes in their ability to process information. Neuroimaging studies show that the brains of individuals with MCI differ from those of normal elders (Ritchie, Artero, & Touchon, 2001).

Clinicians should be alert to the fact that a significant percentage of individuals with MCI will eventually be diagnosed with AD (Flicker, Ferris, & Reisberg, 1991, 1993; O'Neill, Surmon, & Wilcock, 1992). Diagnostic criteria have been developed for MCI and include memory complaints, normal activities of daily living (ADLs), normal general cognitive function, abnormal memory for age, but no dementia.

Preclinical AD

The onset of AD is insidious occurring many years before a clinical diagnosis is typically made. Results of prospective studies reveal that as many as six years before AD is clinically evident, cognitive deterioration has begun (Collie & Maruff, 2000; Grober, Lipton, Hall, & Crystal, 2000; Hodges, 1998). Preclinical deficits have been demonstrated by investigators using a variety of neuropsychological measures: psychomotor speed (Masur, Sliwinski, Lipton, Blau, & Crystal, 1994); perceptual speed (Rainville, Fabrigoule, Amieva, & Dartigues, 1998); abstract reasoning (Fabrigoule, Lafont, Letenneur, Rouch, & Dartigues, 1996); visuospatial performance (Howieson et al., 1997); verbal ability (Jacobs, Sano, Doonief, & Marder, 1995); and episodic memory (Collie & Maruff, 2000; Grober et al., 2000; Hodges, 1998). Preclinical deficits are apparent for verbal and nonverbal information in different retrieval conditions. Elias

and colleagues (2000) reported that lower scores on measures of memory and abstract reasoning are particularly strong predictors of probable AD.

Predictors of Disease Progression

The average duration of Alzheimer's disease is 8 years, though many victims suffer for 12 or more years. More rapid decline in AD is linked to:

- Early age at onset
- Presence of delusions or hallucinations
- Presence of extrapyramidal signs

Effects of AD on Cognitive and Communicative Functions

The ever present features of AD are impairment of episodic and working memory, especially executive functions. Other symptoms are more variable and reflect differences in the distribution of neuropathology (Galton, Patterson, Xuereb, & Hodges, 2000; Perry & Hodges, 2000). Some patients have greater visual spatial than language deficits, for others, the reverse is true (Fisher, Rourke, Bieliauskas, & Giordani, 1996; Martin et al., 1986). Results of longitudinal studies, using the Mini-Mental Status Examination (MMSE), indicate that the average amount of cognitive decline per year is 2 to 4 points (Ballard et al., 2001). On the Alzheimer's Disease Assessment Scale—Cognitive (ADAS-COG, see Chapter 11 for description), the average is 8 points per year (Stern, Mohs, et al., 1994).

Early Stage

The early stage of AD lasts from two to four years (National Alzheimer's Association). When caregivers were asked to specify the earliest changes they observed before the diagnosis of AD was made (Bayles, 1991), they reported:

1. Difficulty handling finances
2. Memory problems
3. Concentration problems
4. Difficulty with complex tasks
5. Forgetting the location of objects
6. Decreased awareness of recent events

Mental Status

In early stage AD, the affected individual is disoriented for time but not place or person. The following chart shows the average score, or range of scores, of early stage AD patients on commonly used mental status tests:

ABCD Mental Status subtest score (Bayles & Tomoeda, 1993)	7.3 to 12.5
Mini-Mental State Examination score (Folstein, Folstein, & McHugh, 1975)	16 to 24
Clinical Dementia Rating Scale (Hughes, Berg, Danziger, Coben, & Martin, 1982)	1.0
Global Deterioration Scale (Reisberg, Ferris, de Leon, & Crook, 1982)	3

Motor Function

Motor function is good and the patient is ambulatory.

Memory Function

The first obvious symptom of AD is a problem with episodic memory: forgetting where the car is parked, getting lost, being repetitious, not remembering having taken medication, and the like. Working memory is also affected early in the progression of the disease, and is manifested by decreased efficiency of encoding and retrieval of information. Individuals have difficulty sustaining attention (Bäckman, Small, & Fratiglioni, 2001; Grady et al., 1988; Morris, 1996; Perry, Watson, & Hodges, 2000) and span memory is modestly attenuated in some individuals, though not all.

Basic ADLs

Individuals in early stage AD are generally able to carry out basic activities of daily living, such as bathing, dressing and feeding themselves and going to the bathroom independently.

Linguistic Communication

Speech is fluent in early AD with no evidence of dysarthria. Spoken language is grammatical though errors of grammar and spelling are common in written language (Blanken, Dittman, Haas, & Wallesch, 1987; Irigaray, 1967). The content of language is noticeably affected and characterized by tangentiality and an increase in the number of "empty words" such as "thing" and "it." Because AD patients often forget what they just heard or thought, their oral discourse contains more sentence fragments and repetitiousness and is less cohesive than the discourse of healthy peers (Bayles, Tomoeda, & Boone, 1985; Bayles, Tomoeda, Kaszniak, Stern, & Eagans, 1985; Tomoeda & Bayles, 1993). Mild dysnomia is common and when a naming error occurs, it is usually semantically related to the target word (e.g., "lime" for "lemon" and "sharp" for "saw") (Bayles & Tomoeda, 1983a). Performance on tests of receptive vocabulary reveal that vocabulary is shrinking.

Language Use. Writing is more affected than oral language and written discourse contains intrusions, perseverations, and more spatial-mechanical disturbances than that of healthy peers (Appell, Kertesz, & Fisman, 1982; Croisile, 1999; Horner, Heyman, Dawson, & Rogers, 1988; Kertesz, Appell, & Fisman, 1986). Although individuals in early stage AD generally comprehend what they hear and read, they quickly forget it (Bayles, Tomoeda, & Trosset, 1992). Mild AD patients often miss the point of a joke or are confused by sarcasm. Some individuals exhibit logorrhea (Gustafson, Hagberg, & Ingvar, 1978; Obler & Albert, 1985), perhaps from disinhibition associated with frontal lobe damage. Early stage patients are able to answer most questions and define words (Bayles & Tomoeda, 1993).

Table 4–1 presents early linguistic communication symptoms (Bayles & Tomoeda, 1991), listed in order of prevalence—from most to least frequent—as reported by 99 primary caregivers of AD patients. The most commonly reported symptom was word-finding difficulty. The least prevalent was an increase in talkativeness.

Discourse Sample of Mild AD Patient. The following discourse sample is typical of early stage AD patients. The individual who produced this sample was instructed to

Table 4–1. Linguistic Communication Symptoms Listed in Order of Prevalence from Most to Least Frequent (Bayles & Tomoeda, 1991)

Most Frequent
Word-finding problems.
Difficulty naming objects.
Difficulty writing a letter.
Impaired comprehension of instructions.
Difficulty sustaining a conversation.
Problem completing sentences.
Tendency to repeat ideas.
Reading comprehension problems.
Production of meaningless sentences.
Decrease in talkativeness.
Inappropriate topics.
Inappropriate to whom said.
Tendency to interpret literally.
Failure to recognize humor.
Increase in talkativeness.
Least Frequent

explain what is happening in the Norman Rockwell picture entitled, "Easter Morning." Rockwell portrays a man sitting in the family living room clad in pajamas and looking sheepish because he is not going to church with his wife and three children on Easter Sunday. Rather, he is staying home to read the newspaper, drink coffee, and smoke cigarettes. His wife and children are lined up behind him ready to go out the door.

> Two, three, four . . . I see we have a one, two, three . . . We have three women, we have a little boy, and we have a rather old male sitting on a chair and reading newspapers, and he also has various newspapers sprawling all over the room. I just . . . what are they doing? What are they doing? The girls seem to be just walking in a sort of a military sort of a way and the little boy follows the girl, the girls in similarly the same way. And of course, in front of the group there is this man, who is probably just got out of bed. And he is dressed like a man who just got out of bed and he's reading the newspaper and these other newspapers that are at the front of his feet, I think so. Is there anything else I could say? Very peculiar. The women seem to be ready to go out of the house, to go somewhere and the male who is sit- sitting there probably for the rest of the day saying, "Oh boy, this is great. I can read all of the newspapers I want now." And I think he even has, if I'm not mistaken, he even has, I don't know. Anyway, so I can't tell what this object is here, I think a lot of my thing is gone now. I better get another pair of eyeglasses. I don't care if it's gonna cost another hundred but I gotta get it.

Notice that the utterances are generally grammatical; however, compared to neurologically normal adults, this mild AD patient is a less efficient communicator. He produced many aborted phrases because of confusion and forgotten linguistic intentions. The volume of discourse produced is not necessarily less than what a healthy elder would produce but it contains fewer ideas. Early stage AD patients tend to repeat ideas as did this gentleman who repeatedly mentioned the newspapers. This phenomenon of *ideational perseveration* occurs more in mild and moderate patients than in severe because by the severe stage, individuals with AD have many fewer ideas.

Middle Stage

The middle stage of AD typically occurs 4 to 10 years after clinical diagnosis (National Alzheimer's Association). During this stage, the patient changes most dramatically becoming more dependent on others for survival.

Mental Status

In mid-stage AD, individuals become disoriented for place as well as time though orientation to self is intact. The following chart shows the average scores of mid-stage individuals on widely used mental status tests.

ABCD Mental Status subtest score (Bayles & Tomoeda, 1993)	1.3 to 7.7
Mini-Mental State Examination score (Folstein, Folstein, & McHugh, 1975)	8 to 15
Clinical Dementia Rating Scale (Hughes, Berg, Danziger, Coben, & Martin, 1982)	2
Global Deterioration Scale (Reisberg, Ferris, de Leon, & Crook, 1982)	4 to 6

Motor Function

Motor function in mid-stage AD patients remains good but restlessness is common.

Memory

Many changes occur in memory in mid-stage AD including worsening of episodic memory, attenuation of span memory, encoding and retrieval deficits, and degradation of semantic memory. Mid-stage patients have difficulty focusing attention, are easily distracted, and can be difficult to engage in activities. Visual-perceptual and visual-constructive deficits are apparent and, in fact, AD patients perform inferiorly to healthy peers on virtually all executive function and cognitive-communicative tests.

Continence

During the latter portion of mid-stage AD, incontinence of bladder becomes a problem.

Basic ADLs

With supervision and environmental support, most mid-stage AD patients can carry out basic ADLs. In contrast, instrumental ADLs such as taking messages and managing finances are problematic. It is in this stage that driving becomes an issue. Although the

---

Definitions

Activities of daily living (ADLs) — activities routinely performed in the course of an average day such as feeding, bathing, dressing, and grooming.

Instrumental activities of daily living (IADLs) — activities related to independent living such as preparing meals, managing finances, shopping, doing housework, and using the telephone.

---

mid-stage AD patient can manipulate the controls and mechanically drive a car, problems with attention, judgment, and memory make them dangerous to themselves and other drivers.

Linguistic Communication

Speech. Speech is fluent though often slower and halting.

Form of Language. The form of language remains generally intact but content is prominently affected (Bayles, Tomoeda, & Trosset, 1992). Oral discourse contains fewer nouns relative to verbs (Blanken et al., 1987; Fung, Chertkow, & Templeman, 2000; Robinson, Rossor, & Cipolotti, 1999), is less cohesive (Critchley, 1964), and can be described as "empty." Performance on vocabulary tests indicates loss of vocabulary and greater degradation of conceptual knowledge (Bayles, Tomoeda, & Trosset, 1992; Hier, Hagenlocker, & Shindler, 1985; Tomoeda & Bayles, 1993). Mid-stage AD patients are significantly impaired relative to healthy peers in generating exemplars of a category (Bayles & Tomoeda, 1983b; Bayles, Salmon, et al., 1989; Hodges, Salmon, & Butters, 1990; Huff, Corkin, & Growdon, 1986) and naming on confrontation (Bayles, Tomoeda, & Trosset, 1992). Written language is replete with errors. Mid-stage patients exhibit diminished comprehension of written and spoken language (Bayles, 1982; Cummings, Benson, Hill, & Read, 1985; Faber-Langendoen et al., 1998; Horner, Dawson, Heyman, & McGorman-Fish, 1992; Kempler, Almor, Tyler, Anderssen, & MacDonald, 1998; Rochon, Waters, & Caplan, 2000) though most do well at the word and phrase level. The mechanics of reading are spared but comprehension is impaired and that which is comprehended is rapidly forgotten.

Language Use. Word finding difficulties are now more obvious in spontaneous speech and on confrontation and generative naming tests (Bayles & Tomoeda, 1983b; Benson, 1979; Kirshner, Webb, & Kelly, 1984; Salmon, Butters, & Chan, 1999). Ideational repetition (Bayles, Tomoeda, Kaszniak, et al., 1985) is frequent in conversation and when individuals are asked to describe a picture or object. Mid-stage patients have poor sensitivity to context (Tomoeda, Bayles, Trosset, Azuma, & McGeagh, 1996) and may miss the point of jokes. Also, they have a tendency to interpret nonliteral language literally. Mid-stage patients can perform the mechanics of reading aloud, comprehend written language at the word level, and follow simple commands but have serious difficulty defining words and repeating phrases (Bayles & Tomoeda, 1993). In terms of writing, mid-stage patients make many spelling errors and mechanical distortions (Neils-Strunjas, Groves-Wright, Mashima, & Harnish, 2006) and their narratives are less complex.

Discourse Sample of Moderately Demented AD Patient

Task: Description of the "Easter Morning" Picture

Yeah, well, this man is, knows that he is, is in the wrong place here. So, but he's hiding away and, and these other people, I don't know whether this boy is ready to do it or not but this man is doing it from someplace over here, but it won't do it. And, ah, these, these, two children are evidently are just very excellent that they are both the same person. And, this man I don't know, would rather . . . He gets his too. And uh, oh, he's got this thing, worried because it's going to have a . . . going up there, you can see it. (Subject points to the cigarette smoke in the picture). And all this stuff is just a mess.

Darn fools got anybody. Darn fools got them walking in it. They want to, I don't think they do. I don't want to go in this place. I don't know what he's for. He's looks like he's getting a ten paper. Here's some more paper. Here's some more, my god! Look at it. He has to be worn down before he can do anything, cause these people don't want to work, work anything with him. Don't you think that's about right?

As is apparent from this description, moderately demented AD patients produce discourse that expresses significantly fewer ideas than that produced by mild AD patients. They are increasingly less concise and more repetitious. As is typical of moderately demented patients, the individual who produced this discourse failed to state the gist of the Rockwell picture. The intention to describe remains but word sequences may have little apparent meaning. Furthermore, there is a lack of self-monitoring and correction.

Late Stage AD

During the late stage, AD patients often become disoriented for person as well as place and time. Their scores on the Mini-Mental State Examination (MMSE) range from 0 to 9 (Folstein et al., 1975). On the Clinical Dementia Rating Scale, they score 3 (Hughes et al., 1982). Motor impairment may be present and, in the very late stage, many are nonambulatory. There is incontinence of bladder and bowel. Intellect is devastated by a global failure of working and declarative memory systems and individuals are unable to carry out basic ADLs.

Linguistic Communication

Speech is typically fluent but generally slower and more halting. In many patients, the form of language remains intact (Bayles, Tomoeda, Cruz, & Mahendra, 2000) though meaningful output is greatly reduced (Appell et al., 1982). Some individuals are mute, others exhibit palilalia (repetition of phrases, words, or syllables that tend to increase in speed at the end of an utterance) (Appell et al., 1982) or echolalia (Irigaray, 1967), or jargon (Obler & Albert, 1984). And yet, other advanced patients can contribute to a conversation, state their name, and retain aspects of social language (Kim & Bayles, 2007). Reading comprehension is severely impaired though some can read single words aloud (Bayles & Tomoeda, 1994; Bayles et al., 2000). Virtually all late-stage patients are unable to express themselves in writing.

Communicative Abilities of Late-Stage AD Patients (Bayles et al., 2000). The verbal communication abilities of 49 late-stage AD patients were evaluated in relation to other markers of late-stage AD (incontinence and ambulatory ability). The authors of two widely used tools, the Global Deterioration Scale (Reisberg et al., 1982) and the Functional Assessment Stages (Reisberg et al., 1984), reported the virtual loss of all verbal abilities in late-stage AD patients. As part of an NIH-supported longitudinal study of individuals with AD, Bayles and colleagues were able to evaluate language in 49 late-stage patients. The *Functional Linguistic Communication Inventory* (FLCI) (Bayles & Tomoeda, 1994) was administered to study participants. The FLCI evaluates greeting and naming, question answering, writing, sign comprehension and object-to-picture matching, word reading and comprehension, ability to reminisce, following commands, pantomime, gesture, and conversation.

Study results revealed that AD patients, who are incontinent only for bladder, have more communication skills than individuals who are bladder and bowel incontinent. They were able to respond appropriately when greeted and to a closing comment and compliment. Several could recognize the written form of their name, state their spouse's name, recognize a common object from a line drawing, follow a one-step command, and even correct misinformation about themselves.

None of the individuals who were incontinent for both bladder and bowel were able to contribute to a conversation. Neither could they state their spouse's name, follow a two-step command, or provide relevant information about a common object. The most limited language was observed in individuals who were bowel and bladder-incontinent and bedridden. However, contrary to what was expected, given previous characterizations of the verbal ability of late-stage patients (Reisberg et al., 1984), 82% of the study participants produced language during the evaluation.

The incontinent but ambulatory patients produced more words than those who were incontinent and nonambulatory. Of the 10 individuals who were incontinent but ambulatory, one AD participant produced 252 words and another produced a single word. Of the 17 individuals who were incontinent and nonambulatory, three individuals were nonverbal, two produced a single word, and one produced 131 words of which 82 were different words.

The following are examples of answers provided by study subjects to questions such as "Where would you like to go on a trip?" and "What is your favorite food?"

"Right now I think I'd like to see Hawaii."

"Fruit of all kind is all right with me, I love fruit."

"I don't think I ought to go anywhere cause I'm in bad shape."

"I eat a lot of things now."

Discourse Sample of Severely Demented AD Patient

Task: Description of a Nail

Severe AD patient:

> Well, that looks just like, uh, uh, hazel. What do they call them, a hazelette. No not a hazelette, that's for outside there. (pause) I could tell you if I knew some of my, uh, father's (laughs) things I could tell you anything other than words because when you been in this business and, uh, had so many things.

As you can see, meaningful verbal output has diminished dramatically. Listeners often have difficulty linking what the AD patient says with the context. However, grammar is often intact.

Summary of Important Points

- Alzheimer's disease (AD) is the most common cause of dementia.
- The key diagnostic criterion for diagnosis is the presence of multiple cognitive deficits sufficient to interfere with social and occupational functioning that are gradual in onset and progressive in nature.
- AD begins in brain areas important to episodic memory and spreads to areas important to working and declarative memory. Procedural memory is spared until late in the disease course.
- The characteristic morphologic changes in the brain are neuritic plaques and neurofibrillary tangles with areas of granulovacuolar degeneration and atrophy.
- AD rarely affects individuals younger than 60 but for every decade after the sixth, the number of individuals with AD doubles.
- A small number of individuals develop familial AD in their 40s, an autosomal dominant form of the disease.
- A type of cholesterol carrying protein has been found to be a major risk factor for late-onset AD, namely, the type 4 allele of apolipoprotein E.
- The average duration of AD after diagnosis is eight years, although some individuals have the disease much longer.
- Communicative ability gradually deteriorates over the disease course. In the early stages, individuals are verbally fluent and able to comprehend most of what they read and hear but rapidly forget it. By end-stage disease, individuals are intellectually devastated and language output is greatly diminished and often nonsensical.
- Semantics and pragmatics are affected early; phonology and syntax are generally preserved well into the disease course.
- Considerable variability exists in the ability of late-stage AD patients to communicate. Some are mute, others produce some meaningful language.

References

American Psychiatric Association (1994). *Diagnostic and statistical manual of mental disorders* (4th ed.). Washington, DC: Author.

Appell, J., Kertesz, A., & Fisman, M. (1982). A study of language functioning in Alzheimer's patients. *Brain and Language, 17,* 73–91.

Bäckman, L., Small, B. J., & Fratiglioni. L. (2001). Stability of the preclinical episodic memory deficit in Alzheimer's disease. *Brain, 124,* 96–102.

Ballard, C., O'Brien, J., Morris, C. M., Barber, R., Swann, A., Neill, D., & McKeith, I. (2001). The progression of cognitive impairment in dementia with Lewy bodies, vascular dementia and

Alzheimer's disease. *International Journal of Geriatric Psychiatry, 16,* 499–503.

Bayles, K. A. (1982). Language function in senile dementia. *Brain and Language, 16,* 265–280.

Bayles, K. A. (1991). Alzheimer's disease symptoms: Prevalence and order of appearance. *Journal of Applied Gerontology, 10,* 419–430.

Bayles, K. A., Salmon, D. P., Tomoeda, C. K., Jacobs, D., Caffrey, J. T., Kaszniak, A. W., et al. (1989). Semantic and letter category naming in Alzheimer's patients: A predictable difference. *Developmental Neuropsychology, 5,* 335–347.

Bayles, K. A., & Tomoeda, C. K. (1983a). Confrontation naming impairment in dementia. *Brain and Language, 19,* 98–114.

Bayles, K. A., & Tomoeda, C. K. (1983b). Confrontation naming and generative naming abilities of dementia patients. In R. Brookshire (Ed.), *Clinical Aphasiology Conference Proceedings 1983* (pp. 304–315). Minneapolis, MN: BRK Publications.

Bayles, K. A., & Tomoeda, C. K. (1991). Caregiver report of prevalence and appearance order of linguistic symptoms in Alzheimer's patients. *The Gerontologist, 31,* 210–216.

Bayles, K. A., & Tomoeda, C. K. (1993). *Arizona Battery for Communication Disorders of Dementia.* Austin, TX: Pro-Ed.

Bayles, K. A., & Tomoeda, C. K. (1994). *Functional Linguistic Communication Inventory.* Austin, TX: Pro-Ed.

Bayles, K. A., Tomoeda, C. K., & Boone, D. R. (1985). A view of age-related changes in language function. *Developmental Neuropsychology, 1,* 231–264.

Bayles, K. A., Tomoeda, C. K., Cruz, R. F., & Mahendra, N. (2000). Communication abilities of individuals with late-stage Alzheimer's disease. *Alzheimer's Disease and Associated Disorders, 14,* 176–181.

Bayles, K. A., Tomoeda, C. K., Kaszniak, A. W., Stern, L. Z., & Eagans, K. K. (1985). Patterns of perseveration of dementia patients. *Brain and Language, 25,* 102–116.

Bayles, K. A., Tomoeda, C. K., & Trosset, M. W. (1992). Relation of linguistic communication abilities of Alzheimer's patients to stage of disease. *Brain and Language, 42,* 454–472.

Benson, D. F. (1979). Neurologic correlates of anomia. In H. Whitaker & H. A. Whitaker (Eds.), *Studies in neurolinguistics* (Vol. 4, pp. 298–328). New York: Academic Press.

Blanken, G., Dittmann, J., Haas, J., & Wallesch, C. (1987). Spontaneous speech in senile dementia and aphasia: Implications for a neurolinguistic model of language production. *Cognition, 27,* 247–274.

Braak, H., Braak, E., & Bohl, J. (1993). Staging of Alzheimer-related cortical destruction. *European Neurology, 33,* 403–408.

Breitner, J. C. S., Gatz, M., Bergem, A. L. M., Christian, J. C., Mortimer, J. A., McClearn, G. E., et al. (1993). Use of twin cohorts for research in Alzheimer's disease. *Neurology, 43,* 261–267.

Cohen, D., Eisdorfer, C., & Leverenz, J. (1982). Alzheimer's disease and maternal age. *Journal of the American Geriatrics Society, 30,* 656–659.

Collie, A., & Maruff, P. (2000). The neuropsychology of preclinical Alzhemier's disease and mild cognitive impairment. *Neuroscience and Biobehavioral Reviews, 24,* 365–374.

Corder, E. H., Saunders, A. M., Strittmatter, W. J., Schmechel, D. E., Gaskell, P. C., Small, G. W., et al. (1993). Gene dose of apolipoprotein E type 4 allele and the risk of Alzheimer's disease in late onset families. *Science, 261,* 921–923.

Critchley, M. (1964). The neurology of psychotic speech. *British Journal of Psychiatry, 110,* 353–364.

Croisile, B. (1999). Agraphia in Alzheimer's disease. *Dementia and Geriatric Cognitive Disorders, 10,* 226–230.

Cummings, J., Benson, F., Hill, M., & Read, S. (1985). Aphasia in dementia of the Alzheimer type. *Neurology, 35,* 394–397.

Elias, M. F., Beiser, A., Wolf, P. A., Au, R., White, R. F., & D'Agostino, R. B. (2000). The preclinical phase of Alzheimer disease: A 22-year prospective study of the Framingham cohort. *Archives of Neurology, 57,* 808–813.

Evans, D. A., Beckett, L. A., Field, T. S., Feng, L., Albert, M. S., Bennett, D. A., et al. (1997). Apolipoprotein epsilon4 and incidence of Alzheimer disease in a community population of older persons. *Journal of the American Medical Association, 277,* 822–824.

Faber-Langendoen, K., Morris, J. C., Knesevich, J. W., LaBarge, E., Miller, J. P., & Berg, L. (1998). Aphasia in senile dementia of the Alzheimer type. *Annals of Neurology, 23*, 365–370.

Fabrigoule, C., Lafont, S., Letenneur, L., Rouch, I., & Dartigues, J. F. (1996). WAIS similarities subtest performance as predictors of dementia in elderly community residents. *Brain and Cognition, 30*, 323–326.

Fabrigoule, C., Rouche, I., Taberly, A., Letenneur, L., Commenges, D., Mazaux, J.-M., et al. (1998). Cognitive process in preclinical phase of dementia. *Brain, 121*, 135–141.

Farkas, T., Ferris, S. H., Wolf, A. P., de Leon, M. J., Christmas, D. R., Reisberg, B., et al. (1982). (18F) F2-deoxy-2-fluoro-D-glucose as a tracer in positron emission tomographic study of senile dementia. *American Journal of Psychiatry, 139*, 352–353.

Fisher, N., Rourke, B., Bieliauskas, L., & Giordani, B. (1996). Neuropsychological subgroups of patients with Alzheimer's disease. *Journal of Clinical and Experimental Neuropsychology, 18*, 349–370.

Flicker, C., Ferris, S. H., & Reisberg, B. (1991). Mild cognitive impairment in the elderly: Predictors of dementia. *Neurology, 41*, 1006–1009.

Flicker, C., Ferris, S. H., & Reisberg, B. (1993). A two-year longitudinal study of cognitive function in normal aging and Alzheimer's disease. *Journal of Geriatric Psychiatry and Neurology, 34*, 294–295.

Folstein, M. F., Folstein, S. E., & McHugh, P. R. (1975). "Mini-mental state": A practical method for grading the mental state of patients for the clinician. *Journal of Psychiatric Research, 12*, 189–198.

Fung, T., Chertkow, H., & Templeman, F. (2000). Pattern of semantic memory impairment in dementia of Alzheimer's type. *Brain and Cognition, 43*, 200–205.

Galton, C., Patterson, K., Xuereb, J., & Hodges, J. (2000). Atypical and typical presentations of Alzheimer's disease: A clinical neuropsychological, neuroimaging and pathological study of 13 cases. *Brain: A Journal of Neurology, 123*, 484–498.

Grady, C., Haxby, J., Horwitz, B., Sundaram, M., Berg, G., Schapiro, M., et al. (1988). Longitudinal study of the early neuropsychological and cerebral metabolic changes in dementia of the Alzheimer type. *Journal of Clinical and Experimental Neuropsychology, 10*, 576–596.

Grober, E., Lipton, R., Hall, C., & Crystal, H. (2000). Memory impairment on free and cued selective reminding predicts dementia. *Neurology, 54*, 827–832.

Gustafson, L., Hagberg, B., & Ingvar, D. (1978). Speech disturbances in presenile dementia related to local cerebral blood flow abnormalities in the dominant hemisphere. *Brain and Language, 5*, 103–118.

Haxby, J., Grady, C., Duara, R., Schlageter, N., Berg, G., & Rapoport, S. I. (1986). Neocortical metabolic abnormalities precede non memory cognitive defects in early Alzheimer-type dementia. *Archives of Neurology, 43*, 882–885.

Haxby, J. V., Grady, C. L., Koss, E., Holtz, B., Heston, L., Shapiro, M., et al. (1990). Longitudinal study of cerebral metabolic asymmetries and associated neuropsychological patterns in early dementia of the Alzheimer type. *Archives of Neurology, 47*, 753–760.

Hebert, L. E., Scherr, P. A., Beckett, L. A., Albert, M. S., Pilgrim, D. M., Chown, M. J., et al. (1995). Age-specific incidence of Alzheimer's disease in a community population. *Journal of the American Medical Association, 273*, 1354–1359.

Hier, D., Hagenlocker, K., & Shindler, A. (1985). Language disintegration in dementia: Effects of etiology and severity. *Brain and Language, 25*, 117–133.

Hodges, J. (1998). The amnestic prodrome of Alzheimer's disease. *Brain: A Journal of Neurology, 121*, 1601–1602.

Hodges, J., Salmon, D., & Butters, N. (1990). Differential impairment of semantic and episodic memory in Alzheimer's and Huntington's diseases: A controlled prospective study. *Journal of Neurology, Neurosurgery and Psychiatry, 53*, 1089–1095.

Horner, J., Dawson, D., Heyman, A., & McGorman-Fish, A. (1992). The usefulness of the Western Aphasia Battery for differential diagnosis of Alzheimer dementia and focal stroke syndromes: Preliminary evidence. *Brain and Language, 42*, 77–88.

Horner, J., Heyman, A., Dawson, D., & Rogers, H. (1988). The relationship of agraphia to the severity of dementia in Alzheimer's disease. *Archives of Neurology, 45,* 760–763.

Howieson, D. B., Dame, A., Camicioli, R., Sexton, G., Payami, H., & Kaye, J. A. (1997). Cognitive markers preceding Alzheimer's dementia in the healthy oldest old. *Journal of the American Geriatrics Society, 45,* 584–589.

Huff, F., Corkin, S., & Growdon, J. (1986). Semantic impairment and anomia in Alzheimer's disease. *Brain and Language, 28,* 235–249.

Hughes, C. P., Berg, L, Danziger, W. L., Coben, L. A., & Martin, R. L. (1982). A new clinical scale for the staging of dementia. *British Journal of Psychiatry, 140,* 566–572.

Irigaray, L. (1967). Approche psycho-linguistique du langage des dements. *Neuropsychologia, 5,* 25–52.

Jack, C. R. Jr., Petersen, R. C., O'Brien, P. C., & Tangalos, E. G. (1992). MR-based hippocampal volumetry in diagnosis of Alzheimer's disease. *Neurology, 42,* 183–188.

Jacobs, D., Sano, M., Dooneief, G., & Marder, K. (1995). Neuropsychological detection and characterization of preclinical Alzheimer's disease. *Neurology, 45,* 957–962.

Jacobs, D., Sano, M., Marder, K., & Bell, K. (1994). Age at onset of Alzheimer's disease: Relation to pattern of cognitive dysfunction and rate of decline. *Neurology, 44,* 1215–1220.

Jagger, C., Clarke, M., & Stone, A. (1995). Predictors of survival with Alzheimer's disease: A community-based study. *Psychological Medicine, 25,* 171–177.

Johnson, S. C., Saykin, A. J., Flashman, L. A., & Riordan, H. J. (1998). Reduction of hippocampal formation in Alzheimer's disease and correlation with memory: A meta-analysis. *Journal of the International Neuropsychological Society, 4,* 22.

Kawas, C. H., & Katzman, R. (1999). Epidemiology of dementia and Alzheimer disease. In R. D. Terry, R. Katzman, K. L. Bick, & S. S. Sisodia (Eds), *Alzheimer disease* (pp. 95–116). Philadelphia: Lippincott Williams & Wilkins.

Kempler, D., Almor, A., Tyler, L., Andersen, E., & MacDonald, M. (1998). Sentence comprehension deficits in Alzheimer's disease: A comparison of off-line vs. on-line sentence processing. *Brain and Language, 64,* 297–316.

Kertesz A., Appell, J., & Fisman, M. (1986). The dissolution of language in Alzheimer's disease. *Canadian Journal of Neurological Science, 13,* 415–418.

Khachaturian, Z. S., & Radebaugh, T. S. (1998). AD: Where are we now? Where are we going? *Alzheimer Disease and Associated Disorders, 12* (Suppl. 3), 24–28.

Kim, E. S., & Bayles, K. A. (2007). Communication in late-stage Alzheimer's disease: Relation to functional markers of disease severity. *Alzheimer's Care Quaterly, 8,* 43–52.

Kirshner, H., Webb, W., & Kelly, M. (1984). The naming disorder of dementia. *Neuropsychologia, 22,* 23–30.

Knopman, D. S., DeKosky, S. T., Cummings, J. L., Chui, H., Corey-Bloom, J., Relkin, N., et al. (2001). Practice parameters: Diagnosis of dementia (an evidence-based review). Report of the Quality Standards Subcommittee of the American Academy of Neurology. *Neurology, 56,* 1143–1153.

Kokmen, E., Chandra, V., & Shoenberg, B. S. (1988). Trends in incidence of dementing illness in Rochester, Minnesota, in three quinquennial periods, 1960–1974. *Neurology, 38,* 975–980.

Krasuski, J. S., Alexander, G. E., Horwitz, B., Daly E. M., Murphy, D. G., Rapoport, S. I., et al. (1998). Volumes of medial temporal lobe structures in patients with Alzheimer's disease and mild cognitive impairment (and in healthy controls). *Biological Psychiatry, 42,* 60–68.

Lovestone, S. (1999). Early diagnosis and the clinical genetics of Alzheimer's disease. *Journal of Neurology, 246,* 69–72.

Martin, A., Brouwers, P., Lalonde, F., Cox, C., Teleska, P., Fedio, P., et al. (1986). Towards a behavioral typology of Alzheimer's patients. *Journal of Clinical and Experimental Neuropsychology, 8,* 594–610.

Masur, D. M., Sliwinski, M., Lipton, R. B., Blau, A. D., & Crystal, H. A. (1994). Neuropsychological prediction of dementia and the absence of dementia in healthy elderly persons. *Neurology, 44,* 1427–1432.

Mayeux, R., Ottman, R., Maestre, G., Ngai, C., Tang, M.-X., Ginsberg, H., et al. (1995). Synergistic effects of traumatic head injury and apolipoprotein-E4 in patients with Alzheimer's disease. *Neurology, 45,* 555–557.

Mayeux, R., Stern, Y., & Spanton, S. (1985). Heterogeneity in dementia of the Alzheimer type: Evidence of subgroups. *Neurology, 35,* 453–461.

McGonigal, G., Thomas, B., McQuade, C., Starr, J. M., MacLennan, W. J., & Whalley, L. J. (1993). Epidemiology of Alzheimer's presenile dementia in Scotland, 1974–88. *British Medical Journal, 306,* 680–683.

McKhann, G., Drachman, D., Folstein, M., Katzman, R., Price, D., & Stadlan, E. M. (1984). Clinical diagnosis of Alzheimer's disease. *Neurology, 34,* 939–944.

Morris, R. G. M. (1996). Attentional and executive dysfunction. In R. G. M. Morris (Ed.), *The cognitive neuropsychology of Alzheimer-type dementia* (pp. 49–70). New York: Oxford University Press.

Myers, R. H., Schaefer, E. J., Wilson, P. W. F., D'Agostino, R., Ordovas, J. M., Espino, A., et al. (1996). Apoliprotein E epsilon 4 association with dementia in a population-based study: The Framingham study. *Neurology, 46,* 673–677.

Neils-Strunjas, J., Groves-Wright, K., Mashima, P., & Harnish, S. (in press). Dysgraphia in Alzheimer's disease: A review for clinical and research purposes. *Journal of Speech Language Hearing Research.*

Obler, L. K. & Albert, M. L. (1984). Language in aging. In M. L. Albert (Ed.), *Clinical neurology of aging* (pp. 245–252). New York: Oxford University Press.

Obler, L. K., & Albert, M. L. (1985). Historical notes: Jules Séglas on language in dementia. *Brain and Language, 24,* 314–325.

O'Neill, D., Surmon, D. J., & Wilcock, G. K. (1992). Longitudinal diagnosis of memory disorders. *Age and Ageing, 21,* 393–397.

Pearlson, G. D., Harris, G. J., Powers, R. E., Barta, P. E., Camargo, E. E., Chase, G. A., et al. (1992). Quantitative changes in mesial temporal volume, regional cerebral blood flow, and cognition in Alzheimer's disease. *Archives of General Psychiatry, 49,* 402–408.

Perry, R. J., & Hodges, J. R. (2000). Relationship between functional and neuropsychological performance in early Alzheimer disease. *Alzheimer Disease and Associated Disorders, 14,* 1–10.

Perry, R., Watson, P., & Hodges, J. (2000). The nature and staging of attention dysfunction in early (minimal and mild) Alzheimer's disease: Relationship to episodic and semantic memory impairment. *Neuropsychologia, 38,* 252–271.

Rainville, C., Fabrigoule, C., Amieva, H., & Dartigues, J. F. (1998). Problem-solving deficits in patients with dementia of the Alzheimer's type on a Tower of London task. *Brain and Cognition, 37,* 135.

Reisberg, G., Ferris, S. H., Anand, R., de Leon, M. J., Schneck, M. K., Buttinger, C., et al. (1984). Functional staging of dementia of the Alzheimer type. *Annals of the New York Academy of Sciences, 435,* 481–483.

Reisberg, B., Ferris, S. H., de Leon, M. J., & Crooke, T. (1982). The global deterioration scale for assessment of primary degenerative dementia. *American Journal of Psychiatry, 139,* 1136–1139.

Ritchie, K., Artero, S., & Touchon, J. (2001). Classification criteria for mild cognitive impairment. A population-based validation study. *Neurology, 56,* 37–42.

Robinson, G., Rossor, M., & Cipolotti, L. (1999). Selective sparing of verb naming in a case of severe Alzheimer's disease. *Cortex, 35,* 443–450.

Rochon, E., Waters, G. S., & Caplan, D. (2000). The relationship between measures of working memory and sentence comprehension in patients with Alzheimer's disease. *Journal of Speech, Language, and Hearing Research, 43,* 395–413.

Salmon, D., Butters, N., & Chan, A. (1999). The deterioration of semantic memory in Alzheimer's disease. *Canadian Journal of Experimental Psychology, 53,* 108–116.

Schoenberg, B. S., Anderson, D. W., & Haeren, A. F. (1985). Severe dementia: Prevalence and clinical features in a biracial US population. *Archives of Neurology, 42,* 740–743.

Selkoe, D. J. (2000). The genetics and molecular pathology of Alzheimer's disease: Roles of amyloid and the presenilins. *Neurologic Clinics, 18,* 903–922.

Soininen, H., Laulumaa, B., Helkala, E. L., Harti-kainen, P., & Riekkinen, P. J. (1992). Extrapyra-midal signs in Alzheimer's disease: A 3-year follow-up study. *Journal of Neural Transmission, 4*, 107–119.

Stern, R. G., Mohs, R. C., Davidson, M., Schmeidler, J., Silverman, J., Kramer-Ginsberg, E., et al. (1994). A longitudinal study of Alzheimer's disease: Measurement, rate and predictors of cognitive deterioration. *American Journal of Psychiatry, 151*, 390–396.

Stern, Y., Albert, M., Brandt, J., Jacobs, D. M., Tang, M. X., Marder, K., et al. (1994). Utility of extrapyramidal signs and psychosis as predic-tors of cognitive and functional decline, nurs-ing home admission and death in Alzheimer's disease: Prospective analyses from the Predic-tors Study. *Neurology, 44*, 2300–2307.

Stern, Y., Mayeux, R., Sano, M., & Hauser, W. (1987). Predictors of disease course in patients with probable Alzheimer's disease. *Neurology, 37*, 1649–1653.

Tomoeda, C. K., & Bayles, K. A. (1993). Longitu-dinal effects of Alzheimer's disease on dis-course production. *Alzheimer Disease and Asso-ciated Disorders, 7*, 223–236.

Tomoeda, C. K., Bayles, K. A., Trosset, M. W., Azuma, T., & McGeagh, A. (1996). Cross-sectional analysis of Alzheimer disease effects on oral discourse in a picture description task. *Alzheimer Disease and Associated Disorders, 10*, 204–215.

van Duijn, C. M., Hofman, A., & Kay, D. W. K. (1991). Risk factors for Alzheimer's disease: A collaborative re-analysis of case-control studies. *International Journal of Epidemiology, 20* (Suppl. 2), S1.

Van Hoesen, G. (1997). Ventromedial temporal lobe anatomy, with comments on Alzheimer's disease and temporal injury. *Journal of Neu-ropsychiatry and Clinical Neurosciences, 9*, 331–341.

Wilson, R. S., Bennet, D. A., Gilley, D. W., Beckett, L. A., Schneider, J. A., & Evans, D. A. (2000). Progression of parkinsonian signs in Alzhei-mer's disease. *Neurology, 54*, 1284–1289.

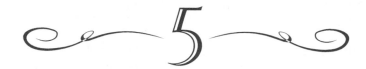

5

Dementia and Down Syndrome

Down syndrome (DS) is a genetic disorder associated with three copies of chromosome 21 and is the most common cause of mental retardation in the United States. The incidence of DS is one in 800 live births (Heller, 1969; Mann, 1988; Steele, 1996) and affected individuals account for approximately 17% of the mentally handicapped population.

Risk of Developing Alzheimer's Disease

Individuals with DS are at high risk for developing Alzheimer's disease (AD). In fact, virtually all individuals with DS over age 40 have the neuropathologic and neurochemical abnormalities that define AD (Burger & Voget, 1973; Figure 5–1). Recall that the

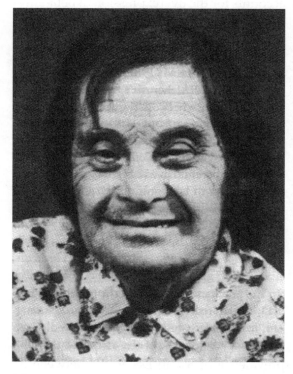

Figure 5–1. Down syndrome and Alzheimer's disease. A photograph of a 55-year-old woman who regressed from a 6- or 7-year mental level to a state in which she cannot speak or comprehend language, is disoriented, and is incontinent. From "Down Syndrome—Alzheimer's Linked," by G. Kolata, *Science, 230,* 1152–1153, by permission. Copyright 1985 by the American Association for the Advancement of Science. (Photo by Krystyna Wisniewski, chief of the Neuropathology Laboratory at New York State's Institute for Basic Research in Developmental Disabilities on Staten Island. Reprinted with permission.)

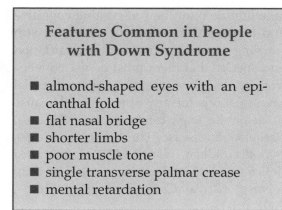

Features Common in People with Down Syndrome

- almond-shaped eyes with an epicanthal fold
- flat nasal bridge
- shorter limbs
- poor muscle tone
- single transverse palmar crease
- mental retardation

neuropathologic features necessary for diagnosis of AD are neuritic plaques and neurofibrillary tangles in sufficient numbers (Kachaturian, 1985; Mirra et al., 1991; National Institute on Aging, 1997). Within the neuritic plaque is beta-amyloid that is derived from the processing of amyloid precursor protein (APP). APP is located on chromosome 21, which is the chromosome that is triplicated in individuals with DS. This triplication likely accounts for the overexpression of beta-amyloid in individuals with DS (Kang et al., 1987; Tanzi et al., 1987) that begins even in childhood (Leverenz & Raskind, 1998).

Other factors also raise the risk of AD in individuals with DS among them accelerated aging. For females with DS, the earlier advent of menopause and associated diminution in endogenous estradiol further increase risk (Schupf et al., 2003; Patel et al., 2004). In addition, those individuals with one or two apolipoprotein E (ApoE) 4 alleles are at even greater risk.

AD pathology accelerates in individuals with DS between the ages of 35 and 45, particularly the formation of neuritic plaques. With plaque proliferation, changes in cognitive function become increasingly apparent (Leverenz & Raskind, 1998). Prasher and Krishnan (1993) reported that the mean age of onset of AD in adults with DS is 51.7 years (range 31–68), significantly lower than for the general population. Dalton and Wisniewski (1990) reviewed published estimates of disease duration in individuals with DS and found they ranged from 3.5 to 10.5 years.

Although AD pathology is virtually omnipresent in individuals with DS, dementia is not. In no longitudinal study of DS adults 50 and older was dementia present in every subject. Answering the question of why some adults with DS develop Alzheimer's dementia, even before the age of 50, whereas others in their 60's do not (Devenny, Krinsky-McHale, Sersen, & Silverman, 2000) is a question of great interest to researchers.

Prevalence of Dementia in DS

As in the general population, the prevalence of dementia in individuals with DS increases with age. Lai and Williams (1989) reported a prevalence of 8% in DS adults between 35 and 49 years, 55% in those between 50 and 59, and 75% in those 60 and older. Zigman, Schupf, Sersen, and Silverman (1995) reported dementia in 50% of DS individuals 50 years of age or older when lenient criteria for dementia were used. When conservative criteria were used, the prevalence dropped to 15%. Other investigators have reported similar findings—a prevalence of dementia between 5% and 22% by the fourth decade and over 50% by the fifth decade (Holland, Hon, Huppert, Stevens, & Watson, 1998; Janicki & Dalton, 2000).

Diagnosing Dementia in Individuals with DS

Recently, consensus criteria were developed for diagnosing dementia in people with intellectual disability (Table 5–1) (Royal College of Psychiatrists, 2001). These criteria take into account the pre-existing cognitive and functional impairments of adults with learning disabilities or mental retardation and specify that there must be no evidence from history, physical examination, or special investigations for any other possible cause of dementia (e.g., cerebrovascular disease, Parkinson's disease, Huntington's disease, hypothyroidism, vitamin B12 or folic acid deficiency, hypercalcaemia, alcohol or drug misuse) (Royal College of Psychiatrists, 2001, p. 31).

Table 5–1. DC-LD Category IIIB1.1 Unspecified Dementia

A	The symptoms/signs must be present for at least a 6-month duration.
B	They must not be a direct consequence of other psychiatric or physical disorders.
C	The symptoms/signs must represent a change from the person's premorbid state.
D	Impaired memory must be present.
E	Impairment of other cognitive skills, judgment, and thinking must be present.
F	Items D and E above must not be solely attributed to clouding of consciousness as in delirium (i.e., the person must demonstrate clear consciousness).
G	Reduced emotional control or motivation or change in social behavior must be present.

Source: From Royal College of Psychiatrists, 2001, "*DC-LD: Diagnostic Criteria for Psychiatric Disorders for Use with Adults with Learning Disabilities/Mental Retardation.*" London: Gaskell. Copyright 2001 Royal College of Psychiatrists; reprinted with permission.

Because mental impairment is an inherent feature of DS, the diagnosis of *early* dementia is challenging. Detecting small changes in cognitive function is a difficult enterprise in and of itself but is further complicated by age effects on cognition. Clinicians must be able to tease apart cognitive deficits associated with DS and normal aging from those caused by early AD.

Guidelines have been published that can help clinicians better recognize the presence of dementia in adults with DS (Alyward, Burt, Thorpe, Lai, & Dalton, 1995). First, obtain a baseline of cognitive and behavioral functioning by the time the individual is 25 years of age. Use standardized instruments and assess cognition, health, and functional skills. Periodically thereafter, but especially by the time the individual has reached age 40, assessments should be readministered and family and caregivers interviewed about possible changes in cognitive function and behavior. If change is reported, the individual should be referred to a physician to evaluate whether the cause of mental and or behavioral decline is treatable. When early Alzheimer's dementia is suspected, the individual should be periodically evaluated, ideally every six months but at least annually.

Cognitive and Behavioral Measures Appropriate for Individuals with DS

Several standardized cognitive and behavioral measures have been developed for use with adults with intellectual impairment. Table 5–2 contains descriptions of some of the commonly used measures.

Table 5–2. Measures of Cognitive Function and Behavior Commonly Used with Adults with Down Syndrome

Observer Rating Scales of Cognitive Function
Modified CAMDEX Informant Interview (Roth, Huppert, Mountjoy, & Tym, 1998) • Includes an informant interview, client interview, and an objective examination of cognitive function • Has demonstrated validity and reliability (Ball et al., 2004)
Dementia Questionnaire for Persons with Mental Retardation (DMR) (Evenhuis, 1992) • Comprises 50 questions that respondents answer "normally yes," "sometimes," or "normally no" • Provides a summary of cognitive scores and a summary of social scores • A cutoff score is provided for diagnosis of dementia in people with differing levels of intellectual disability • Has good sensitivity (.92) and specificity (.92)
Dementia Scale for Down's Syndrome (DSDS) (Gedye, 1995) • Contains questions in three categories: early, middle, late-stage dementia • Places emphasis on change in function • Distinguishes between new and typical behaviors • Diagnosis is based on reaching a global numerical threshold at each level of severity • Has good sensitivity (.85) and specificity (.89)
Measures of Functional and Vocational Abilities
Scales of Independent Behavior (Thase, Liss, Smeltzer, & Maloon, 1982)
Vineland Adaptive Behavior Scales (Sparrow, Balla, & Cicchetti, 1984)
Disability Assessment Schedule (Holmes et al., 1982)

Cognitive Profiles of DS Adults With and Without Dementia

Studies comparing the neuropsychological profiles of young DS adults (<age 35), older nondemented DS adults (>age 35) and older demented DS adults (>age 35) indicate that the cognitive profiles of *older nondemented* adults reflect relatively spared language and short-term memory span but impairment of the ability to form new long-term memories and perform visuoconstruction (Haxby, 1989; Schapiro, Haxby, & Grady, 1992). Haxby (1989) observed that this profile is similar to

that of patients with early to intermediate AD. The *older demented* DS adults had more global cognitive decline like adults with severe AD.

A Study of the Cognitive-Communicative Profiles of DS Adults With and Without Dementia

Moss, Tomoeda, and Bayles (2000) investigated the relation of age to neuropsychological test performance in 22 nondemented DS adults and two with dementia and compared their performance to individuals with mild and moderate AD. The average chronologic age of the individuals with DS was 42.9 years (range 32–65) and their average mental age was 5.5 years. The Arizona Battery for Communication Disorders of Dementia (ABCD) (Bayles & Tomoeda, 1993), comprising 14 subtests of 5 constructs, was administered to study participants. An inverse correlation was obtained between ABCD total score and chronologic age ($r = -.57, p = .002$), that is, older age in the DS group (demented and nondemented) was associated with lower mental age and lower performance on the ABCD. The two oldest individuals with DS (ages 62 and 65) had the lowest mental ages and ABCD overall score and met the diagnostic criteria for dementia in DS.

Comparison of Performance of DS Readers with DS Nonreaders

Because study participants with DS were heterogeneous in cognitive development, their performance data were grouped by mental age and whether they could read at the single word level. The nondemented adults with DS, who could read ($N = 13$), had higher scores on ABCD subtests that did not involve reading than DS adults who could not read ($N = 9$). For nine of the 14 subtests, the scores of the readers were significantly higher (Mental Status, Story-Retelling Immediate, Comparative Questions, Word Learning—Free Recall, Word Learning-Total Recall, Word Learning Recognition, Repetition, Object Description, and Story-Retelling Delayed). Differences between the readers and nonreaders were particularly noticeable on the three components of the Word Learning subtest in which the ability to read can aid performance although reading is not required. Thus, Moss et al. (2000) cautioned that the scores of nonreaders on the Word Learning subtest likely did not accurately reflect their ability to encode and remember verbal stimuli.

Comparison of Nondemented Adults with DS with Individuals with Mild AD

The nondemented adults with DS had lower scores than AD patients on two measures of linguistic comprehension and two measures of visuospatial construction ability. The only subtest on which the nondemented DS subjects had higher scores than the AD patients was Story Retelling—Delayed, an episodic memory test.

Comparison of Demented DS Individuals with AD Subjects

The construct scores of the two DS adults with dementia were compared to those of mild and moderate AD patients in the ABCD standardization study and to the group of nondemented DS adults with mental ages of six or less. The demented DS individuals scored lower on all five ABCD constructs than individuals with AD and they scored lower on Episodic Memory and Linguistic Expression than the nondemented DS adults with mental ages of six or less.

Language and Communication in Adults with DS

Compared to nondemented age mates in the general population, individuals with DS perform poorer on tests of language and have shorter mean length of utterance and use simpler grammar (Rondal, 1988; Rondal & Lambert, 1983; Sabsay & Kernan, 1993). Some evidence exists that adults with DS experience loss of communication skills as they age (Carter Young, & Kramer, 1991; Collacott & Cooper, 1997; Haxby, 1989; Rasmussen & Sobsey, 1994) particularly in receptive language. Cooper and Collacott (1995) reported that the receptive language skills of DS adults 40 to 49 years of age were significantly inferior to those of younger DS adults. An issue in interpreting these reports is whether declines represent the effect of aging or aging plus the onset of Alzheimer's dementia. However, data from functional neuroimaging studies of young adults with DS and age- and sex-matched peers in the general population show reduced cerebral glucose metabolism in brain areas important to language (Azari et al., 1994).

Roeden and Zitman (1997) followed 28 individuals with DS, 14 of whom had dementia. They reported progressive declines in receptive and expressive language skills in those with dementia. Declines in communication skills also were reported by caregivers of four individuals with DS in a study by Rasmussen and Sobsey (1994). All four were confirmed as having AD pathology at postmortem examination. In a case study of confrontation naming in an individual with DS and dementia, Kledaras, McIlvane, and Mackay (1989) reported significant longitudinal decline over a 20-month period. The types of naming errors made by the individual were like those of individuals with AD— naming items related to the target (visually and/or semantically) or the category of the target item rather than the item.

In sum, young adults with DS have language skills that reflect their intellectual ability. With advancing age, language skills are likely to be affected. Without a baseline profile of language abilities, derived when the individual was a young adult, it is difficult to determine the effect of aging and dementia on language in the early stages of AD. Nonetheless, when dementia is clearly present, communicative function will be compromised.

Summary of Important Points

- Clinicians need to be mindful of the high incidence of AD in individuals with DS, particularly those older than 50.

- Because evidence of decline in function is the prominent sign of emerging AD, obtain a profile of cognitive abilities when the individual with DS is in young adulthood. This profile serves as a baseline that will facilitate later detection of cognitive decline.
  - Use standardized measures of cognitive and functional abilities including tests of language comprehension and expression.
  - Identify whether the individual can read and take that into account when selecting and interpreting test performance.
- When the individual reaches the age of 40, begin periodic evaluations and interview family about possible changes in function.
- When using the ABCD with DS adults, pay attention to performance on episodic memory tests. If the individual's score is equal to or less than the average of AD subjects in the standardization sample, consider the possibility of dementia.
- If you detect a change in function, refer the individual with DS to a neurologist and include information about the nature of the change with your referral.
- When dementia is apparent, continue to periodically re-evaluate the individual and provide counseling to family about accommodations that will enable the individual to function maximally and have quality of life.

References

Alyward, E., Burt, D., Thorpe, L., Lai, F., & Dalton, A.J. (1995). *Diagnosis of dementia in individuals with intellectual disability: Report of the AAMR-IASSID Working Group for Establishment of Criteria for the Diagnosis of Dementia in Individuals with Intellectual Disability*. Washington, DC: American Association on Mental Retardation.

Azari, N. P., Horwitz, B., Pettigrew, K. D., Grady, C. L., Haxby, J. V., Giacometti, K. R., et al. (1994). Abnormal pattern of cerebral glucose metabolic rates involving language areas in young adults with Down syndrome. *Brain and Language, 46*, 1–20.

Ball, S. L., Holland, A. J., Huppert, F. A., Treppner, P., Watson, P., & Hon, J. (2004). The modified CAMDEX informant interview is a valid and reliable tool for use in the diagnosis of dementia in adults with Down's syndrome. *Journal of Intellectual Disability Research, 48*, 611–620.

Bayles, K. A., & Tomoeda, C. K. (1993). *Arizona Battery for Communication Disorders of Dementia*. Austin, TX: Pro-Ed.

Burger, P. C., & Voget, F. S. (1973). The development of pathologic changes of Alzheimer's disease and senile dementia in patients with Down's syndrome. *American Journal of Pathology, 73*, 457–476.

Carter Young, E., & Kramer B. (1991). Characteristics of age-related language decline in adults with Down's syndrome. *Mental Retardation, 29*, 75–79.

Collacott, R. A., & Cooper, S. A. (1997). A five-year follow-up study of adaptive behaviour in adults with Down syndrome. *Journal of Intellectual and Developmental Disability, 22*, 187–197.

Cooper, S. A., & Collacott, R. A. (1995). The effect of age on language in people with Down's syndrome. *Journal of Intellectual Disability Research, 39*, 197–200.

Dalton, A. J., & Wisniewski, H. M. (1990). Down syndrome and the dementia of Alzheimer's disease. *International Review of Psychiatry, 2*, 41–50.

Devenny, D. A., Krinsky-McHale, S. J., Sersen, G., & Silverman, W. P. (2000). Sequence of cognitive decline in dementia in adults with Down's syndrome. *Journal of Intellectual Disability Research, 44*, 654–665.

Evenhuis, H. M. (1992). Evaluation of a screening instrument for dementia in ageing mentally retarded persons. *Journal of Intellectual Disability Research, 36*, 337–347.

Gedye, A. (1995). *Dementia Scale for Down's Syndrome*. Vancouver, BC: Gedye Research and Consulting.

Haxby, J. V. (1989). Neuropsychological evaluation of adults with Down's syndrome: Patterns of selective impairment in non-demented old adults. *Journal of Mental Deficiency Research, 33*, 193–210.

Heller, J. H. (1969). Human chromosome abnormalities as related to physical and mental dysfunction. *Journal of Heredity, 60*, 239–252.

Holland, A. J., Hon, J., Huppert, F. A., Stevens, F., & Watson, P. (1998). Population-based study of the prevalence and presentation of dementia in adults with Down's syndrome. *British Journal of Psychiatry, 172*, 493–498.

Holmes, N., Shah, A., & Wing, L. (1982). The Disability Assessment Schedule: A brief screening device for use with the mentally retarded. *Psychological Medicine, 12*, 879–890.

Janicki, M. P., & Dalton, A. J. (2000). Prevalence of dementia and impact on intellectual disability services. *Mental Retardation, 38*, 276–288.

Kang, J., Lemaire, H. G., Unterbeck, A., Salbaum, J. M., Masters, C. L., Grzeschik, K. H., et al. (1987). The precursor of Alzheimer's disease amyloid A4 protein resembles a cell-surface receptor. *Nature, 325*, 733–736.

Khachaturian, Z. S. (1985). Diagnosis of Alzheimer's disease. *Archives of Neurology, 421*, 1097–1106.

Kledaras, J. B., McIlvane, W. J., & Mackay, H. A. (1989). Progressive decline of picture naming in an ageing Down syndrome man with dementia. *Perceptual and Motor Skills, 69*, 1091–1100.

Lai, F., & Williams, R. S. (1989). A prospective study of Alzheimer disease in Down syndrome. *Archives of Neurology, 46*, 849–853.

Leverenz, J. B., & Raskind, M. A. (1998). Early amyloid deposition in the medial temporal lobe of young Down syndrome patients: A regional quantitative analysis. *Experimental Neurology, 150*, 296–304.

Mann, D. M. A. (1988). The pathological association between Down syndrome and Alzheimer disease. *Mechanisms of Ageing and Development, 43*, 99–136.

Mirra, S. S., Heyman, A., McKeel, D., Sumi, S. D., Crain, B. J., Brownlee, L. M., et al. (1991). The Consortium to Establish a Registry for Alzheimer's Disease (CERAD). Part II. Standardization of the neuropathologic assessment of Alzheimer's disease. *Neurology, 41*, 479–486.

Moss, S. E., Tomoeda, C. K., & Bayles, K. A. (2000). Comparison of the cognitive-linguistic profiles of Down syndrome adults with and without dementia to individuals with Alzheimer's disease. *Journal of Medical Speech-Language Pathology, 8,* 69–81.

National Institute on Aging, and Reagan Institute Working Group on Diagnostic Criteria for the Neuropathological Assessment of Alzheimer's disease. (1997). Consensus recommendations for the post mortem diagnosis of Alzheimer's disease. *Neurobiology of Aging, 18*(S4), 1–2.

Patel, B. N., Pang, D., Stern, Y., Silverman, W., Kiline, J. K., Mayeux, R., et al. (2004). Obesity enhances verbal memory in postmenopausal women with Down syndrome. *Neurobiology of Aging, 25,* 159–166.

Prasher, V. P., & Krishan V. H. R. (1993). Age of onset and duration of dementia in people with Down syndrome: Integration of 98 reported cases in the literature. *International Journal of Geriatric Psychiatry, 8,* 915–922.

Rasmussen, D. E., & Sobsey, D. (1994). Age, adaptive behaviour, and Alzheimer disease in Down syndrome: Cross-sectional and longitudinal analysis. *American Journal on Mental Retardation, 99,* 151–165.

Roeden, J. M., & Zitman, F. G. (1997). A longitudinal comparison of cognitive and adaptive changes in participants with Down's syndrome and an intellectually disabled control group. *Journal of Applied Research in Intellectual Disabilities, 10,* 289–302.

Rondal, J. A. (1988). Language development in Down's syndrome: A life-span perspective. *International Journal of Behavioural Development, 11,* 21–36.

Rondal, J. A. & Lambert, J. L. (1983). The speech of mentally retarded adults in a dyadic communication situation: Some formal and informative aspects. *Psychologic Belgica, 23,* 49–56.

Roth, M., Huppert, F., Mountjoy, C., & Tym, E. (1998). *CAMDEX-R: The Cambridge Examination for Mental Disorder of the Elderly* (Rev. ed.). Cambridge: Cambridge University Press.

Royal College of Psychiatrists. (2001). *DC-LD: Diagnostic criteria for psychiatric disorders for use with adults with learning disabilities/mental retardation.* London: Gaskell.

Sabsay, S., & Kernan, K. T. (1993). On the nature of language impairment in Down syndrome. *Topics in Language Disorders, 13,* 20–35.

Schapiro, M. B., Haxby, J. V., & Grady, C. L. (1992). Nature of mental retardation and dementia in Down syndrome: Study with PET, CT, and neuropsychology. *Neurobiology of Aging, 13,* 723–734.

Schupf, N., Pang, D., Patel, B. N., Silverman, W., Schubert, R., Lai, F., et al. (2003). Onset of dementia is associated with age at menopause in women with Down's syndrome. *Annals of Neurology, 54,* 433–438.

Sparrow, S. S., Balla, D. A., Cicchetti, D. V. (1984). *Vineland Adaptive Behavior Scales.* Circle Pines, MN: American Guidance Service.

Steele, J. (1996). Epidemiology: incidence, prevalence and size of the Down's syndrome population. In B. Stratford & P. Gunn (Eds.), *New approaches to Down syndrome* (pp. 45–72). London: Cassell.

Tanzi, R. E., Gusella, J. F., Watkins, P. C., Bruns, G. A., St. George-Hyslop, P., Van Keuren, M. L., et al. (1987). Amyloid b protein genes: cDNA, mRNA distribution and genetic linkage near the Alzheimer locus. *Science, 235,* 880–884.

Thase, M. E., Liss, L., Smeltzer, D., & Maloon, J. (1982). Clinical evaluation of dementia in Down's syndrome: A preliminary report. *Journal of Mental Deficit Research, 26,* 239–244.

Zigman, W. B., Schupf, N., Sersen, E., & Silverman, W. (1995). Prevalence of dementia in adults with and without Down syndrome. *American Journal on Mental Retardation, 100,* 403–412.

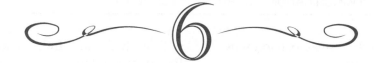

Vascular Dementia

Cerebrovascular disease can cause dementia and, in fact, is its second most common cause (Doody et al., 2001; Rockwood et al., 2000). Worldwide, it accounts for approximately 20% of the cases and is more common in men (Dubois & Herbert, 2001). The median survival time after onset of vascular dementia is 3.3 years (Wolfson et al., 2001) and individuals with cerebrovascular disease and dementia are at greater risk for morbidity and mortality than those with Alzheimer's disease (Bennett, 2001).

A widely used term for the presence of cerebrovascular disease and dementia is multi-infarct dementia (Hachinski, Lassen, & Marshall, 1974). However, in the recent past, the term vascular dementia has become more popular because individuals with dementia secondary to cerebrovascular disease do not always have multiple infarctions.

Neuropathology

Vascular dementia (VaD) is the *"loss of cognitive functions to a degree that interferes with ADLs, resulting from ischemic or hemorrhagic cerebrovascular disease (CVD) or from cardiovascular or circulatory disturbances that injure brain regions important for memory, cognition, and behavior"* (Román, 2005, p. 7). The clinical presentation of VaD varies by etiology and no one pattern of cognitive impairment is associated with the term. The type of vascular disease, its location, and the amount of brain damage, dictate the clinical presentation of dementia. The major etiologic subtypes of vascular dementia are:

1. Large vessel disease associated with multiple infarcts in cortex, white matter, and basal ganglia

---

Definitions (Blumenfeld, 2002)

Ischemic—the process in which there is inadequate blood supply to a region of the brain for enough time to cause infarction (death) of brain tissue.

Lacunar—lacunes are small, deep, ischemic infarcts that resemble small lakes or cavities when the brain is examined on pathologic section.

Hypoperfusion—decreased blood flow.

Granular—granules are types of cells found both in cortex and throughout the body.

Encephalopathy—a term for any diffuse disease of the brain that alters brain function or structure. http://www.ninds.nih.gov/disorders/encephalopathy/encephalopathy.htm

2. Small vessel disease associated with multiple infarcts
3. Multilacunar state (Figure 6–1)
4. Hypoperfusion in border zones and granular cortical atrophy
5. Postischemic encephalopathy

Risk Factors for VaD

Researchers have identified numerous risk factors for vascular disease, some associated with aging and genetics, others that reflect lifestyle choices. Both the incidence and prevalence of VaD increase with age and tend to be higher in males (Ruitenberg, Ott, van Swieten, Hofman, & Breteler, 2001). After age 55, the incidence of stroke doubles with each decade. Individuals who have a first-degree relative (parent or sibling) with a history of stroke are themselves at greater risk for stroke. According to epidemiologic data, prevalence of stroke is higher in black populations than white, and more common in Asia than in Western Europe and the United States.

Risk factors associated with lifestyle choices include dietary habits, lack of physical exercise, alcohol abuse, and smoking. Many individuals with VaD have a history of hypertension. In fact, *hypertension* is the single most important risk factor for VaD, particularly when left untreated for a long period of time. Diabetes is another important risk factor. Luchsinger, Tang, Stern, Shea, and Mayeux (2001) found that individuals with diabetes were three times more likely to de-

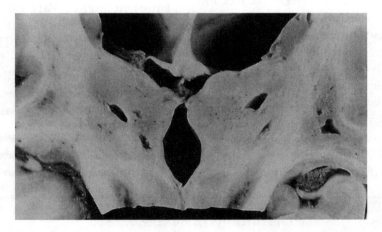

Figure 6–1. Lacunar state in this patient who suffered from a stepwise cognitive decline; there are at least seven lacunes of varying sizes in this plane of section of the thalamus and posterior putamen. Other planes of section in this case showed additional lacunes with very little focal vascular disease elsewhere in the brain. From "Vascular Dementias," by J. H. Morris, H. Kalimo, & M. Viitanen, 2004. In M. M. Esiri, V. M.-Y. Lee, and J. Q. Trajanowski (Eds.), *The Neuropathology of Dementia* (2nd ed., pp. 289–329). Cambridge: Cambridge University Press. Copyright 2004 Cambridge University Press. Reprinted with permission of Cambridge University Press.

velop stroke-associated dementia than those without diabetes. In individuals with cerebrovascular disease, the risk of developing dementia is increased if lesions are multiple and bilateral and located in frontosubcortical and limbic structures (Erkinjuntti et al., 1999; O'Brien, Erkinjuntti, et al., 2003, O'Brien, Reisberg, & Erkinjutti, 2003; Román, Erkinjuntti, Pantoni, Wallin, & Chui, 2002).

In short, the risk of stroke and VaD increase as a function of the number of risk factors an individual has. Management of hypertension and healthful lifestyle choices significantly reduce the risk of stroke and, therefore, VaD.

Course of VaD

Lechner, Bertha, and Ott (1988) conducted a five-year prospective study of 94 patients with VaD and reported that the appearance of cognitive disturbances was identified in 77 of the 94 patients at the onset of stroke. Depression and loss of motivation and attention were often part of the clinical picture. These same cognitive disturbances were present at follow-up but more pronounced. The annual mortality rate ranged between 7% and 13% over the five years of the study. By the end of the study, 43% of study subjects had died, two-thirds from cardiovascular events. In six patients the symptoms of dementia resolved with recovery from a strategic infarct (an infarct in a brain area that affects many cognitive functions). Each of these individuals had a strategic infarct.

Desmond et al. (2000) also conducted a study of the course of cognitive decline in 453 patients who were 60 years or older and hospitalized with acute ischemic stroke. Patients were given a neuropsychological examination three months poststroke. One hundred and nineteen patients, or 26.3% of the sample, were demented three months poststroke. Of these, 57% had dementia that was directly attributable to stroke or vascular disease; 38.7% had dementia due to the co-occurrence of stroke and AD; and 4.2% had dementia for other reasons such as alcohol abuse.

Similar epidemiologic studies were conducted in Finland by Pohjasvaara et al. (1998) and in Spain by Barba et al. (2000). Results from these studies, together with those from the Lechner and Desmond studies, strongly suggest that between one-quarter to one-third of elderly individuals who suffer a stroke meet the criteria for dementia within three months.

Diagnostic Criteria

The diagnosis of VaD requires evidence of deterioration in memory and two or more other cognitive domains that is sufficient to interfere with social and occupational functioning. The deterioration in cognitive function must represent a significant decline from the patient's previous level of functioning and be objectively verifiable from history, neuroimaging, and neuropsychological testing. The NINDS-AIREN (Román et al., 1993) criteria for *probable* vascular dementia are as follows:

1. *Dementia*

NINDS-AIREN

NINDS-AIREN is the acronym used to refer to the National Institute of Neurological Disorders and Stroke— Association International pour la Recherché et l'Enseignement en Neurosciences.

2. *Cerebrovascular disease*, defined by the presence of focal signs on neurologic examination such as hemiparesis, lower facial weakness, Babinski sign, sensory deficit, hemianopsia, and dysarthria consistent with stroke (with and without history of stroke), and evidence of relevant cerebrovascular disease by brain imaging (CT or MRI) including *multiple large-vessel infarcts or a single strategically placed infarct* (angular gyrus, thalamus, basal fore-brain, posterior communicating arteries, or anterior communicating arteries territories), as well as *multiple basal ganglia* and *white matter lacunes or extensive periventricular white matter lesions*, or combinations thereof.
3. *A relationship between the above two disorders*, manifested or inferred by the presence of one or more of the following:
   a. Onset of dementia within 3 months following a recognized stroke;
   b. Abrupt deterioration in cognitive functions; or fluctuating, stepwise progression of cognitive deficits. (Román et al., 1993, p. 257)

The clinical features consistent with the diagnosis of *probable* vascular dementia include the following:

A. early presence of a gait disturbance (small-step gait, or marche à petits pas, or magnetic, apraxic-ataxic, or parkinsonian gait);
B. history of unsteadiness and frequent, unprovoked falls;
C. early urinary frequency, urgency, and other urinary symptoms not explained by urologic disease;
D. pseudobulbar palsy; and
E. personality and mood changes, abulia, depression, emotional incontinence, other subcortical deficits including

psychomotor retardation and abnormal executive function (Román et al., 1993, p. 257).

Certain clinical features make the diagnosis of vascular dementia uncertain or unlikely and include:

A. early onset of memory deficit and progressive worsening of memory and other cognitive functions such as language (transcortical sensory aphasia), motor skills (apraxia), and perception (agnosia), in the absence of corresponding focal lesions on brain imaging;
B. absence of focal neurologic signs, other than cognitive disturbances;
C. absence of cerebrovascular lesions on brain CT or MRI. (Román et al., 1993, p. 257)

Criteria for diagnosis of *definite* vascular dementia are:

A. clinical criteria for *probable* vascular dementia;
B. histopathologic evidence of cerebrovascular disease obtained from biopsy or autopsy;
C. absence of neurofibrillary tangles and neuritic plaques exceeding those appropriate for age; and
D. absence of other clinical or pathologic disorder capable of producing dementia. (Román et al., 1993, p. 257).

Effects on Cognitive Functioning

Because dementia is associated with many types of vascular disease, there is no one pattern of cognitive decline. However, the cognitive profile of VaD patients, without concomitant AD pathology, generally differs from that of individuals with AD because memory dysfunction is not the most prominent feature. Damage to frontal-subcortical circuits is commmon, particularly the circuit involving the dorsolateral prefrontal cortex, and executive dysfunction is the most commonly reported clinical characteristic of individuals with VaD (Breteler et al., 1994; Fukuda, Kobayashi, Okada, & Tsunematsu, 1990; Hom & Reitan, 1990; Kertesz & Clydesdale, 1994; Tatemichi et al., 1994; Traykov et al., 2002; Wolfe, Linn, Babikian, Knoefel, & Albert, 1990). Desmond and Pasquier (2002) in their review of the literature on cognitive functioning in VaD draw the following conclusions:

■ Executive dysfunction is the most frequent cognitive consequence of cerebrovascular disease, whereas memory impairment is typically associated with Alzheimer's disease. Memory impairment can occur as a primary manifestation of cerebrovascular disease, however, when there are infarcts in the posterior cerebral artery territory involving the medial temporal lobe, or as a secondary consequence of deficits in executive function, such as inattention.

■ Patients with cerebrovascular disease restricted to subcortical regions frequently exhibit executive dysfunction due to the involvement of frontalsubcortical pathways. Patients with cortical lesions may present with one or more focal cognitive syndromes (e.g., aphasia, spatial neglect), the features of which may or may not be sufficient to fulfill dementia criteria, whereas other patients may exhibit more generalized cognitive deficits (e.g., patients with hypoperfusion dementia).

■ The stereotypic stepwise course of cognitive decline is most frequently evident in patients with subcortical disease due to recurrent subcortical ischemic strokes, whereas other subtypes of vascular dementia may exhibit an insidious onset and a gradually progressive course of decline mimicking Alzheimer's disease.

■ Alzheimer's disease may act in combination with cerebrovascular disease to impair cognitive function or it may serve as the primary basis for cognitive impairment, with a concomitant stroke being of little or no clinical importance (Desmond & Pasquier, 2002, p. 199).

Effects on Communicative Functioning

Communicative function is affected in most individuals with VaD but varies with type of vascular disease. Those individuals with large vessel disease that significantly damages left perisylvian cortex exhibit frank aphasia (Erkinjuntti, 1987; Erkinjuntti, Haltia, Palo, Sulkava, & Paetau, 1988). Other individuals, whose pathology in perisylvian cortex is insufficient to produce aphasia, nonetheless have communication disorders secondary to executive function deficits that result in less efficient processing of linguistic information. Sections of the left dorsolateral frontal lobe that are frequently damaged in vascular disease, work with posterior cortices and subcortical structures to support language formulation and comprehension (Damasio & Anderson, 1993). Thus, damage in any of these brain areas can compromise language formulation and expression.

Subcortical ischemic disease can produce multiple lacunar infarcts (lacunar state) and Binswanger's disease (subacute arteriosclerotic encephalopathy). Individuals with subcortical ischemic disease frequently have the following clinical characteristics: dysarthria, motor weakness, gait disturbance, bulbar signs, deficits in executive functioning

(Babikian & Ropper, 1987; Erkinjuntti, 2005; Ishii, Nishihara, & Imamura, 1986; Román, 1987) and alterations in the melody, pitch, and the rate of articulation of language (Powell, Cummings, Hill, & Benson, 1988).

Mixed Dementia: AD and VaD

Dementia caused solely by vascular pathology, or pure VaD, is quite uncommon. In the famous "Nun study" (Snowdon et al., 1997), pure VaD was found in only 2.5% of the cases. In this study, elderly nuns from the same Catholic order agreed to postmortem examination of their brains. What Snowdon et al. discovered was that many had AD pathology but were not demented based on results of a clinical examination that occurred prior to their death. What differentiated those with AD pathology and dementia from those with AD who were nondemented was the presence of vascular lesions in the brain. A similarly low incidence of vascular dementia (i.e., 1.6%) was also found when the results of 11 European population-based studies, of individuals over 65, were pooled and analyzed (Lobo et al., 2000).

The term "mixed dementia" (MD) refers to the presence of both AD pathology and vascular disease. Mixed dementia is far more common than previously thought. In most autopsy studies of demented elders, 20 to 60% of AD brains also show cerebrovascular lesions (Jellinger, 2002; Lee, Olichney, Hansen, Hofstetter, & Thal, 2000; Neuropathology Group of the Medical Research Council Cognitive Function and Ageing Study, 2001). Similarly, most individuals diagnosed with VaD have evidence of AD (Korczyn, 2005). Vascular pathology appears to deleteriously interact with AD pathology to produce earlier and more severe cognitive impairment (Pasquier & Leys, 1997) and shorter length of survival (Lopez et al., 2000).

Interest in cognitive impairment secondary to vascular disease is significant, and physicians and researchers are debating various terms and taxonomies for characterizing the cognitive deficits of individuals with vascular disease with and without AD pathology. The term "vascular cognitive impairment" (VCI) is increasingly popular and refers to all causes of ischemic cerebrovascular disease and all levels of cognitive impairment ranging from nondemented but cognitively impaired to frank dementia (Bowler, Steenhuis, & Hachinski, 1999; Erkinjuntti, 2005; O'Brien, Erkinjuntti, et al., 2003; O'Brien, Reisberg, et al., 2003). Likely you will witness an evolution of terminology over the next decade as research provides a better understanding of the vascular burden of cognition and the relation of vascular disease to AD (Erkinjuntti, 2005; Kalaria & Ballard, 1999; Skoog, Kalaria, & Breteler, 1999).

Summary of Important Points

- Cerebrovascular disease is the second most common cause of dementia.
- The term "vascular dementia" has replaced the term "multi-infarct dementia" because individuals with dementia secondary to cerebrovascular disease do not always have multiple infarctions.
- Vascular dementia is the loss of cognitive function sufficient to interfere with ADLs and is the consequence of ischemic or hemorrhagic cerebrovascular disease or cardiovascular or circulatory disorders.
- The type of vascular disease, its location, and the amount of brain damage dictate the clinical presentation of dementia.
- The major subtypes of vascular dementia are: large vessel disease, small vessel disease, deep ischemic infarcts, hypoperfusion in border zones and granular cortical atrophy, and postischemic encephalopathy.

- The incidence and prevalence of vascular disease increase with age and tend to be higher in men.
- Hypertension is the single most important risk factor, especially when untreated for a long period of time.
- In individuals with cerebrovascular disease, risk of developing dementia is increased if lesions are multiple, bilateral, and located in frontosubcortical and limbic structures.
- Executive dysfunction is the most commonly reported clinical characteristic of individuals with vascular dementia.
- Communicative function is affected in most individuals with vascular disease but varies with type of disease.
- Pure vascular disease with dementia is uncommon. "Mixed dementia" is a term used by many to refer to the presence of AD pathology and vascular disease.
- The term "vascular cognitive impairment" is becoming a popular term for referring to all causes of ischemic cerebrovascular disease and all levels of cognitive impairment ranging from nondemented but cognitively impaired to frank dementia.

References

Babikian, V., & Ropper, A. H. (1987). Binswanger's disease: A review. *Stroke, 18*, 2–12.

Barba, R., Martinez-Espinosa, S., Rodriguez-Garcia, E., Pondal, M., Vivancos, J., & Del Ser, T. (2000). Poststroke dementia: Clinical features and risk factors. *Stroke, 31*, 1494–1501.

Bennett, D. (2001). Public health importance of vascular dementia and Alzheimer's disease with cerebrovascular disease. *International Journal of Clinical Practice Supplementary, 120*, 41–48.

Blumenfeld, H. (2002). *Neuroanatomy through clinical cases*. Sunderland, MA: Sinauer Associates.

Bowler, J. V., Steenhuis, R., & Hachinski, V. (1999). Conceptual background to vascular cognitive impairment. *Alzheimer Disease and Associated Disorders, 13*(Suppl. 3), S30–S37.

Breteler, M. M., van Swieten, J. C., Bots, M. L., Grobbee, D. E., Claus, J. J., van den Hout, J. H., et al. (1994). Cerebral white matter lesions, vascular risk factors, and cognitive function in a population-based study: The Rotterdam Study. *Neurology, 44*, 1246–1252.

Damasio, A. R., & Anderson, S. W. (1993). The frontal lobes. In K. H. Heilman & E. Valenstein (Eds.), *Clinical neuropsychology* (pp. 409–460). New York: Oxford University Press.

Desmond, D. W., Moroney, J. T., Paik, M. C., Sano, M., Mohr, J. P., Aboumatar, S., et al. (2000). Frequency and clinical determinants of dementia after ischemic stroke. *Neurology, 54*, 1124–1131.

Desmond D. W., & Pasquier, F. (2002). Global cognitive syndromes. In T. Erkinjuntti & S. Gautheir (Eds.), *Vascular cognitive impairment* (pp. 189–204). London: Martin Dunitz.

Doody, R. S., Stevens, J. C., Beck, C., Dubinsky, R. M., Kaye, J. A., Gwyther, L., et al. (2001). Practice parameter: Management of dementia (an evidence-based review). Report of the Quality Standards Subcommittee of the American Academy of Neurology. *Neurology, 56*, 1154–1166.

Dubois, M. F., & Herbert, R. (2001). The incidence of vascular dementia in Canada: A comparison with Europe and East Asia. *Neuroepidemiology, 20*, 179–187.

Erkinjuntti, T. (1987). Types of multi-infarct dementia. *Acta Neurologica Scandinavica, 75*, 391–399.

Erkinjuntti, T. (2005). Vascular cognitive impairment. In A. Burns, J. O'Brien, & D. Ames (Eds.), *Dementia* (3rd ed., pp. 529–545). London: Hodder Arnold.

Erkinjuntti, T., Bowler, J. V., DeCarli, C., Fazekas, F., Inzitari, D., O'Brien, J. T., et al. (1999). Imaging of static brain lesions in vascular dementia: implications for clinical trials. *Alzheimer Disease and Associated Disorders, 13*(Suppl. 3), S81–S90.

Erkinjuntti, T., Haltia, M., Palo, J., Sulkava, R., & Paetau, A. (1988). Accuracy of the clinical diagnosis of vascular dementia: A retrospective clinical and post-mortem neuropathological study. *Journal of Neurology, Neurosurgery, and Psychiatry, 51,* 1037–1044.

Fukuda, H., Kobayashi, S., Okada, K., & Tsunematsu, T. (1990). Frontal white matter lesions and dementia in lacunar infarction. *Stroke, 21,* 1143–1149.

Hachinski, V. C., Lassen, N. A., & Marshall, J. (1974). Multi-infarct dementia. A cause of mental deterioration in the elderly. *Lancet, 2,* 207–210.

Hom, J., & Reitan, R. M. (1990). Generalized cognitive function after stroke. *Journal of Clinical and Experimental Neuropsychology, 12,* 644–654.

Ishii, N., Nishihara, Y., & Imamura, T. (1986). Why do frontal lobe symptoms predominate in vascular dementia with lacunes? *Neurology, 36,* 340–345.

Jellinger, K. A. (2002). Alzheimer disease and cerebrovascular pathology: An update. *Journal of Neural Transmission, 109,* 813–836.

Kalaria, R. N., & Ballard, C. (1999). Overlap between pathology of Alzheimer disease and vascular dementia. *Alzheimer Disease and Associated Disorders, 13*(Suppl. 3), S115–S123.

Kertesz, A., & Clydesdale, S. (1994). Neuropsychological deficits in vascular dementia vs Alzheimer's disease. Frontal lobe deficits prominent in vascular dementia. *Archives of Neurology, 51,* 1226–1231.

Korczyn, A. D. (2005). The underdiagnosis of the vascular contribution to dementia. *Journal of the Neurological Sciences, 229–230,* 3–6.

Lechner, H., Bertha, G., & Ott, E. (1988). Results of a five-year prospective study of 94 patients with vascular and multi-infarct dementia. In J. S. Meyer, H. Lechner, J. Marshall, & J. F. Toole (Eds.), *Vascular and multi-infarct dementia* (pp. 101–111). Mount Kisco, NY: Future Publishing.

Lee, J. H., Olichney, J. M., Hansen, L. A., Hofstetter, C. R., & Thal, L. J. (2000). Small concomitant vascular lesions do not influence rates of cognitive decline in patients with Alzheimer disease. *Archives of Neurology, 57,* 1474–1479.

Lobo, A., Launer, L. J., Fratiglioni, L., Andersen, K., Di Carlo, A., Breteler, M. M., et al. (2000). Prevalence of dementia and major subtypes in Europe: A collaborative study of population-based cohorts. Neurologic diseases in the elderly research group. *Neurology 54,* S4–S9.

Lopez, O. L., Becker, J. T., Klunk, W., Saxton, J., Hamilton, R. L., Kaufer, D. I., et al. (2000). Research evaluation and diagnosis of possible Alzheimer's disease over the last two decades: II. *Neurology, 55,* 1863–1869.

Luchsinger, J. A., Tang, M. X., Stern, Y., Shea, S., & Mayeux, R. (2001). Diabetes mellitus and risk of Alzheimer's disease and dementia with stroke in a multiethnic cohort. *American Journal of Epidemiology, 154,* 635–641.

Neuropathology Group of the Medical Research Council Cognitive Function and Ageing Study (MRC CFAS). (2001). Pathological correlates of late-onset dementia in a multicentre, community-based population in England and Wales. *Lancet, 357,* 169–175.

O'Brien, J. T., Erkinjuntti, T., Reisberg, B., Román, G., Sawada, T., Pantoni, et al. (2003). Vascular cognitive impairment. *Lancet Neurology, 2,* 89–98.

O'Brien, J., Reisberg, B., & Erkinjuntti, T. (2003). Vascular burden of the brain. *International Psychogeriatrics, 15*(Suppl. 1), 11–13.

Pasquier, F., & Leys, D. (1997). Why are stroke patients prone to develop dementia? *Journal of Neurology, 244,* 135–142.

Pohjasvaara, T., Erkinjuntti, T., Ylikoski, R., Hietanen, M., Vataja, R. & Kaste, M. (1998). Clinical determinants of poststroke dementia. *Stroke, 29,* 75–81.

Powell, A. L., Cummings, J. L., Hill, M. A, & Benson, D. F. (1988). Speech and language alterations in multi-infarct dementia. *Neurology, 38,* 717–719.

Rockwood, K., Wenzel, C., Hachinski, V., Hogan, D. B., MacKnight, C., & McDowell, I. (2000). Prevalence and outcomes of vascular cognitive impairment. *Neurology, 54,* 447–451.

Román, G. C. (1987). Senile dementia of the Binswanger type. A vascular form of dementia in the elderly. *JAMA: Journal of the American Medical Association, 258,* 1782–1788.

Román, G. C. (2005). Clinical forms of vascular dementia. In R. H. Paul, R. Cohen, B. R. Ott, & S. Salloway (Eds.), *Vascular dementia: Cerebrovascular mechanisms and clinical management* (pp. 7–21). Totowa, NJ: Humana Press.

Román, G. C., Erkinjuntti, T., Pantoni, L., Wallin, A., & Chui, H. C. (2002). Subcortical ischaemic vascular dementia. *Lancet Neurology, 1,* 426–436.

Román, G. C., Tatemichi, T. K., Erkinjuntti, T., Cummings, J. L., Masdeu, J. C., Garcia, J. H., et al. (1993). Vascular dementia: Diagnostic criteria for research studies. Report of the National Institute of Neurological Disorders and Stroke-Association Internationale pour la Recherche et l'Enseignement en Neurosciences (NINDS-AIREN) International Workshop. *Neurology, 43,* 250–260.

Ruitenberg, A., Ott, A., van Swieten, J. C., Hofman, A., & Breteler, M. M. (2001). Incidence of dementia: Does gender make a difference? *Neurobiology of Aging, 22,* 575–580.

Skoog, I., Kalaria, R. N., & Breteler, M. M. (1999). Vascular factors and Alzheimer's disease. *Alzheimer Disease and Associated Disorders, 13*(Suppl. 3), S106–S114.

Snowdon, D. A., Greiner, L. H., Mortimer, J. A., Riley, K. P., Greiner, P. A., & Markesbery, W. R. (1997). Brain infarction and the clinical expression of Alzheimer disease. The nun study. *JAMA: The Journal of the American Medical Association, 277,* 813–817.

Tatemichi, T. K., Desmond, D. W., Stern, Y., Paik, M., Sano, M. & Bagiella, E. (1994). Cognitive impairment after stroke: Frequency, patterns, and relationship to function abilities. *Journal of Neurology, Neurosurgery, and Psychiatry, 57,* 202–207.

Traykov, L., Baudic, S., Thibaudet, M. C., Rigaud, A. S., Smagghe, A., & Boller, F. (2002). Neuropsychological deficit in early subcortical vascular dementia: Comparison to Alzheimer's disease. *Dementia and Geriatric Cognitive Disorders, 22,* 445–454.

Wolfe, N., Linn, R., Babikian, V. L., Knoefel, J. E., & Albert, M. L. (1990). Frontal systems impairment following multiple lacunar infarcts. *Archives of Neurology, 47,* 129–132.

Wolfson, C., Wolfson, D. B., Asgharian, M., M'Lan, C. E., Ostbye, T., Rockwood, K., et al. (2001). A reevaluation of the duration of survival after the onset of dementia. *New England Journal of Medicine, 344,* 1111–1116.

7

Parkinson's Disease and Dementia

Parkinsonism and Parkinson's Disease

Parkinsonism is a syndrome characterized by rigidity, tremor, and, bradykinesia (slowness of movement). It is associated with many disorders, the most common being Parkinson's disease (PD) named after James Parkinson, who first described it in 1817. Although PD is better understood today, its cause remains a mystery. Several causes have been considered, primarily genetic and environmental factors. However, Parkinsonism that is solely genetic in origin is unusual (Farrer et al., 1998; Papadimitriou et al., 1999). Studies of twins have not produced convincing evidence of a genetic effect; in fact, the rate in monozygotic twins is not greater than that in dizygotic twins (Tanner et al., 1999). Likely genetic and environmental factors are interrelated such that genetic makeup creates a vulnerability to certain environmental factors.

Several neurodegenerative diseases result in parkinsonism, among them progressive supranuclear palsy, Alzheimer's disease, Lewy body disease, multiple system atrophy, and cortical-basal ganglionic degeneration. Parkinsonism is also a known sequela of encephalitis and vascular disease. Nonetheless, the vast majority of individuals with parkinsonism have what is known as idiopathic PD, meaning the cause is unknown. Within North America, between 500,000 and a million individuals carry the PD diagnosis and 50,000 new cases are diagnosed yearly (Lozano & Kalia, 2005). With the growth in the elderly population, these figures are expected to double by the year 2040.

Symptoms of PD

As previously mentioned, three classic features define PD: slowness of movement, rigidity, and rest tremor. A fourth feature, manifesting later in the disease course, is postural instability. The common initial complaints of PD patients include aching pains, paresthesia (a sensation such as burning or tingling in the absence of external stimulation), numbness, and coldness. These are followed by presentation of one or more of the classic motor symptoms.

Neuropathology of PD

The signature neuropathology of PD is loss of dopaminergic neurons in the substantia nigra pars compacta, and the presence of neuronal Lewy bodies (neuronal intracytoplasmic inclusions) and Lewy neurites in the substantia nigra (Aarsland & Janvin, 2005). The substantia nigra is one of a collection of structures referred to as the basal ganglia that are important in the modulation and coordination of movement. When half or more of the dopaminergic cells in the substantia nigra disappear, parkinsonian symptomatology develops (Lozano & Kalia, 2005). Figure 7–1 shows the substantia nigra of (A) an individual with idiopathic PD compared to (B) a normal individual.

Lewy bodies are also found in many other regions of the nervous system along with nerve cell loss (Braak & Braak, 2000;

Hirsh, 2000). The widespread distribution of Lewy bodies in the brain suggests that PD is a multisystem neurodegenerative disorder affecting both the central and peripheral nervous systems (Takahashi & Wakabayashi, 2005). For those interested in learning more about the cellular events that produce PD, see Lozano and Kalia (2005).

Diagnostic Criteria

Making an early clinical diagnosis of PD is challenging because no confirmatory laboratory test exists. Thus, physicians use the fol-

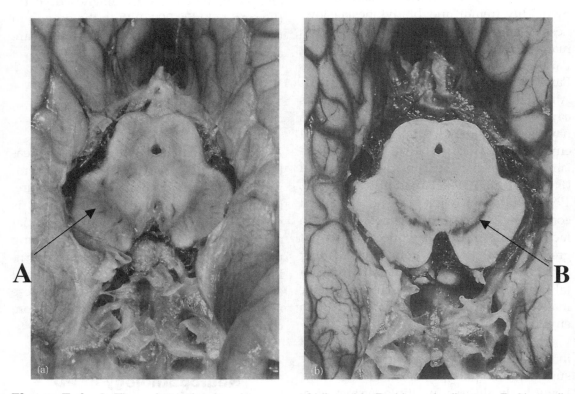

Figure 7–1. A. The substantia nigra in a case of idiopathic Parkinson's disease. **B.** Normally pigmented mesencephalon. From Esiri, M. M., & Morris, J. H., 2004. "Practical Approach to Pathological Diagnosis." In M. M. Esiri, V. M.-Y. Lee, and J. Q. Trojanowski (Eds.), *The Neuropathology of Dementia* (2nd ed., pp. 48–74). Cambridge: Cambridge University Press. Reprinted with permission of Cambridge University Press. Arrows added.

lowing criteria for designating the degree of their certainty about the diagnosis (Calne, Snow, & Lee, 1992):

Clinically *possible* idiopathic Parkinson's disease: presence of one of the following: resting or postural tremor, rigidity, or bradykinesia. Impaired postural reflexes is not included because it is judged to be nonspecific.

Clinically *probable* idiopathic Parkinson's disease: any two of the cardinal features: resting tremor, rigidity, bradykinesia, or impaired postural reflexes. Alternatively, asymmetric resting tremor, rigidity, or bradykinesia are sufficient.

Clinically *definite* idiopathic Parkinson's disease: any combination of three of the four cardinal features. Alternatively, two of these features are sufficient with one of the first three displaying asymmetry.

Risk Factors

Age is the primary and undisputed risk factor for PD. With advancing age the incidence and prevalence increase (Chen et al., 2001; de Rijk, 1995; Morens et al., 1996). Being male may also increase risk. Several investigators, though not all, have reported higher incidence and prevalence in males (Fall et al., 1996; Kuopio, Marttila, Helenius, & Rinne, 1999; Mayeux et al., 1995). In a small percentage of people, genetics is a risk factor and most genetic parkinsonism occurs in individuals younger than age 50. Finally, results of case-controlled studies indicate an association between PD and exposure to pesticides (Gorell et al., 1998; Seidler et al. 1996; Semchuk, Love, & Lee, 1992), rural living (Koller et al. 1990; Wong, Gray, Has-

sanein, & Koller, 1991), consumption of well water (Koller et al., 1990; Wong et al., 1991), and certain metals (Gorell et al., 1997).

PD and Depression

Depression is common in individuals with PD affecting approximately 43% of patients (Cummings, 1992). Usually the depression is mild, but in 5 to 7% of cases, it is severe. Depression appears to be more common in patients who are younger, female, and in the early stage of illness (Wengel, Bohac, & Burke, 2005). Generally the depression is treatable, and if suspected, the patient should be referred to a specialist for treatment. Clinicians need to be aware of the high frequency of depression because its presence can worsen memory and executive functioning causing a misdiagnosis of dementia.

Effects of PD on Cognitive Function

PD Without Dementia

Cognitive dysfunction can occur even in the earliest stages of the disease (Emre, 2003) and most individuals with PD have demonstrable cognitive deficits (Janvin, Aarsland, & Larsen, 2005). With disease progression, many develop dementia. The most commonly observed deficits are in executive function, memory, and visuoperceptual and visuomotor skills (Dubois & Pillon, 1997; Girotti et al., 1988; Stern, Richards, Sano, & Mayeux, 1993).

Executive Functions

Executive function skills enable individuals to process sensory information, make decisions, and carry out goal-directed behavior. In nondemented PD patients, executive function deficit is common and most apparent on tasks of temporal ordering, sequencing, planning, and the ability to shift sets (Bondi, Kaszniak, Bayles, & Vance, 1993; Emre, 2003; Lees & Smith, 1983; Owen et al., 1992; Taylor, Saint-Cyr, & Lang, 1986).

Memory

In nondemented PD patients memory dysfunction is most often observed on procedural learning tasks (Harrington, Haaland, Yeo, & Marder, 1990; Hochstadt, Nakano, Lieberman, & Friedman, 2006; Stefanova, Kostic, Ziropadja, Markovic, & Ocic, 2000) and tests involving the free recall of information, particularly in the delayed condition (Girotti et al., 1988). Although performance on free-recall tasks differs from that of normal elders, performance on recognition tasks generally does not (Breen, 1993; Buytenhuijs et al., 1994; Taylor et al., 1986).

Visual Function

PD affects visual function in myriad ways (Bodis-Wollner, 2002; Rodnitzky, 1998). Most frequently reported are diminished visual acuity (Repka, Claro, Loupe, & Reich, 1996), abnormal color discrimination (Buttner et al., 1993; Buttner et al, 1995), and reduced visual contrast sensitivity (Bulens, Meerwaldt, & van der Wildt, 1988; Regan & Maxner, 1987; Struck, Rodnitzky, & Dobson, 1990). Also, visual hallucinations commonly occur in individuals with late stage PD. Considerable evidence exists that visual system dysfunction is linked to dopamine deficiency, the most compelling of which is improvement with dopaminergic therapy (Rodnitzky, 2005).

Cortical Regions of the Brain Are Affected in Late Stage PD

Jagust, Reed, Martin, Eberling, and Nelson-Abbott (1992) used single photon emission computed tomography to study late stage, nondemented, but cognitively impaired PD patients and reported diminished temporal and parietal perfusion. Peppard et al. (1992) used positron emission tomography to study brain metabolism in both nondemented and demented PD patients. They reported cortical glucose hypometabolism involving mostly frontal lobe but also left temporal and parietal regions in nondemented patients. In contrast, PD patients with dementia had more severe and widespread hypometabolism and reduction bilaterally in temporoparietal areas.

PD with Dementia

Some individuals with PD develop multiple cognitive deficits that are of sufficient severity to meet the criteria for dementia. When dementia develops, it typically occurs late in the disease course (Tröster & Woods, 1987). Janvin and colleagues (2005) conducted a prospective study in a community-based population and determined prevalence of dementia in PD at baseline and after 4 and 8 years (mean duration of disease was 9 years). At baseline, the rate of dementia was 26%; at 4 years, 52%; and 78% at 8 years. Several investigators have examined the influence of age on preva-lence of dementia in PD and reported a significantly higher prevalence in patients older than 70 years of age compared to those who are younger (Martilla & Rinne, 1976; Mayeux et al., 1992; Reid, 1992). Using strict criteria for a diagnosis of PDD in a population-based sample, Mayeux et al. (1992) reported prevalence to be 42.3% overall and 68.7% in patients over 80 years of age. Zakanis and Freedman (1999) did a metaanalysis of the results of studies of the neuropsychological characteristics of individuals with PD and suggest that they are best conceptualized as a continuum with normal cognitive function at one end and frank dementia at the other.

Cognitive Profile of PD Patients with Dementia

A deficit in delayed recall develops early and over time, deficits in cognitive flexibility, manual dexterity, and abstraction emerge (Girotti et al., 1988). Particularly characteristic of PDD are slowness in processing information (Rippon & Marder, 2005) and executive dysfunction. PDD patients have difficulty problem-solving, shifting sets, and planning and regulating their behavior. Visuoperceptual and visuomotor deficits also are common and exacerbated by executive function deficits (Levin et al. 1991; Stern, Mayeux, Rosen & Ilson, 1983). Ultimately, working, episodic, semantic, and procedural memory are all compromised (Helkala, Laulumaa, Soininen, & Riekkinen, 1989; Litvan, Mohr, Williams, Gomez, & Chase, 1991; Pillon, Deweer, Agid, & Dubois, 1993; Pillon, Dubois, Ploska, & Agid, 1991; Stern et al., 1993).

Comparison of the Dementia of PD and AD

The dementia associated with PD and AD can be studied cross-sectionally or longitudinally. In cross-sectional research, groups of PD and AD patients with dementia, who are similar in severity, are compared at a point in time. Results of cross-sectional studies indicate no distinct pattern of neuropsycho-

logical test performance that differentiates the two groups (Brown & Marsden, 1988; Kuzis et al., 1999; Mayeux, Stern, Rosen, & Benson, 1983). In longitudinal research, the two groups are followed over time and compared. Stern and colleagues (1998) studied 40 well-matched pairs of AD and PD participants over a period of 1 to 3 years prior to their diagnosis of dementia. Stern et al. found that at the time of dementia diagnosis, the AD and PD patients performed similarly on a number of different language and memory measures with few exceptions. Over time, the PD patients with dementia experienced more rapid decline on tests of naming and delayed recall than the AD patients. In addition, the demented PD patients performed worse on category fluency measures at the time of diagnosis and at follow-up, which Stern and colleagues interpreted to mean that the demented PD group had a pre-existing performance deficit in executive function. The AD group performed more poorly on a delayed recognition measure consistent with an encoding deficit.

Communicative Function in Nondemented PD Patients

The ability to communicate depends on having knowledge of phonology, syntax, semantics, pragmatics, *and* nonlinguistic cognitive abilities such as attention, memory, and perception. An individual can have a communication disorder without a language deficit, and in nondemented PD patients, that is the case. Whereas it is true that these individuals may score below normal elders on some linguistically-oriented tasks, their language performance scores generally reflect disease effects on memory, attention, or the ability to switch sets (Bayles, 1990).

Hochstadt et al. (2006) administered tests of verbal working memory span, cognitive set switching, and sentence comprehension to 41 PD patients. Although there was evidence of impairment in sentence comprehension, Hochstadt and colleagues attributed it to observed deficits in cognitive set-switching, verbal working memory, and articulatory rehearsal. Hochstadt et al. argued that comprehension errors on sentences containing relative clauses result from cognitive inflexibility.

Historically, language processing has been considered the province of neocortical regions, principally Broca's and Wernicke's areas and adjacent cortex. However, in recent years evidence has accumulated that subcortical regions modulate linguistic function (Lieberman, 2000, 2002) and PD patients have subcortical pathology. The circuitry that runs from the cortex to the striatum and back to cortex has been shown to be involved in planning, motor control, dual task performance, and mood (Brainard & Doupe, 2000; Cools, Barker, Sahakian, & Robbins, 2001; Mesulam, 1990; Monchi, Petrides, Petre, Worsley, & Dagher, 2001). Cortico-striato-cortical circuitry is also important in speech production and sentence comprehension (Caplan & Waters, 1999; Friederici, Kotz, Werheid, Hein, & von Cramon, 2003; Grossman, 1999; Grossman et al., 2001; Stowe, Paans, Wijers, & Zwarts, 2004). Thus, the diminished performance of nondemented PD patients on linguistically oriented neuropsychologic tasks likely reflects cognitive rather than linguistic deficits.

Communicative Function in Demented PD Patients

Bayles et al. (1997) conducted a study of the effect of idiopathic PD on language function in 74 individuals with PD and 32 normal elderly control subjects. Individuals with PD were subdivided according to performance on the Mini-Mental State Examination (MMSE) (Folstein, Folstein, & McHugh, 1975). PD patients with MMSE scores of 27 to 30 were classified as nondemented ($N = 42$), those with MMSE scores of 24 to 26 were defined as questionably demented ($N = 25$), and those with MMSE scores 16 to 23 were designated as mildly demented ($N = 7$). All study participants were given 15 linguistic communication tasks to assess linguistic competence and performance. The four measures of linguistic competence were: Semantic Judgment, Semantic Correction, Syntactic Judgment, Syntactic Correction. The 11 measures of linguistic performance were:

Repetition of Phrases

Confrontation Naming

Definitions

Generative Naming/Fruit

Generative Naming/Animals

Following Commands

Picture Description

Reading Comprehension of Words

Reading Comprehension of Sentences

Comparative Questions

Object Description

The performances of each participant group on the linguistic communication tasks are presented in Table 7–1. The only measures on which the questionably demented PD participants achieved significantly lower scores than normal control participants were the generative naming tests. Mildly demented PD participants performed significantly poorer than the control and nondemented PD groups on six tasks: Confrontation Nam-

Table 7–1. Mean Scores and Standard Deviations (SD) for Normal Elderly Control (NC), Nondemented PD (NPD), Questionably Demented PD (QPD), and Mildly Demented PD (MPD) Participants on 15 Linguistic Communication Tasks

Task	Group (n)			
	NC (32) M (SD)	NPD (42) M (SD)	QDPD (25) M (SD)	MPD (7) M (SD)
Semantic Judgment	18.9 (0.9) 19.0	18.5 (1.4) 18.5	17.9 (2.0) 17.9	18.0 (1.6) 18.0
Semantic Correction	9.7 (0.6) 9.6	9.3 (1.0) 9.2	9.0 (1.5) 9.0	7.0 (1.2) 7.2
Syntactic Judgment	18.4 (2.0) 19.4	19.8 (0.5) 19.8	18.9 (2.2) 18.9	19.7 (0.5) 19.8
Syntactic Correction	9.8 (1.1) 9.8	9.9 (0.3) 9.9	9.4 (1.6) 9.4	9.9 (0.4) 9.9
Repetition	177.9 (5.5) 177.4	177.7 (6.0) 177.4	177.3 (3.9) 177.0	164.6 (11.9) 165.6
Confrontation Naming	17.7 (0.7) 17.6	17.5 (0.8) 17.4	17.3 (1.2) 17.3	15.0 (3.7) 15.2
Generative Naming—Fruit	15.6 (4.2) 15.3	13.0 (3.2) 12.8	11.3 (2.7) 11.1	8.6 (4.2) 9.3
Generative Naming—Animals	16.5 (3.7) 16.2	13.8 (3.6) 13.6	12.5 (2.9) 12.3	7.1 (3.7) 7.9
Picture Description	32.0 (7.3) 31.2	33.7 (7.5) 33.1	33.3 (10.2) 32.8	29.7 (9.3) 31.6
Definitions	35.1 (1.6) 35.0	34.4 (2.5) 34.3	33.1 (3.4) 33.0	30.1 (4.8) 30.5
Comparative Questions	6.0 (0.0) 6.0	5.9 (0.3) 5.9	5.6 (1.1) 5.6	5.3 (1.5) 5.3
Object Description	9.4 (2.3) 9.2	8.5 (2.6) 8.3	7.2 (3.0) 7.0	6.9 (3.5) 7.3
Reading Comprehension—Words	8.0 (0.2) 8.0	8.0 (0.2) 8.0	7.9 (0.3) 7.9	7.0 (0.4) 7.9
Reading Comprehension—Sentences	6.4 (1.0) 6.4	6.4 (1.0) 6.3	6.0 (1.6) 6.0	5.3 (2.1) 5.5
Following Commands	9.0 (0.2) 9.0	8.9 (0.4) 8.9	8.5 (1.1) 8.5	8.3 (1.1) 8.3

Note: First row = raw means; second row = means adjusted for age.

From "The Effect of Parkinson's Disease on Language," by K. Bayles, K. Tomoeda, J. A. Wood, R. F. Cruz, T. Azuma, and E. B. Montgomery in *Journal of Medical Speech–Language Pathology*, edited by L. LaPointe, Ed., 1997. *Vol 5*, 157–166. Reprinted with permission of Delmar Learning, a division of Thomson Learning.

ing, Generative Naming—Fruits, Generative Naming—Animals, Definitions, Repetition, and Semantic Correction. The mildly demented PD participants had significantly lower scores than the questionably demented PD participants on five of the six aforementioned tasks, the exception being Generative Naming—Fruits. Based on these findings, Bayles and colleagues (1997) concluded that although individuals with PD and mild dementia performed more poorly on some linguistic communication tasks, their performance was more indicative of a cognitive problem rather than a language competence problem. Indeed, mildly demented PD patients did not perform significantly more poorly on 9 of the 15 tasks.

PD with Dementia Compared to AD on Language Measures

The Arizona Battery of Communication Disorders of Dementia (Bayles & Tomoeda, 1993) was administered to eight PD patients with dementia, 62 nondemented PD patients, 86 AD patients, and 86 age-matched normal elders. The eight PD patients with dementia had scores similar to those of mildly demented AD patients on most subtests. For the five subtests (Object Description, Comparative Questions, Generative Naming, and Figure Copying) in which significant differences were observed, mildly demented AD patients obtained *better* scores than the demented PD patients. The demented PD patients obtained higher scores than the mildly demented AD patients on Word Learning Total Recall.

Discourse Sample of PD patient with Dementia

The following is a sample of the discourse produced by a PD patient with dementia on the Object Description test. It is similar to that produced by AD patients. The sentences are grammatical but content is aberrant and reflects disordered perception and thinking.

Examiner: Tell me about this (marble).

Subject: It's like candy and it's nearly as light. You can feel it. It's light. Some liquid in it. It hasn't been used. That's the way it looks to me. Orange color, or orange colored candy. Orange colored candy that you put in your mouth. That's all I can think of.

Examiner: What does it mean, "to advise"?

Subject: Oh, asking questions. I was able to ask me questions.

Examiner: What does it mean, "to predict"?

Subject: There's moisture on a big plant object.

Summary of Important Points

- Parkinsonism is a syndrome.
- It is associated with rigidity, tremor, and slowness of movement.
- Many disorders are associated with parkinsonism among them Alzheimer's disease, Lewy body disease, multiple system atrophy, and cortical-basal ganglionic degeneration.
- Idiopathic Parkinson's disease (PD) is the most prevalent form of parkinsonism.
- The loss of dopaminergic neurons in the substantia nigra pars compacta and the presence of neuronal Lewy bodies and Lewy neurites in the substantia nigra and

other brain areas are the defining pathology of PD.

- Age is the primary risk factor and incidence and prevalence of PD increase with advancing age.

- Depression is common in individuals with PD and can diminish cognitive functioning and result in the misdiagnosis of dementia and its severity.

- Most individuals with PD have cognitive deficits. In many individuals cognitive deficits worsen and dementia becomes apparent.

- The most common cognitive deficits associated with PD are in executive function, memory, and visuoperceptual and visuomotor skills.

- The communicative functioning of non-demented PD patients is affected primarily by executive function deficits. Their language does not reflect lack of linguistic knowledge but rather nonlinguistic cognitive deficits.

- The communicative functioning of PD patients with dementia is similar to that of AD patients.

References

Aarsland, D., & Janvin, C. (2005). Cognitive impairment and dementia in Parkinson's disease. In A. Burns, J. O'Brien, & D. Ames (Eds.). *Dementia* (3rd ed., pp. 657–663). London: Hodder Arnold.

Bayles, K. A. (1990). Language and communication in Parkinson's disease. *Alzheimer's Disease and Associated Disorders, 4,* 171–180.

Bayles, K. A., & Tomoeda, C. K. (1993). *Arizona Battery for Communication Disorders of Dementia.* Austin, TX: Pro-Ed.

Bayles, K., Tomoeda, C. K., Wood, J. A., Cruz, R. F., Azuma, T., & Montgomery, E. B. (1997). The effect of Parkinson's disease on language.

Journal of Medical Speech-Language Pathology, 5, 157–166.

Bodis-Wollner, I. (2002). Visualizing the next steps in Parkinson disease. *Archives of Neurology, 59,* 1233–1234.

Bondi, M. W., Kaszniak, A. W., Bayles, K. A., & Vance, K. T. (1993). Contributions of frontal system dysfunction to memory and perceptual abilities in Parkinson's disease. *Neuropsychology, 7,* 89–102.

Braak, H., & Braak, E. (2000). Pathoanatomy of Parkinson's disease. *Journal of Neurology, 247*(Suppl. 2), II3–II10.

Brainard, M. S, & Doupe, A. J. (2000). Interruption of a basal ganglia-forebrain circuit prevents the plasticity of learned vocalizations. *Nature, 404,* 762–766.

Breen, E. K. (1993). Recall and recognition in Parkinson's disease. *Cortex, 29,* 91–102.

Brown, R. G., & Marsden, C. D. (1988). "Subcortical dementia": The neuropsychological evidence. *Neuroscience, 25,* 363–387.

Bulens, C., Meerwaldt, J. D., & van der Wildt, G. J. (1988). Effect of stimulus orientation on contrast sensitivity in Parkinson's disease. *Neurology, 38,* 76–81.

Buttner, T., Kuhn, W., Klotz, P., Steinberg, R., Voss, L., Bulgaru, D., et al. (1993). Disturbance of color perception in Parkinson's disease. *Journal of Neural Transmission Parkinson's Disease and Dementia Section, 6,* 11–15.

Buttner, T., Kuhn, W., Muller, T., Patzold, T., Heidbrink, K., & Przuntek, H. (1995). Distorted color discrimination in "de novo" parkinsonian patients. *Neurology, 45,* 386–387.

Buytenhuijs, E. L., Berger, H. J. C., Van Spaendonck, K. P. M., Horstink, M. W. I., Borm, G. F., & Cools, A. R. (1994). Memory and learning strategies in patients with Parkinson's disease. *Neuropsychologica, 32,* 335–342.

Calne, D. B., Snow, B. J., & Lee, C. (1992). Criteria for diagnosing Parkinson's disease. *Annals of Neurology, 32,* S125–S127.

Caplan, D., & Waters, G. S. (1999). Verbal working memory and sentence comprehension. *Behavioral and Brain Sciences, 22,* 77–126.

Chen, R. C., Chang, S. F., Su, C. L., Chen, T. H., Yen, M. F., Wu, H. M., et al. (2001). Prevalence, incidence, and mortality of PD: A door-to-door survey in Ilan County, Taiwan. *Neurology, 57,* 1679–1686.

Cools R., Barker R. A., Sahakian, B. J., & Robbins, T. W. (2001). Enhanced or impaired cognitive function in Parkinson's disease as a function of dopaminergic medication and task demands. *Cerebral Cortex, 11,* 1136–1143.

Cummings, J. L. (1992). Depression and Parkinson's disease: A review. *American Journal of Psychiatry, 149,* 443–454.

de Rijk, M. C., Breteler, M. M. B., Graveland, G. A., Ott, A., Grobbee, D. E., van der Meche, F. G. A., et al. (1995). Prevalence of Parkinson's disease in the elderly: The Rotterdam Study. *Neurology, 45,* 2143–2146.

Dubois, B., & Pillon, B. (1997). Cognitive deficits in Parkinson's disease. *Journal of Neurology, 244,* 2–8.

Emre, M. (2003). What causes mental dysfunction in Parkinson's disease? *Movement Disorders, 18*(Suppl 6), S63–S71.

Fall, P., Axelson, O., Fredriksson, M., Hansson, G., Lindvall, B., Olsson, J., et al. (1996). Age-standardized incidence and prevalence of Parkinson's disease in a Swedish community. *Journal of Clinical Epidemiology, 49,* 637–641.

Farrer M., Wavrant-De-Vrieze, F., Crook, R., Boles, L., Perez, T. J., Hardy, J., et al. (1998). Low frequency of alpha-synuclein mutations in familial Parkinson's disease. *Annals of Neurology, 43,* 394–397.

Folstein, M. F., Folstein, S. E., & McHugh, P. R. (1975). Mini-mental state. A practical method for grading the cognitive state of patients for the clinician. *Journal of Psychiatric Research, 12,* 189–198.

Friederici, A. D., Kotz, S. A., Werheid, K., Hein, G., & von Cramon, D. Y. (2003). Syntactic comprehension in Parkinson's disease: Investigating early automatic and late integrational processes using event-related brain potentials. *Neuropsychology, 17,* 133–142.

Girotti, F., Soliveri, P., Carella, F., Piccolo, I., Caffarra, P., Musicco, M., et al. (1988). Dementia and cognitive impairment in Parkinson's disease. *Journal of Neurology, Neurosurgery, and Psychiatry, 51,* 1498–1502.

Gorell, J. M., Johnson, C. C., Rybicki, B. A., Peterson, E. L., Kortsha, G. X., Brown, G. G., et al. (1997). Occupational exposures to metals as risk factors for Parkinson's disease. *Neurology, 48,* 650–658.

Gorell, J. M., Johnson, C. C., Rybicki, B. A., Peterson, E. L., & Richardson, R. J. (1998). The risk of Parkinson's disease with exposure to pesticides, farming, well water and rural living. *Neurology, 50,* 1346–1350.

Grossman, M. (1999). Sentence processing in Parkinson's disease. *Brain and Cognition, 40,* 387–413.

Grossman, M., Glosser, G., Kalmanson, J., Morris, J., Stern, M. B., & Hurtig, H. I. (2001). Dopamine supports sentence comprehension in Parkinson's disease. *Journal of the Neurological Sciences, 184,* 123–130.

Harrington, D. L., Haaland, K. Y., Yeo, R. A., & Marder, E. (1990). Procedural memory in Parkinson's disease: Impaired motor but not visuoperceptual learning. *Journal of Clinical and Experimental Neuropsychology, 12,* 323–339.

Helkala, E. L., Laulumaa, V., Soininen, H., & Riekkinen, P. J. (1989). Different error pattern of episodic and semantic memory in Alzheimer's disease and Parkinson's disease with dementia. *Neuropsychologia, 27,* 1241–1248.

Hirsh, E. C. (2000). Glial cells and Parkinson's disease. *Journal of Neurology, 247*(Suppl. 2), II58–II62.

Hochstadt, J., Nakano, H., Lieberman, P., & Friedman, J. (2006). The roles of sequencing and verbal working memory in sentence comprehension deficits in Parkinson's disease. *Brain and Language, 97,* 243–257.

Jagust, W. J., Reed, B. R., Martin, E. M., Eberling, J. L., & Nelson-Abbott, R. A. (1992). Cognitive function and regional cerebral blood flow in Parkinson's disease. *Brain, 115,* 521–537.

Janvin, C. C., Aarsland, D., & Larsen, J. P. (2005). Cognitive predictors of dementia in Parkinson's disease: A community-based, 4-year longitudinal study. *Journal of Geriatric Psychiatry and Neurology, 18,* 149–154.

Koller, W., Vetere-Overfield, B., Gray, C., Alexander, C., Chin, T., Dolezal, J., et al. (1990). Environmental risk factors in Parkinson's disease. *Neurology, 40,* 1218–1221.

Kuzis, G., Sabe, L., Tiberti, C., Merello, M., Leiguarda, R., & Starkstein S E. (1999). Explicit and implicit learning in patients with Alzheimer disease and Parkinson disease with dementia. *Neuropsychiatry, Neuropsychology, and Behavioral Neurology, 12*, 265–269.

Kuopio, A. M., Marttila, R. J., Helenius, H., & Rinne, U. (1999). Changing epidemiology of Parkinson's disease in southwestern Finland. *Neurology, 52*, 302–308.

Lees, A. J., & Smith, E. (1983). Cognitive deficits in the early stages of Parkinson's disease. *Brain, 106*, 257–270.

Levin, B. E., Llabre, M. M., Resiman, S., Weiner, W. J., Sanchez-Ramos, J., Singer, C. et al. (1991). Visuospatial impairment in Parkinson's disease. *Neurology, 41*, 365–369.

Lieberman, P. (2000). *Human language and our reptilian brain: The subcortical bases of speech, syntax, and thought.* Cambridge, MA: Harvard University.

Lieberman, P. (2002). On the nature and evolution of the neural bases of human language. *Yearbook of Physical Anthropology, 45*, 36–62.

Litvan, I., Mohr, E., Williams, J., Gomez, C., & Chase, T. N. (1991). Differential memory and executive functions in demented patients with Parkinson's and Alzheimer's disease. *Journal of Neurology, Neurosurgery and Psychiatry, 54*, 25–29.

Lozano, A. M. & Kalia, S. K. (2005). New movement in Parkinson's. *Scientific American, 293*, 68–75.

Martilla, R. J., & Rinne, U. K. (1976). Dementia in Parkinson's disease. *Acta Neurologica Scandinavia, 54*, 431–441.

Mayeux, R., Denaro, J., Hemenegildo, N., Marder, K., Tang, M-X., Cote, L. J., et al. (1992). A population-based investigation of Parkinson's disease with and without dementia: Relationship to age and gender. *Archives of Neurology, 49*, 492–497.

Mayeux, R., Marder, K., Cote, L. J., Denaro, J., Hemenegildo, N., Mejia, H., et al. (1995). The frequency of idiopathic Parkinson's disease by age, ethnic group, and sex in northern Manhattan: 1988-1993. *American Journal of Epidemiology, 142*, 820–827.

Mayeux, R., Stern, Y., Rosen, J., & Benson, F. (1983). Is "subcortical dementia" a recognizable clinical entity? *Annals of Neurology, 14*, 278–283.

Mesulam, M. M. (1990). Large-scale neurocognitive networks and distributed processing for attention, language, and memory. *Annals of Neurology, 28*, 597–613.

Monchi, O., Petrides, M., Petre, V., Worsley, K., & Dagher, A. (2001). Wisconsin Card Sorting revisited: Distinct neural circuits participating in different stages of the task identified by event-related functional magnetic resonance imaging. *Journal of Neuroscience, 21*, 7733–7741.

Morens, D. M., Davis, J. W., Grandinetti, A., Ross, G. W., Popper, J. S., & White, L. R. (1996). Epidemiologic observations on Parkinson's disease: Incidence and mortality in a prospective study of middle-aged men. *Neurology, 46*, 1044–1050.

Owen, A. M., James, M., Leigh, P. N., Summers, B. A., Marsden, C. D., Quinn, N. P., et al. (1992). Fronto-striatal cognitive deficits at different stages of Parkinson's disease. *Brain, 115*, 1727–1751.

Papadimitriou A., Veletza, V., Hadjigeorgious, G.M., Patrikiou, A., Hirano, M., & Anastasopoulos, I. (1999). Mutated alpha-synuclein gene in two Greek kindreds with familial PD: Incomplete penetrance? *Neurology, 52*, 651–654.

Peppard, R. F., Martin, W. R., Carr, G. D, Grochowski, E., Schulzer, M., Guttman, M., et al. (1992). Cerebral glucose metabolism in Parkinson's disease with and without dementia. *Archives of Neurology, 49*, 1262–1268.

Pillon, B., Deweer, B., Agid, Y., & Dubois, B. (1993). Explicit memory in Alzheimer's, Huntington's, and Parkinson's diseases. *Archives of Neurology, 50*, 374–379.

Pillon, B., Dubois, B., Ploska, A., & Agid, Y. (1991). Severity and specificity of cognitive impairment in Alzheimer's, Huntington's, and Parkinson's diseases and progressive supranuclear palsy. *Neurology, 41*, 634–643.

Regan, D., & Maxner, C. (1987). Orientation-selective visual loss in patients with Parkinson's disease. *Brain, 110*, 415–432.

Reid, W. G. (1992). The evolution of dementia in idiopathic Parkinson's disease: Neuropsychological and clinical evidence in support of subtypes. *International Psychogeriatrics, 4,* 147–160.

Repka, M. X., Claro, M. C., Loupe, D. N, & Reich, S. G. (1996). Ocular motility in Parkinson's disease. *Journal of Pediatric Ophthalmology and Strabismus, 33,* 144–147.

Rippon, G. A., & Marder, K. S. (2005). Dementia in Parkinson's disease. *Advances in Neurology, 96,* 95–113.

Rodnitzky, R. L. (1998). Visual dysfunction in Parkinson's disease. *Clinical Neuroscience, 5,* 102–106.

Rodnitzky, R. L. (2005). Visual dysfunction. In R. F. Pfieffer & I. Bodis-Wollner (Eds.), *Parkinson's disease and nonmotor dysfunction* (pp. 221–232). Totowa, NJ: Humana Press.

Seidler, A., Hellenbrand, W., Robra, B.-P., Vieregge, P., Nischan, P., Joerg, J., et al. (1996). Possible environmental, occupational, and other etiologic factors for Parkinson's disease: A case-control study in Germany. *Neurology, 46,* 1275–1284.

Semchuk, K. M., Love, E. J, & Lee R.G. (1992). Parkinson's disease and exposure to agricultural work and pesticide chemicals. *Neurology, 42,* 1328–1335.

Stefanova, E. D., Kostic, V. S., Ziropadja, L., Markovic, M., & Ocic, G. G. (2000). Visuomotor skill learning on serial reaction time task in patients with early Parkinson's disease. *Movement Disorders, 15,* 1095–1103.

Stern, Y., Mayeux, R., Rosen, J., & Ilson, J. (1983). Perceptual motor dysfunction in Parkinson's disease: A deficit in sequential and predictive voluntary movement. *Journal of Neurology Neurosurgery and Psychiatry, 46,* 145–151.

Stern, Y., Richards, M., Sano, M., & Mayeux, R. (1993). Comparison of cognitive changes in patients with Alzheimer's and Parkinson's disease. *Archives of Neurology, 50,* 1040–1045.

Stern, Y., Tang, M-X., Jacobs, D. M., Sano, M., Marder, K., Bell, K., et al. (1998). Prospective comparative study of the evolution of proba-

ble Alzheimer's disease and Parkinson's disease dementia. *Journal of the International Neuropsychological Society, 4,* 279–284.

Stowe, L. A., Paans, A. M. J., Wijers, A. A., & Zwarts, F. (2004). Activations of "motor" and other non-language structures during sentence comprehension. *Brain and Language, 89,* 290–299.

Struck, L. K., Rodnitzky, R. L., & Dobson, J. K. (1990). Circadian fluctuations of contrast sensitivity in Parkinson's disease. *Neurology, 40,* 467–470.

Takahashi, H., & Wakabayashi, K. (2005). Controversy: Is Parkinson's disease a single disease entity? Yes. *Parkinsonism & Related Disorders, 11,* S31–S37.

Tanner, C. M., Ottman, R., Goldman, S. M., Ellenberg, J., Chan, P., Mayeux, R., et al. (1999). Parkinson disease in twins: An etiologic study. *Journal of the American Medical Association, 281,* 341–346.

Taylor, A. E., Saint-Cyr, J. A., & Lang, A. E. (1986). Frontal lobe dysfunction in Parkinson's disease: The cortical focus of neostriatal outflow. *Brain, 109,* 845–883.

Tröster, A. I., & Woods, S. P. (1987). Neuropsychological aspects of Parkinson's disease and parkinsonian syndromes. In R. Pahwa, K. E. Lyons & W. C. Koller (Eds.), *Handbook of Parkinson's disease* (3rd ed., pp. 127–157). New York: Marcel Dekker.

Wengel, S. P., Bohac, D., & Burke, W. J. (2005). Depression in Parkinson's disease. In M. Ebadi & R. F. Pfeiffer (Eds.), *Parkinson's disease* (pp. 329–338). Boca Raton, FL: CRC Press.

Wong, G. F., Gray, C. S., Hassanein, R. S., & Koller, W. C. (1991). Environmental risk factors in siblings with Parkinson's disease. *Archives of Neurology, 48,* 287–289.

Zakanis, K. K., & Freedman, M. A. (1999). A neuropsychological comparison of demented and nondemented patients with Parkinson's disease. *Applied Neuropsychology, 6,* 129–146.

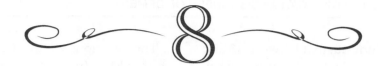

Dementia and Lewy Body Disease

Lewy Body Disease

Originally thought to be rare, Lewy body dementia (LBD) may be the second most common type of dementia (Jellinger, 1996). In 1923 Fredrich Heinrich Lewy, a contemporary of Alois Alzheimer, observed the round lumps of protein in the cell processes of neurons that characterize LBD (Holdorff, 2002; Figure 8–1). However, it was not until 1961 that much attention was paid to the neuro-

pathology and behavioral changes associated with LBD. In 1961 two individuals with progressive dementia and widespread cortical Lewy bodies were described by Okazaki, Lipton, and Aronson and rekindled interest in the disease. Subsequently, Kosaka (1978) detailed the characteristics and distribution of cortical Lewy bodies. Today, the literature contains many reports of individuals with progressive dementia who had extensive Lewy body formation in the cortex (Lowe et al., 1988). In fact, autopsy studies of elderly individuals

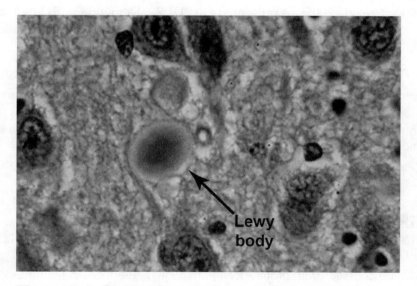

Figure 8–1. Brain cells containing a Lewy body, which is an abnormal aggregation of protein. Photo courtesy of Kondi Wong, Armed Forces Institute of Pathology. http://www.genome.gov

with dementia indicate that between 15 and 25% of dementia patients have diffuse cortical Lewy bodies (Hansen et al., 1990; Perry, Irving, Blessed, Perry, & Fairbairn, 1989; Perry, Irving, Blessed, Fairbairn, & Perry, 1990).

Three patterns of Lewy body disease have been identified (McKeith et al., 2005): nigrostriatal involvement; cortical involvement; and sympathetic nervous system involvement. Lewy bodies often occur in individuals with AD and are typically present in individuals with Parkinson's disease (Cummings & Mega, 2003; Reichman & Cummings, 1999). They also occur in individuals with Down syndrome (Lippa, Schmidt, Lee, & Trojanowski, 1999; Simard & van Reekum, 2001).

Diagnostic Criteria

Consensus criteria for the clinical diagnosis of probable and possible dementia with Lewy bodies were developed in 1996 by the Consortium on DLB (dementia with Lewy bodies) (McKeith et al., 1996) and have been reviewed, tested for predictive validity, and modified (McKeith et al., 2005), as presented in Table 8–1.

The revisions of the Consortium are such that REM (rapid eye movement) sleep disorders, severe neuroleptic (antipsychotic) sensitivity, and reduced striatal dopamine transporter activity on functional neuroimaging are given greater diagnostic weight as features *suggestive* of a DLB diagnosis. REM sleep behavior disorder is characterized as "vivid and often frightening dreams during REM sleep" (McKeith et al., 2005, p. 1866) in which patients vocalize, flail their limbs, and move around violently. Often, the patient has limited recollection of these episodes; however, the bed partner reports their presence as well as excessive daytime drowsiness. Severe neuroleptic sensitivity refers to an adverse reaction to antipsychotic drugs, typically the exacerbation of parkinsonism and impaired consciousness. Low striatal dopamine transporter activity in functional imaging studies occurs in DLB and can help differentiate DLB from AD in which striatal dopamine transporter activity is normal.

LBD = Lewy body disease
DLB = Dementia with Lewy bodies

Table 8–1. Revised Criteria for the Clinical Diagnosis of Dementia with Lewy bodies (DLB)

1. *Central feature* (essential for a diagnosis of possible or probable DLB)

   Dementia defined as progressive cognitive decline of sufficient magnitude to interfere with normal social or occupational function.

   Prominent or persistent memory impairment may not necessarily occur in the early stages but is usually evident with progression.

   Deficits on tests of attention, executive function, and visuospatial ability may be especially prominent.

2. *Core features* (two core features are sufficient for a diagnosis of probable DLB, one for possible DLB)

   Fluctuating cognition with pronounced variations in attention and alertness.

   Recurrent visual hallucinations that are typically well formed and detailed.

   Spontaneous features of parkinsonism.

Table 8–1. *continued*

3. *Suggestive features* (If one or more of these is present in the presence of one or more core features, a diagnosis of probable DLB can be made. In the absence of any core features, one or more suggestive features is sufficient for possible DLB. Probable DLB should not be diagnosed on the basis of suggestive features alone.)

   REM sleep behavior disorder.

   Severe neuroleptic sensitivity.

   Low dopamine transporter uptake in basal ganglia demonstrated by SPECT or PET imaging.

4. *Supportive features* (commonly present but not proven to have diagnostic specificity)

   Repeated falls and syncope.

   Transient, unexplained loss of consciousness.

   Severe autonomic dysfunction (e.g., orthostatic hypotension, urinary incontinence).

   Hallucinations in other modalities.

   Systematized delusions.

   Depression.

   Relative preservation of medial temporal lobe structures on CT/MRI scan.

   Generalized low-uptake on SPECT/PET perfusion scan with reduced occipital activity.

   Abnormal (low-uptake) MIBG myocardial scintigraphy.

   Prominent slow-wave activity on EEG with temporal lobe transient sharp waves.

5. A diagnosis of DLB is *less likely*

   In the presence of cerebrovascular disease evident as focal neurologic signs or on brain imaging.

   In the presence of any other physical illness or brain disorder sufficient to account in part or in total for the clinical picture.

   If parkinsonism only appears for the first time at a stage of severe dementia.

6. *Temporal sequence* of symptoms

   DLB should be diagnosed when dementia occurs before or concurrently with parkinsonism (if it is present). The term Parkinson disease dementia (PDD) should be used to describe dementia that occurs in the context of well-established Parkinson disease. In a practice setting the term that is most appropriate to the clinical situation should be used and generic terms such as LB disease are often helpful. In research studies in which distinction needs to be made between DLB and PDD, the existing 1-year rule between the onset of dementia and parkinsonism DLB continues to be recommended. Adoption of other time periods will simply confound data pooling or comparison between studies. In other research settings that may include clinicopathologic studies and clinical trials, both clinical phenotypes may be considered collectively under categories such as LB disease or alpha-synucleinopathy.

Reprinted with permission from: "Diagnosis and Management of Dementia with Lewy Bodies", by I. G. McKeith et al., 2005. *Neunology, 65*, 1863–1872.

Clinical Features Helpful in the Diagnosis of LBD

LBD is often confused with Parkinson's disease because Lewy bodies occur in both diseases and commonly used brain imaging techniques do not differentiate PD and LBD (Jagust, 2000). In fact, many pathologists question whether they are separate disease entities (Benecke, 2003; Tsuboi & Dickson, 2005). Sulkava (2003) specified the core clinical features of PD and LBD (Table 8–2). Notice that extrapyramidal symptoms (tremor, rigidity, and bradykinesia) often occur in LBD and

are always present in PD. When patients with LBD do not have, or report, visual hallucinations, they can easily be misdiagnosed as having PD. Mistaking LBD for PD can be serious because of the extreme sensitivity of LBD patients to treatment with neuroleptic medications that are tolerated by individuals with PD.

An important defining feature of LBD is fluctuation in cognitive symptoms. It occurs in more than half the cases but is uncommon in PD. Response to levodopa is another differentiating feature. More than half the patients with LBD do not respond to treatment with

Table 8–2. Clinical Features Helpful in the Differential Diagnosis of Early Parkinson's Disease (PD) and Dementia with Lewy bodies (DLB)

	PD	DLB
Impairment of psychomotor functions	mild	more marked
Executive dysfunction	often	often
Visuospatial impairment	seldom	often
Visual hallucinations	no	often
Other hallucinations, (e.g. auditory)	no	sometimes
Extrapyramidal symptoms	always	often
Effect of levodopa	good	variable
Fluctuations of symptoms	not marked	marked
Symptoms of depression	often	often
Delusions	no	often
Absence of rest tremor	sometimes	often
Syncopal attacks	no	sometimes
Episodes of unresponsiveness	no	sometimes
Balance disorders	sometimes	seldom

From "Differential Diagnosis Between Early Parkinson's Disease and Dementia with Lewy Bodies," by R. Sulkava. In A. Gordin, S. Kaakkda, & H. Teravainen (Eds.), *Parkinson's Disease: Advances in Neurology* (Vol. 91, 411–413), 2003. Reprinted with permission from Lippincott, Williams & Wilkins.

levodopa (Louis, Klatka, Liu, & Fahn, 1997). Early presentation of dementia also differentiates LBD and PD. In LBD, dementia precedes parkinsonism; in PD, parkinsonism is usually apparent before dementia. Finally, the psychiatric symptoms of visual hallucinations and delusions differentiate LBD from individuals with PD.

Age at onset of LBD varies and has been reported to range from 50 to 83 years (Papka, Rubio, & Schiffer, 1998). Disease duration was originally thought to be shorter than in AD because of reports of individuals in whom disease progression was very rapid (Armstrong et al., 1991); however, recent reports suggest otherwise (McKeith, 2005). The incidence and prevalence of LBD by sex and age and other demographic factors have not been established with large epidemiologic studies.

Cognition and Communication in LBD

LBD begins insidiously over several years during which time affected individuals experience periodic episodes of forgetfulness, distractibility, and executive dysfunction. With disease progression, cognitive impairment is omnipresent although its severity fluctuates. Hallucinations are common. Daytime drowsiness, apathy, and sleep disorders develop. A gait disorder may be present along with slowness of movement. In later stages, help is generally sought for severe behavioral disturbances. Aphasia and apraxia are reported as late stage features (McKeith, 2005).

As can be seen, early symptoms of DLB can be similar to those associated with Alzheimer's dementia: memory loss, attention deficits, constructional dyspraxia, and executive dysfunction (Byrne, Lennox, Lowe,

& Godwin-Austen, 1989; Gibb, Esiri, & Lees, 1985; Salmon & Hamilton, 2005). Rigorous neuropsychological testing reveals differences, however. Pure LBD patients with dementia have greater deficits in visuoconstructive ability, verbal fluency, psychomotor speed, and some executive functions (Galasko, Salmon, Lineweaver, Hansen, & Thal, 1998; Hamilton, Salmon, Galasko, & Hansen, 2004; Salmon, Lineweaver, Galasko, & Hansen, 1998). Investigators who have compared individuals with LBD to those with AD report that a "double discrimination" can help differentiate the two diseases. Individuals with LBD tend to have relative preservation of confrontation naming and better recall and recognition memory but greater impairment on verbal fluency (category naming) and visual perception tasks (Connor, Salmon, Sandy, Galasko, Hansen, & Thal, 1998; McKeith et al., 2005; Mormont, Grymonprez, Baisset-Mouly, & Pasquier, 2003; Walker, Allan, Shergill, & Katona, 1997). Conversely, individuals with AD have prominent recall and recognition memory deficits and comparatively less difficulty with verbal fluency and visual perception. Nonetheless, individuals with LBD, like those with AD, ultimately develop severe dementia.

A Case of Pure LBD

Few descriptions exist of the effects on communication of "pure" LBD, that is, LBD without coexistent Alzheimer's pathology. However, Gurd, Herzberg, Joachim, and Marshall (2000) described a 68-year-old man who was examined neuropsychologically and neuroradiologically several times in life and had autopsy confirmation of pure LBD. This contribution to the literature is valuable because it confirms reports of earlier investigations and adds new information about communicative functioning.

Early in the disease, Gurd et al.'s patient experienced periods of forgetfulness and described himself as having trouble putting thoughts into words. He sought advice from his general practitioner who referred him to specialists who followed him for two years. Gurd and colleagues reported that the patient was unable to shop with a list, sometimes forgot the beginning of a sentence by the end and occasionally made comments that were out of context. At the time of first neuropsychological evaluation, cognitive impairment was obvious and he scored 15 of 30 on the MMSE. His attention was poor, and he was disoriented for time and space. Furthermore, he was anosognosic for his cognitive deficits. Over the disease course the patient complained of visual hallucinations, confusion upon waking and nightmares. He became depressed, irritable, stubborn, and preoccupied with death which occurred 2.5 years after diagnosis.

In conversation, Gurd et al.'s patient made several tangential departures from topic and was extremely poor on semantic and letter category naming. Gurd et al. described him as having difficulty remembering and maintaining the semantic category as evident from several out-of-category errors. He could write his name and address and draw a house, man, and flower. One year after his initial examination, his spontaneous speech was grammatical but he was described as aphasic although he did not display obvious language comprehension problems. His descriptions of a picture were plausible though he confabulated at the end of picture description. Stress and intonation patterns were normal but he was mildly deficient in word retrieval, articulation, and phrase completion. Word retrieval was often labored with long, frequent pauses. Some articulatory errors were noted and occasionally he "mumbled" his words. Although he named 18 of 21 pictured objects at his first test session, his object naming score diminished to 10 of 21 a year and a half later.

Neuroimaging (CT and SPECT) in life revealed progressive medial temporal lobe atrophy. Postmortem pathologic analysis documented Lewy bodies, degeneration in the substantia nigra, nucleus basalis of Meynert, and locus ceruleus, but none of the neuritic plaques and neurofibrillary tangles that characterize AD.

Definition of Terms

anosognosia—unawareness of cognitive, linguistic, sensory, and or motor deficits after brain disease or injury.

neuroleptic drugs—tranquilizers used to treat psychotic conditions.

syncope—fainting or temporary loss of consciousness due to inadequate blood flow to the brain.

hallucination—a false perception; sensory experience of stimuli that are not actually present.

Summary of Changes in Communicative Functioning Observed in Gurd et al.'s (2000) Patient

Early Features

Grammatical speech

Mild anomia on confrontation naming

Forgot what he intended to say

Some tangential comments

Could write name and address

Severe impairment in semantic and letter category naming

Later Features

Speech grammatical

Normal stress and intonation

Occasional articulation error

Occasional confabulation

Slow in word retrieval

Deficit in phrase completion

Long, frequent pauses

No obvious comprehension problems

Summary of Important Points

- Little attention was paid to Lewy body disease until 1961. Since then it has gained recognition as a common cause of dementia.
- Lewy bodies are round lumps of protein in the cell processes of neurons.
- Between 15 to 25% of dementia patients have diffuse cortical Lewy bodies.
- Lewy bodies commonly occur in individuals with Alzheimer's disease and are generally present in those with Parkinson's disease.
- An important defining feature of Lewy body disease is fluctuation in cognitive symptoms which is uncommon in Parkinson's and Alzheimer's diseases.
- Visual hallucinations are also a common differentiating feature of the disease.
- Because individuals with Lewy body disease often have extrapyramidal symptoms, they may be misdiagnosed as having Parkinson's disease.
- The early symptoms of the disease are memory loss, attentional deficits, constructional dyspraxia, and executive dysfunction.
- With disease progression, severe behavioral problems and dementia develop.

- Changes in communicative functioning include: anomia, tangentiality, impaired letter and category naming, and forgetting of intentions.

References

Armstrong T. P., Hansen, L. A., Salmon, D. P., Masliah, E., Pay, M., Kunin, J. M., et al. (1991). Rapidly progressive dementia in a patient with the Lewy Body variant of Alzheimer's disease. *Neurology, 41*, 1178–1180.

Benecke, R. (2003). Diffuse Lewy body disease–a clinical syndrome or a disease entity? *Journal of Neurology, 250* (Suppl. 1). I39–I42.

Byrne, E. J., Lennox, G., Lowe, J., & Godwin-Austen, R. B. (1989). Diffuse Lewy body disease: Clinical features in 15 cases. *Journal of Neurology, Neurosurgery, and Psychiatry, 52*, 709–717.

Connor, D. J., Salmon, D. P., Sandy, T. J., Galasko, D., Hansen, L. A., & Thal, L. J. (1998). Cognitive profiles of autopsy-confirmed Lewy body variant vs pure Alzheimer disease. *Archives of Neurology 55*, 994–1000.

Cummings, J. L., & Mega, M. S. (2003). *Neuropsychiatry and behavioral neuroscience.* New York: Oxford University Press.

Galasko, D., Salmon, D. P., Lineweaver, T., Hansen, L., & Thal, L. J. (1998). Neuropsychological measures distinguish patients with Lewy body variant from those with Alzheimer's disease. *Neurology, 50*, A181.

Gibb, W. R. G., Esiri, M. M., & Lees, A. J. (1985). Clinical and pathological features of diffuse cortical Lewy body disease (Lewy body dementia). *Brain, 110*, 1131–1153.

Gurd, J. M., Herzberg, L., Joachim, C., & Marshall, J. C. (2000). Dementia with Lewy bodies: A pure case. *Brain and Cognition, 44*, 307–323.

Hamilton, J. M., Salmon, D. P., Galasko, D., & Hansen, L. A. (2004). Distinct memory deficits in dementia with Lewy bodies and Alzheimer's disease. *Journal of the International Neuropsychological Society, 10*, 689–697.

Hansen, L., Salmon D., Galasko D., Masliah, E., Katzman, R., DeTeresa, R., et al. (1990). The

Lewy body variant of Alzheimer's disease: A clinical and pathological entity. *Neurology, 40,* 1–8.

Holdorff, B. (2002). Friedrich Heinrich Lewy (1885–1950) and his work. *Journal of the History of Neuroscience, 11,* 19–28.

Jagust, W. J. (2000). Neuroimaging in dementia. *Neurologic Clinics, 18,* 885–902.

Jellinger, K.A. (1996). Structural basis of dementia in neurodegenerative disorders. *Journal of Neural Transmission Supplement, 47,* 1–29.

Kosaka, K. (1978). Lewy bodies in cerebral cortex: Report of three cases. *Acta Neuropathologica, 42,* 127–134.

Lippa, C. F., Schmidt, M. L., Lee, V. M., & Trojanowski, J. Q. (1999). Antibodies to alpha-synuclein detect Lewy bodies in many Down syndrome brains with Alzheimer's disease. *Annals of Neurology, 45,* 353–357.

Louis, E. D., Klatka, L. A., Liu, Y., & Fahn, S. (1997). Comparison of extrapyramidal features in 31 pathologically confirmed cases of diffuse Lewy body disease and 34 pathologically confirmed cases of Parkinson's disease. *Neurology, 48,* 376–380.

Lowe, J., Blanchard A., Morrell K., Lennox, G., Reynolds, L., Billett, M., et al. (1988). Ubiquitin is a common factor in intermediate filament inclusion bodies of diverse type in man, including those of Parkinson's disease, Pick's disease, and Alzheimer's disease, as well as Rosenthal fibres in cerebellar astrocytomas, cytoplasmic bodies in muscle, and Mallory bodies in alcoholic liver disease. *Journal of Pathology, 155,* 9–15.

McKeith, I. G. (2005). Dementia with Lewy bodies: A clinical overview. In A. Burns, J. O'Brien, & D. Ames (Eds.), *Dementia* (3rd ed., pp. 603–614). London: Hodder Arnold.

McKeith, I. G., Dickson, D. W., Lowe, J., Emre, M., O'Brien, J. T., Feldman, et al. (2005). Diagnosis and management of dementia with Lewy bodies: Third report of the DLB consortium. *Neurology, 65,* 1863–1872.

McKeith, I. G., Galaska, D., Kosaka, K., Perry, E. K., Dickson, D. W., Hansen, L. A., et al. (1996). Consensus guidelines for the clinical and pathologic diagnosis of dementia with Lewy bodies (DLB): Report of the consortium on DLB international workshop. *Neurology, 47,* 1113–1124.

Mormont, E., Grymonprez, L. L., Baisset-Mouly, C., & Pasquier, F. (2003). The profile of memory disturbance in early Lewy body dementia differs from that in Alzheimer's disease. *Review Neurologique, 159,* 762–766.

Okazaki, H., Lipton, L. S., & Aronson, S. M. (1961). Diffuse intracytoplasmic ganglionic inclusions (Lewy type) associated with progressive dementia and quadriparesis in flexion. *Journal of Neurology, Neurosurgery, and Psychiatry, 20,* 237–244.

Papka M., Rubio, A., & Schiffer R. B. (1998). A review of Lewy body disease: An emerging concept of cortical dementia. *Journal of Neuropsychiatry and Clinical Neuroscience, 10,* 267–279.

Perry, R. H., Irving, D., Blessed, G. Perry, E. K., & Fairbairn, A. F. (1989). Clinically and neuropathologically distinct form of dementia in the elderly. *Lancet, 1,* 166.

Perry, R. H., Irving, D., Blessed, G., Fairbairn, A., & Perry, E. K.(1990). Senile dementia of Lewy body type: A clinically and neuropathologically distinct form of Lewy body dementia in the elderly. *Journal of Neurological Sciences, 95,* 119–139.

Reichman, W. E., & Cummings, J. L. (1999). Dementia. In E. H. Duthie & P. R. Katz (Eds.), *Practice of geriatrics* (3rd ed., pp. 295–304). Philadelphia: W. B. Saunders.

Salmon, D. P., & Hamilton, J. M. (2005). Neuropsychological changes in dementia with Lewy bodies. In A. Burns, J. O'Brien, & D. Ames (Eds.), *Dementia* (3rd ed., pp. 634–647). London: Hodder Arnold.

Salmon, D. P., Lineweaver, T. T., Galasko, D., & Hansen, L. (1998). Patterns of cognitive decline in patients with autopsy-verified Lewy body variant of Alzheimer's disease. *Journal of the International Neuropsychological Society, 4,* 228.

Simard, M., & van Reekum, R. (2001). Dementia with Lewy bodies in Down syndrome. *International Journal of Geriatric Psychiatry, 16,* 311–320.

Sulkava, R. (2003). Differential diagnosis between early Parkinson's disease and dementia with

Lewy bodies. In A. Gordin, S. Kaakkola, & H. Teravainen (Eds.), *Parkinson's disease: Advances in neurology* (Vol. 91., pp. 411–413). Philadelphia: Lippincott, Williams, & Wilkins.

Tsuboi, Y., & Dickson, D. W. (2005). Dementia with Lewy bodies and Parkinson's disease with dementia: Are they different? *Parkinsonism and Related Disorders, 11,* S47–S51.

Walker, A., Allan, R. L., Shergill, S., & Katona, C. L. E. (1997). Neuropsychological performance in Lewy body dementia and Alzheimer's disease. *British Journal of Psychiatry, 170,* 156–158.

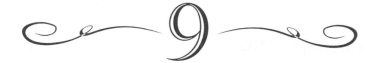

Dementia and Huntington's Disease

Overview and Genetics

Huntington's disease (HD), also known as Huntington's chorea, is an inherited degenerative disease of the nervous system characterized by dementia and uncontrollable dancelike movements known as chorea. It is named for George Huntington who in 1872 described its characteristics in members of a Long Island, New York family. Because of the uncoordinated movements of the affected family members, he called the disease a "chorea," from the Greek word *choros* for "dance."

The mutant gene that causes HD is called huntingtin and is autosomal dominant (Chua & Chiu, 2005). "Autosomal" means that the gene is located on a chromosome other than the sex chromosome and therefore the disease is not sex-linked; males and females are equally likely to be affected. "Dominant" means that the defective gene dominates its normal partner gene from the unaffected parent. Each child of an affected parent has a 50% chance of inheritance. If a child has not received the Huntington's gene from a parent, the child and his or her children will be free of the disease but children who inherit the gene will develop the dis-

ease if they live long enough. HD affects roughly one person in every 10,000.

The median age at onset of HD is the late 40s or early 50s (Kremer, 2003); however, it can begin in childhood. Young et al. (1986) reported that 94% of individuals with HD developed it as adults and only 6% developed it as juveniles. In the large majority of individuals with juvenile onset (90%), the gene was inherited from the father (Harper, 1996).

In 1983 the gene that causes HD was identified by a team of scientists from around the world (Gusella et al., 1983). It lies at one end of chromosome 4 and makes a mutant form of huntingtin protein in which the same amino acid, glutamine, repeats dozens of time (Cattaneo, Rigamonti, & Zuccato, 2002). Mutant huntingtin appears to be toxic to certain nerve cells and lacks the ability to trigger the production of a necessary growth factor. Tragically, there is no known cure for HD. However, soon after the discovery of huntingtin, genetic tests were developed enabling individuals with a family member with HD to determine whether they carry the HD gene. Many individuals at risk for developing HD have taken advantage of genetic testing.

Neuropathology of HD

The signs and symptoms of HD result from brain atrophy and neurochemical deficiencies. Atrophy is most prominent in the head of the caudate nucleus but exists to a lesser extent in the putamen and globus pallidus (Bamford, Caine, Kido, Cox, & Shoulson, 1995; Bamford, Caine, Kido, Plassche, & Shoulson, 1989; Zakzanis,1998), the cortex, and the substantia nigra. The atrophy of the caudate nucleus and putamen is the most striking neuropathologic feature of HD. Atrophy of the frontal lobes also is apparent in 80% of HD brains (Vonsattel, Myers, Stevens, Ferrante, Bird, & Richardson, 1985). Other regions of the brain often show atrophy that varies in severity. Typically, the brains of individuals who have suffered with HD weigh 10 to 20% less than the brains of age-matched controls (Lange, Thorner, Hofp, & Schroder, 1976; MacMillan & Quarrell, 1996).

To understand the movement disorder of HD, it is necessary to appreciate that components of the basal nuclei are part of reverberating neuronal networks that control body movements. These networks rely upon specific neurotransmitters and a particular balance between them. In HD an imbalance occurs within the caudate nucleus in which dopamine is excessive in relation to acetylcholine and gamma amino butyric acid (GABA). When the balance between these three neurotransmitters is restored, choreiform movements are reduced (Stipe, White, & Van Arsdale, 1979).

Early Symptoms

Most individuals who carry the HD gene develop and function normally into early adulthood before experiencing a change in mood, cognition, or motor function that signals the onset of the disease. *Early mood changes* include sadness, irritability, depression, and occasionally an episode of verbal or physical abuse (Kirkwood, Su, Conneally, & Foroud, 2001). *Early motor symptoms* include facial grimaces, abnormal eye movements, impaired finger tapping, excessive movements of the fingers or hands, and sometimes a mild dysarthria (Penney et al., 1990). These lesser abnormalities usually precede the more obvious signs of extrapyramidal dysfunction by several years (Penney et al., 1990). *Early cognitive changes* include deficits in psychomotor, attentional, and executive functions (Kirkwood et al., 2001), verbal fluency, verbal learning (Hahn-Barma et al., 1998) and visual working memory (Ho et al., 2003; Lemiere, Decruyenaere, Evers-Kiebooms, Vandenbussche, & Dom, 2002).

Diagnosing HD on the basis of these early symptoms can be difficult especially when the individual is not known to be at risk for HD. However, as the disease progresses and clear extrapyramidal signs appear, such as chorea (Figure 9–1), hypokinesia, rigidity, or dystonia, the diagnosis of HD becomes definitive. Inexorably, the dancelike movements of chorea increase in severity and eventually become disabling. Similarly, cognitive deficits become increasingly pronounced (Brandt et al., 1996; Butters, Wolfe, Granholm & Martone, 1986; Claus & Mohr, 1996; Sprengelmeyer et al., 1996) and dementia results.

Definitions

Hypokinesia—abnormally decreased motor function

Dystonia—impairment of voluntary movement

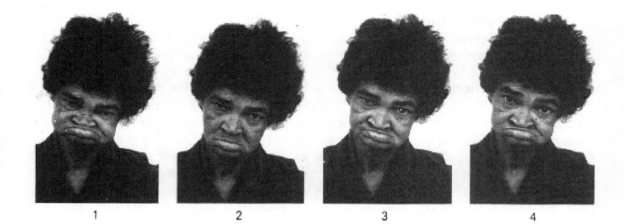

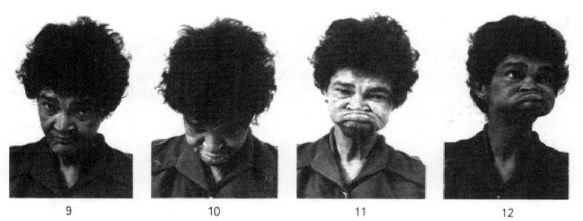

Figure 9–1. Sequential photographs taken at one-second intervals showing choreiform movements of face and neck. From Hayden, M. R. (1981). *Huntington's Chorea*. New York: Springer-Verlag. Reprinted with kind permission of Springer Science and Business Media.

Progression of Cognitive Deficits

Executive Function

Executive function and attention are most vulnerable to the effects of HD (Lemiere, Decruyenaere, Evers-Kiebooms, Vandenbussche, & Dom, 2004). Affected individuals may be disorganized, have difficulty planning (Watkins et al., 2000), and use poor judgment. As the ability to self-monitor deteriorates, errors go unnoticed. Lack of self-monitoring often leads to problems in relationships with other people. Psychomotor slowing also contributes to the poor performance of HD patients on executive function tasks (Dubois, Pillon, Legault, Agid, & Lhermitte, 1988). Lemiere et al. (2004) report that the Symbol Digit Modalities Test (Smith, 1982), a test of attention, was the most important of a large neuropsychological battery for evaluating the onset and progression of HD.

Memory

Lemiere et al. (2004) found that memory tasks differentiated individuals who were asymptomatic carriers of the mutated HD gene from those with clinically verified HD. Subjects with clinically verified HD had deficits in the learning of new information and retrieval of previously acquired information and recognition memory was superior to free recall. However, as the disease progressed, the superiority of recognition memory over free recall in individuals with confirmed HD was lost. Bayles & Kaszniak (1987) reported episodic memory deficits in individuals with HD but of lesser severity than in AD.

As might be predicted by HD's effects on basal nuclei, individuals with HD have trouble learning new motor skills involving a repeated sequence of movements (Gabrieli, Stebbins, Singh, Willingham, & Goetz, 1997; Heindel, Butters, & Salmon, 1988). Willingham, Koroshetz, and Peterson (1996) reported that HD patients had no difficulty learning to track a moving target with a joystick on a computer screen, provided the target moved randomly. However, when the target moved in a repeated sequence, HD patients were impaired.

Effects on Language

Individuals with early HD typically do not show impairment in everyday language (Brandt, 1991); however, if given linguistically-based neuropsychological tests, deficits can be demonstrated and are proportional to task difficulty. In fact, the literature on HD and language contains reports of impaired confrontation naming, repetition, decreased conversational initiative, syntactic deficits in spontaneous speech, and decreased language output in written narratives in individuals with early HD (Bayles & Tomoeda, 1983; Caine, Bamford, Schiffer, Shoulson, & Levy, 1986; Podoll, Caspary, Lange, & Noth, 1988; Wallesch & Fehrenbach, 1988). At issue is whether these reports of impaired performance reflect deficits in language knowledge or other neuropsychological deficits. Likely executive function deficits have affected performance but there is, nonetheless, some evidence of a "signature profile" (Chenery, Copland, & Murdoch, 2002) of impaired language function in individuals who have damage to the nonthalamic subcortex as a consequence of HD or stroke. Chenery and colleagues (2002) compared the language abilities of 13 individuals with

HD to those of age- and education-matched patients with chronic non-thalamic subcortical pathology following stroke and 13 non-neurologically impaired individuals. Study participants were given a variety of language tests to assess primary and complex language abilities including:

- Western Aphasia Battery (Kertesz, 1982)
- Boston Naming Test (Kaplan, Goodglass, & Weintraub, 1983)
- Test of Language Competence—Expanded (Wiig & Secord, 1989)
- Selected subtests from the Test of Word Knowledge (Wiig & Secord, 1992), and
- Word Test—Revised (Huisingh, Barrett, & Zachman, 1990).

Individuals with HD performed similarly to normal control subjects on many of the tests from the Western Aphasia Battery but were significantly inferior to normal control subjects on the Boston Naming Test and other *lexico-semantic* tasks including providing definitions, word and sentence-level generation, interpreting ambiguity, and deriving figurative and inferential meaning. The profile of performance of the HD patients was strikingly similar to the language profile of the individuals with nonthalamic subcortical pathology secondary to stroke. Chenery et al. (2002) concluded that whereas language deficits in individuals with HD may reflect other cognitive impairments, results of their study raise the possibility that "a signature language profile exists in both HD and non-thalamic subcortical patients" (p. 471).

Teichmann and colleagues (2005) tested the hypothesis that the left caudate is involved in the application of grammatical rules as theorized by Ullman (2001). In the Teichmann et al. study, 30 HD patients and 20 control subjects were administered a verb conjugation task, a sentence-picture matching task, and arithmetic tasks. HD patients were found to be impaired in rule application in both the linguistic and nonlinguistic domains (morphology, syntax, and subtraction).

Bayles and Kaszniak (1987) observed impairment of object recognition and semantic processing in 11 individuals with HD and mild or moderate dementia as can be seen from the following language sample of an HD subject with moderate dementia.

Sample of Language from Individual with HD and Moderately Severe Dementia

The examiner has asked the HD patient to describe a button and define two words.

Examiner: What is this? (button)

Subject: Oh, that's a needle. But . . . button hole scissors. And they go ahead they put buttons or they put, ss, that's how they put buttons your coat with it, I guess.

Examiner: What does it mean to describe?

Subject: Well like you're a buttoning your blouse would be an example.

Examiner: What does it mean to guarantee?

Subject: Guarantee you're gonna get it. I guess we're gonna have company
Something. That would be a guarantee, wouldn't it?

In sum, individuals with HD have cognitive-communicative impairments that are proportional to the severity of their dementia. Results of structural neuroimaging studies support a relation between degree of striatal and cortical atrophy and performance on tests of attention, working memory, and executive functions. Striatal hypoperfusion and decreased glucose uptake correlate with degree of executive dysfunction. Cortical hypometabolism correlates with impairment on recognition memory, language, and perceptual tests (see Montoya, Price, Menear, & Lepage, 2006 for a review of brain imaging and cognitive dysfunction in Huntington's disease). Thus, early in the disease when neuropathology is less extensive and cognitive deficits are mild, everyday language functioning is good but as pathology increases and deficits in executive function, attention, memory, and perceptual processing worsen, communication is markedly affected. The cognitive-communicative disorders of individuals with HD, together with the dysarthria that commonly develops and the not uncommon occurrence of dysphagia, provide the SLP with a prominent role in patient management.

Summary of Important Points

- Huntington's disease (HD) is an inherited degenerative disease of the nervous system characterized by dementia and uncontrollable dancelike movements known as chorea.
- The mutant gene that causes HD is called huntingtin and is autosomal dominant.
- Most individuals with HD develop and function normally until mid-life. The mean age at onset is 40 years.
- The gene that causes HD was identified in 1993 and genetic tests were developed that enable at-risk individuals to determine if they are carriers.
- The signs and symptoms of HD result from brain atophy and neurochemical deficiencies. Atophy is most pronounced in the head of the caudate nucleus but exists to a lesser extent in the putamen and globus pallidus.
- In HD an imbalance occurs between the neurochemicals needed to control movement.
- As HD progresses, cognitive deficits become increasingly pronounced and dementia always develops.
- Executive functions are those most vulnerable to the effects of HD.
- Episodic memory deficits are apparent in HD but not to the extent they exist in individuals with AD.
- Recognition memory is better than recall in early AD.
- HD patients have trouble learning new motor skills involving a repeated sequence of movements.
- Many reports exist of diminished performance of individuals with HD on linguistic tasks such as naming, sentence comprehension, and discourse production.
- At issue is whether language knowledge is disrupted by the disease because the cognitive deficits associated with the disease also impair communicative functioning.
- However, it may be that individuals with HD have a "signature language" impairment that causes disruption of lexical-semantic processing and the application of grammatical rules that is caused by striatal pathology.
- Overall, communicative functioning reflects the degree of dementia severity.

References

Bamford, K. A., Caine, E. D., Kido, D. K., Cox, C., & Shoulson, I. (1995). A prospective evaluation of cognitive decline in early Huntington's disease: Functional and radiographic correlates. *Neurology*, 45, 1867–1873.

Bamford, K. A., Caine, E. D., Kido, D. K., Plassche, W. M., & Shoulson, I. (1989). Clinical-pathologic correlation in Huntington's disease: A neuropsychological and computer tomography study. *Neurology*, 39, 796–801.

Bayles, K. A., & Kaszniak, A. W. (1987). *Communication and cognition in normal aging and dementia*. Austin, TX: Pro-Ed.

Bayles K. A. & Tomoeda, C. K. (1983). Confrontation naming impairment in dementia. *Brain and Language*, 19, 98–114.

Brandt, J. (1991). Cognitive impairments in Huntington's disease: Insights into the neuropsychology of the striatum. In F. Boller & J. Grafman (Eds.), *Handbook of neuropsychology* (Vol. 5, pp. 241–264). New York: Elsevier Science.

Brandt, J., Bylsma, F. W., Gross, R., Stine, O. C., Ranen, N., & Ross, C. A. (1996). Trinucelotide repeat length and clinical progression in Huntington's disease. *Neurology*, 46, 527–531.

Butters, N., Wolfe, J, Granholm, E., & Martone, M. (1986). An assessment of verbal recall, recognition and fluency abilities in patients with Huntington's disease. *Cortex*, 22, 11–32.

Caine, E. D., Bamford, K. A., Schiffer, R. B., Shoulson, I., & Levy, S., (1986). A controlled neuropsychological comparison of Huntington's disease and multiple sclerosis. *Archives of Neurology*, 43, 249–254.

Cattaneo E., Rigamonti, D., & Zuccato, D. (2002). Huntington's disease. *Scientific American*, 287, 93–97.

Chenery, H. J., Copland, D. A., & Murdoch, B. E. (2002). Complex language functions and subcortical mechanisms: Evidence from Huntington's disease and patients with non-thalamic subcortical lesions. *International Journal of Language and Communication Disorders*, 37, 459–474.

Chua P., & Chiu, E. (2005). Huntington's disease. In A. Burns, J. O'Brien, & D. Ames (Eds.), *Dementia* (3rd ed., pp. 754–762). London: Hodder Arnold.

Claus, J. J., & Mohr, E. (1996). Attentional deficits in Alzheimer's, Parkinson's and Huntington's diseases. *Acta Neurologica Scandinavia*, 93, 346–351.

Dubois, B., Pillon, B., Legault, F., Agid, Y., & Lhermitte, F. (1988). Slowing of cognitive processing in progressive supranuclear palsy: A comparison with Parkinson's disease. *Archives of Neurology*, 45, 1194–1199.

Gabrieli, J. D. E., Stebbins, G. T., Singh, J., Willingham, D. B., & Goetz, C. G. (1997). Intact mirror-tracing and impaired rotary-pursuit skill learning in patients with Huntington's disease. *Neuropsychology*, 11, 272–281.

Gusella J., Wexler, N. S., Conneally, P. M., Naylor, S. L., Anderson, M. A., Tanzi, R. E., et al. (1983). A polymorphic DNA marker genetically linked to Huntington's disease. *Nature*, 306, 234–238.

Hahn-Barma, V., Deweer, B., Durr, A., Dode, C., Feingold, J., Pillon, B., et al. (1998). Are cognitive changes the first symptoms of Huntington's disease? A study of gene carriers. *Journal of Neurology, Neurosurgery and Psychiatry*, 64, 172–177.

Harper, P. S. (1996). *Huntington's disease. Major problems in neurology* (2nd ed.). London: W. B. Saunders.

Heindel, W. C., Butters, N., & Salmon, D. P. (1988). Impaired learning of a motor skill in patients with Huntington's disease. *Behavioural Neuroscience*, 102, 141–147.

Ho, A. K., Sahakian, B. J., Brown, R. G., Barker, R. A., Hodges, J. R., Ané, M.-N., et al, for the NEST-HD Consortium. (2003). Profile of cognitive progression in early Huntington's disease. *Neurology*, 61, 1702–1706.

Hiusingh, R., Barret, M., & Zachman, L. (1990). *The Word Test—Revised*. Moline, IL: LinguiSystems.

Kaplan E., Goodglass H., & Weintraub, S. (1983). *The Boston Naming Test*. Philadelphia: Lea & Febiger.

Kertesz A. (1982). *The Western Aphasia Battery*. New York: Grune & Stratton.

Kirkwood, S. C., Su, J. L., Conneally, P., & Foroud, T. (2001). Progression of symptoms in the early and middle stages of Huntington disease. *Archives of Neurology*, 58, 273–278.

Kremer B. (2003). Clinical neurology of Huntington's disease. In G. Bates, P. Harper, & L. Jones (Eds.), *Huntington's disease* (3rd ed., pp. 28–61). Oxford: Oxford University Press.

Lange, H., Thorner, G., Hofp, A., & Schroder, K. F. (1976). Morphometric studies of the neuropathological changes in choreatic diseases. *Journal of Neurological Science, 28,* 401–425.

Lemiere, J., Decruyenaere, M., Evers-Kiebooms, G., Vandenbussche, E., & Dom, R. (2002). Longitudinal study evaluating neuropsychological changes in so-called asymptomatic carriers of the Huntington's disease mutation after 1 year. *Acta Neurologica Scandinavia, 106,* 131–141.

Lemiere, J., Decruyenaere, M., Evers-Kiebooms, G., Vandenbussche, E., & Dom R. (2004). Cognitive changes in patients with Huntington's disease (HD) and asymptomatic carriers of the HD mutation: A longitudinal follow-up study. *Journal of Neurology, 251,* 935–942.

MacMillan J., & Quarrell O. (1996). The neurobiology of Huntington's disease. In P. S. Harper (Ed.), *Huntington's disease* (2nd ed., pp. 317–357). London: WB Saunders.

Montoya, A. L., Price, B. H., Menear, M., & Lepage, M. (2006). Brain imaging and cognitive dysfunctions in Huntington's disease. *Journal of Psychiatry and Neuroscience, 31,* 21–29.

Penney, J. B., Jr., Young, A. D., Shoulson, I., Starosta-Rubenstein, S., Snodgrass, S. R., Sanchez-Ramos, J., et al. (1990). Huntington's disease in Venezuela: 7 years of follow-up on symptomatic and asymptomatic individuals. *Movement Disorders, 5,* 93–99.

Podoll, K., Caspary, P., Lange, H. S., & Noth, J. (1988). Language functions in Huntington's disease. *Brain, 111,* 1475–1503.

Smith, A. (1982). *Symbol Digit Modalities Test (SDMT) Manual Revised.* Los Angeles: Western Psychological Services

Sprengelmeyer, R., Young, A. W., Calder, A. J., Karnat, A., Lange, H., Homberg, V., et al. (1996). Loss of disgust. Perception of faces and emotions in Huntington's disease. *Brain, 119,* 1647–1665.

Stipe, J., White, D., & Van Arsdale, E. (1979). Huntington's disease. *American Journal of Nursing, 79,* 1428–1433.

Teichmann, M., Dupoux, E., Kouider, S., Brugieres, P., Boisse, M. F., Baudic, S., et al. (2005). The role of the striatum in rule application: The model of Huntington's disease at early stage. *Brain, 128,* 1155–1167.

Ullman, M. T. (2001). The declarative/procedural model of lexicon and grammar. *Journal of Psycholinguistic Research, 30,* 37–69.

Vonsattel, J. P. G., Myers, R. H., Stevens, T. J., Ferrante, R. J., Bird, E. D., & Richardson, E. P., Jr. (1985). Neuropathological classification of Huntington's disease. *Journal of Neuropathology and Experimental Neurology, 44,* 559–577.

Wallesch, C. W., & Fehrenbach, R. A. (1988). On the neurolinguistic nature of language abnormalities in Huntington's disease. *Journal of Neurology, Neurosurgery and Psychiatry, 51,* 367–373.

Watkins, L.H., Rogers, R.D., Lawrence, A.D., Sahakian, B.J., Rosser, A.E., & Robbins, T.W. (2000). Impaired planning but intact decision making in early Huntington's disease: Implications for specific frontostriatal pathology. *Neuropsychologia, 38,* 1112–1125.

Wiig, E. H., & Secord, W. (1989). *Test of Language Competence—Expanded.* New York: Psychological Corporation.

Wiig, E. H., & Secord, W. (1992). *Test of Word Knowledge.* San Antonio, TX: Psychological Corporation.

Willingham, D. B., Koroshetz, W. J., & Peterson, E. W. (1996). Motor skills have diverse neural bases: Spared and impaired skill acquisition in Huntington's disease. *Neuropsychology, 10,* 315–321.

Young, A. B., Shoulson, I., Penney, J. B., Starosta-Rubinstein, S., Gomez, F., Travers, H., et al. (1986). Huntington's disease in Venezuela: Neurologic features and functional decline. *Neurology, 36,* 244–249.

Zakzanis, K. K. (1998). The subcortical dementia of Huntington's disease. *Journal of Clinical and Experimental Neuropsychology, 20,* 565–578.

10

Frontotemporal Dementia

The term frontotemporal dementia describes a clinical syndrome associated with various degenerative conditions (McKhann et al., 2001). Those likely to be seen by the SLP include Pick's disease, primary progressive aphasia, semantic dementia, and amyotrophic lateral sclerosis.

The first paper describing an individual with frontotemporal dementia (FTD) was written by Arnold Pick in 1892. The individual was a 71-year-old man with a history of progressive mental deterioration and severe aphasia whose postmortem examination revealed atrophy of the left temporal cortex. In subsequent years Pick described several other patients with similar symptoms and temporal or frontotemporal atrophy (Pick, 1901, 1904, 1906). In 1911, Alois Alzheimer identified the microscopic brain changes that caused the clinical profile described earlier by Pick. Alzheimer found intraneuronal inclusions (later called Pick bodies), circumscribed atrophy, and ballooned cortical neurons. In 1922, Gans used the name Pick's disease to refer to individuals with the morphologic changes first noted by Pick and later described by Alzheimer, and usage of the term became widespread.

Subsequently, many clinicians reported individuals with dementia and prominent language and personality changes but whose neuropathology *did not match* that described by Pick. Confusion developed over whether to label them as having Pick disease (now preferred instead of Pick's disease) and, indeed, whether Pick disease was a spectrum of disorders. Various terms were used to refer to these patients, as can be seen in Table 10–1, and the need developed for consensus terminology and clinical criteria for differentiating Pick disease cases from those with similar clinical features but different neuropathology.

Table 10–1. Terms Used to Refer to Individuals with Frontotemporal Dementia

Pick complex
Frontal lobe degeneration
Frontal lobe dementia
Frontal lobe degeneration of the non-Alzheimer type
Frontotemporal lobar degeneration
Dementia lacking distinct histopathologic features
Semantic dementia
Primary progressive aphasia
Progressive nonfluent aphasia

After Kertesz, 2004.

Diagnostic Criteria

The National Institutes of Health responded to the need for consensus terminology and diagnostic criteria for frontotemporal dementia by forming an international workgroup composed of basic and clinical scientists. The group was charged with proposing *clinical* criteria that would enable clinicians worldwide to recognize patients with frontotemporal dementia and terminology for describing them. The workgroup's recommended clinical criteria for FTD were published in 2001 (McKhann et al., 2001, p. 1805) and include the following:

1. The development of behavioral or cognitive deficits manifested by either:
   A. early and progressive change in personality, characterized by difficulty in modulating behavior, often resulting in inappropriate responses or activities or
   B. early and progressive change in language, characterized by problems with expression of language or severe naming difficulty and problems with word meaning.
2. The deficits outlined in 1A or 1B cause significant impairment in social or occupational functioning and represent a significant decline from a previous level of functioning.
3. The course is characterized by a gradual onset and continuing decline in function.
4. The deficits outlined in 1A or 1B are not due to other nervous system conditions (e.g., cerebrovascular disease), systemic conditions (e.g., hypothyroidism), or substance-induced conditions.
5. The deficits do not occur exclusively during a delirium.
6. The disturbance is not better accounted for by a psychiatric diagnosis (e.g., depression).

Notice that a distinction is made between individuals with FTD who *present* with progressive changes in behavior and those who *present* with progressive changes in language function, (Figure 10–1). Those

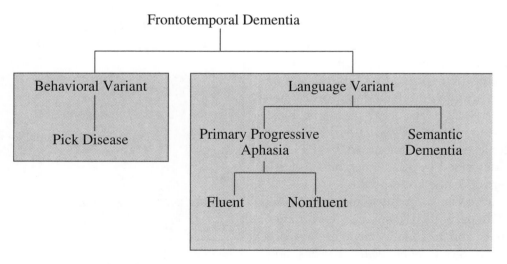

Figure 10–1. Categorization of frontotemporal dementias.

with behavioral presentation include individuals with Pick disease (who therefore have Pick bodies in cortex). Those with language presentation include individuals with primary progressive aphasia and those with semantic dementia. The word "present" is emphasized because a behavioral presentation does not mean that language and communicative function are necessarily spared throughout the disease course but rather that the *early* symptoms involve notable changes in behavior and personality. Similarly, a language presentation does not mean that cognitive, behavioral, and personality changes will not be part of the syndrome.

Behavioral Presentation

Pick Disease

Pick disease is a rare disorder that affects women more than men. It typically manifests when individuals are in their 50s, although it has been reported to occur as early as 21 (Lowenberg, Boyd, & Salon, 1939). Disease duration can vary from 3 to 17 years (Gustafson, Brun, & Risberg, 1990). Because of frontal pathology, Pick disease patients exhibit changes in personality, character, and comportment. These changes often appear before brain abnormalities can be detected with neuroimaging (Gregory, Serra-Mestres, & Hodges, 1999). Lack of concern about the disease process is common in Pick patients as are poor judgment, emotional blunting, compulsive exploration of environmental stimuli, hyperorality, altered dietary preferences, changes in sexual behavior, and visual and auditory agnosia (Cummings & Benson, 1983). Most Pick patients exhibit repetitive behaviors, 78% according to Ames, Cummings, Wirshing, Quinn, and Mahler (1994).

Cognitive Changes

The cognitive deficits of Pick patients reflect frontal lobe dysfunction and include deficits in attention, difficulty shifting mental set, and executive dysfunction including poor performance on category fluency tests (Elfgren, Passant, & Risberg, 1993; Hodges et al., 1999). Although memory disturbance is demonstrable with neuropsychological testing (Elfgren et al., 1993; Gregory et al., 1999; Hodges et al., 1999; Rahman, Sahakian, Hodges, Rogers, & Robbins, 1999), Pick patients do not have a true amnestic syndrome and can track day-to-day events until late in the disease (Hodges et al., 1999; McKhann et al., 2001; Rascovsky et al., 2002). A striking feature of these patients is preservation of visuospatial abilities (Hodges, 2001).

Language and Communication

Although the majority of individuals with Pick disease do not have aphasia early in the disease (Hodges et al., 1999; Karbe, Kertesz, & Polk, 1993; Mesulam, 2001; Siri, Benaglio, Frigerio, Binetti, & Cappa, 2001; Weintraub & Mesulam, 1993), many develop communication disorders (Snowden & Neary, 1993) that take the form of nonfluent aphasia with phonological and articulatory impairment and agrammatism.

Holland, McBurney, Moossy, and Reinmuth (1985) published a comprehensive account of the deterioration of language in an individual with Pick disease, a man known as Mr. E. They conducted a retrospective study of his communicative functioning from the time of his first speaking difficulty in 1967 until his death 12 years later. Upon postmortem examination, Mr. E. was found to have the neuropathologic features typical of Pick disease and neurofibrillary tangles but no neuritic plaques. Recall that in AD, both neurofibrillary tangles and neuritic plaques are present. In the earlier stages, Mr. E's speech slowed, became more deliberate, and was interspersed with inordinately long pauses. Thereafter, he began to substitute lower frequency words for words of higher frequency, a tendency that continued throughout the language dissolution process. In a speech-language evaluation in 1971, Mr. E was observed to have language formulation and word-finding problems although his responses were clear and concise. Particularly troublesome was what appeared to be a progressive auditory agnosia. After 1971, he became more and more reluctant to talk, preferring to communicate in writing. From letters written in his last years of life, it is apparent that Mr. E retained memory for names of people and environments. In his final 24 months, marked personality changes occurred; he became increasingly passive, impulsive, and exhibited poor judgment. Thus, unlike individuals with AD, Mr. E. first lost the formal syntactic elements of language but retained access to semantic memory throughout the disease course, a fact clearly revealed in letters he wrote.

Diagnosing Pick Disease

Before routine use of neuroimaging, individuals with Pick disease often were misdiagnosed as having AD. Today, evidence of focal atrophy in younger persons (individuals in their 50s), who have relatively preserved memory makes Pick disease easier to diagnose. A comparison of AD and Pick disease was carried out by Mendez, Selwood, Mastri, and Frey (1993) who compared 21 pathologically confirmed cases of Pick disease to 42 pathologically confirmed cases of AD. The two groups of patients were matched by sex and duration of dementia. All the Pick patients, but none of the AD patients, had onset before age 65. The Pick patients had early change in personality (roaming, disin-

hibition, and hyperorality), and a tendency toward reiterative and other speech disturbances such as decreased verbal output, poor articulation, verbal stereotypies, and echolalia. These characteristics contrasted with the fluent speech and impaired memory of AD patients. Lobar atrophy of temporal and frontal lobes, or both, was apparent on CT scans in 44% of the Pick patients but not on the scans of AD patients.

Language Presentation

Primary Progressive Aphasia

The diagnosis of primary progressive aphasia (PPA) is made when an individual presents with progressive aphasia in the absence of other cognitive or behavioral problems. The progressive aphasia predates other behavioral changes by at least two years (Mesulam, 1987, 2001). Although the aphasia may interfere negatively with performance on memory and reasoning tests, the PPA patient has no difficulty recalling day-to-day events or in problem-solving.

Language Characteristics

The characteristics of PPA are variable. Some researchers assert the existence of PPA subtypes distinguished by fluency (nonfluent PPA and fluent PPA). Others suggest that fluency varies as a function of the evolution of neuropathology (Kertesz, Davidson, McCabe, Takagi, & Munoz, 2003) and does not distinguish subtypes. In a series of 67 patients with PPA, Kertesz and colleagues found that most patients were fluent initially but became agrammatic and nonfluent later in their disease. Some clinical researchers recommend the term PPA for only those individuals with nonfluent aphasia (Hodges et al., 1992) and the term "semantic dementia" for individuals with fluent aphasia and comprehension problems. Others object to the term semantic dementia because the clinical syndrome is associated with more than a deficit in semantic processing (Mesulam, Grossman, Hillis, Kertesz, & Weintraub, 2003). In fact, individuals with semantic dementia have a combination of language deficits and difficulty recognizing objects and faces, tastes and smells (Neary et al., 1998). Clearly, consensus is lacking about the best terminology for referring to the different types of PPA. Because fluency differences are apparent clinically, we review reported characteristics of individuals with PPA who are nonfluent and those who are fluent.

Nonfluent PPA

Patients with nonfluent PPA exhibit anomia and effortful, agrammatic spontaneous speech that lacks function words (Clark, Charuvastra, Miller, Shapira, & Mendez, 2005; Mesulam, 2001). Comprehension typically is good except for grammatically complicated sentences (Mesulam, 2001). Some patients have been reported to have oral apraxia, stuttering, impaired repetition, dyslexia, dysgraphia and, late in the course of the disease, mutism (Neary et al., 1998). Grossman (2002) speculated about the existence of an underlying grammatical disorder that produces difficulty in constructing and decoding complex grammar.

Fluent PPA

Patients with fluent PPA are anomic and often have language comprehension deficits but their articulation is relatively normal as are speech rate and phrase length. With disease progression, comprehension worsens, reading and spelling often deteriorate, paraphasias are evident, and their language becomes increasingly empty (Mesulam, 2001).

Neuropathology of PPA

Neuroimaging reveals left perisylvian atrophy as the most common pathology (Abe, Ukita, & Yanagihara, 1997; Hodges, 2001) in individuals with PPA. The atrophy is generally in anterior perisylvian areas in contrast to the posterior perisylvian atrophy associated with semantic dementia (Abe et al., 1997). Many cases have histologic features of neuronal loss, gliosis, and spongiosis in layers II and III of the cortex (Kirshner, Tanridag, Thurman, & Whetsell, 1987; Turner, Kenyon, Trojanowski, Gonatas, & Grossman, 1996).

Nonfluent PPA patients have pathology in the inferior portion of the frontal lobes as well as in the anterior portion of the temporal lobe that is greater in the left than right hemisphere; fluent PPA patients have pathology in the parietal lobe and anterolateral portion of the temporal lobe that is greater in the left than right hemisphere (Warren, Harvey, & Rossor, 2005).

Semantic Dementia

Semantic dementia (SD) is an uncommon but distinctive syndrome in which individuals progressively lose their semantic (conceptual) knowledge. Consequently, they have difficulty understanding the meaning of words, objects, faces, nonverbal sounds, tastes, and smells. In contrast, the nonsemantic aspects of cognition remain intact. Their problem is not one of perception but of assigning meaning to perception. Typically preserved are visuoperceptual and spatial abilities, nonverbal reasoning, executive functions, and episodic memory (Hodges et al., 1999).

SD presents most often in individuals between 50 and 65 years of age. The median duration of illness approximates 8 years and ranges from 3 to 15 years (Snowden, 2005). Although Pick reported the syndrome much earlier, it was not until 1975 that the behavioral symptoms of semantic dementia were fully characterized (Warrington, 1975) as a loss of semantic memory. In 1975 Warrington published a report of three individuals with progressive anomia without phonologic or syntactic deficits who had difficulty comprehending verbal and pictorial presentations of the same stimuli. Her patients had preserved episodic memory and intact perceptual and visuospatial abilities. Warrington hypothesized that these individuals were exhibiting deterioration in semantic memory. In 1982 Mesulam published a description of six patients who experienced progressive deterioration of spoken language but who did not have frank dementia. This publication generated considerable interest in the dementias and in the next decade many papers appeared in the literature with descriptions of individuals who presented with various types of language problems. Snowden, Goulding, and Neary (1989) drew attention to the similarity between patients with a progressive fluent aphasia and Warrington's cases and introduced the term "semantic dementia" to define what Warrington believed to be the underlying deficit. In 1998 Neary and colleagues published clinical criteria to aid in the identification of semantic dementia (Table 10–2).

Language Characteristics

Individuals with SD come to the clinic complaining of a loss of memory for words. They are verbally fluent with intact grammar and syntax. Testing reveals the presence of anomia that is greater for nouns than verbs. Also present is a comprehension deficit for single words and difficulty providing definitions. Occasionally their word finding problems in conversation are masked by circumlocution (Garrard & Hodges, 1999). They perform poorly when asked to identify the correct referent for a word when the target and foils are from the same semantic category. As might be expected, they struggle to perform category fluency tests in which they must think of as many examples as possible from the same semantic category (Rosser & Hodges, 1994). Often they have difficulty with reading and spelling irregular words and make regularization errors (Graham, Patterson, & Hodges, 2000; Jeffries, Lambon Ralph, Jones, Bateman, & Patterson, 2004; Macoir & Bernier, 2002).

Individuals with SD also have a loss of semantic knowledge about objects. When presented with an object, for example, a key, they are unable to provide its name, explain the object's use, nor can they provide appropriate associations for the object such as "a key is used to open doors." A clue that deterioration of semantic memory is causing the communication problem is the fact that SD patients also perform poorly on nonverbal tests of conceptual knowledge (Howard & Patterson, 1992). Garrard and Hodges (1999) published examples of the spontaneous speech of an individual with SD and an individual with nonfluent aphasia (Table 10–3). Compare these examples to better understand how to differentiate individuals with SD from those with nonfluent aphasia.

Neuropathology of SD

Results of MRI scans indicate bilateral but asymmetric pathology of the temporal lobes with the left more affected. Within the temporal lobes, the areas most involved are the middle and inferior gyri particularly in the polar and inferolateral regions (Hodges et al., 1992). It is also common for the pathology to extend to the frontal lobes.

Table 10–2. Clinical Diagnostic Features of Semantic Dementia

Core diagnostic features

A. Insidious onset and gradual progression

B. Language disorder characterized by
    i. progressive, fluent, empty spontaneous speech
    ii. loss of word meaning, manifest by impaired naming and comprehension
    iii. semantic paraphasias and/or

C. Perceptual disorders characterized by:
    i. prosopagnosia and/or
    ii. associative agnosia: impaired recognition of object identity

D. Preserved perceptual matching and drawing reproduction

E. Preserved single word repetition

F. Preserved ability to read aloud and write to dictation orthographically regular words.

Other features that support the diagnosis of semantic dementia

A. Speech and language
    i. press of speech
    ii. idiosyncratic word usage
    iii. absence of phonemic paraphasias
    iv. surface dyslexia and dysgraphia
    v. preserved calculation

B. Behavior
    i. loss of sympathy and empathy
    ii. narrowed preoccupations
    iii. parsimony

C. Physical signs
    i. absent or late primitive reflexes
    ii. akinesia, rigidity, and tremor

D. Neuropsychological testing
    i. profound semantic loss, manifest in failure of word comprehension and naming and/or face and object recognition
    ii. preserved phonology and syntax, elementary perceptual processing, spatial skills, and day-to-day memorizing

E. Electrophysiology
    i. Normal

F. Brain imaging (structural or functional)
    i. predominant anterior temporal abnormality (symmetric or asymmetric)

From "Frontotemporal Lobar Degeneration," by D. Neary et al., 1998. *Neurology, 51*, 1546–1554.

Table 10–3. Language Samples from an Individual with Semantic Dementia (SD) Compared to an Individual with Primary Progressive Aphasia

---

Individual with SD

(On being shown a picture of a soldier): Oh gosh, this seems to be, oh come on, try to remember the name; I know what they are cause there's three of these so it's not the two and three, it's the one which, er . . . Some of them will be in Britain because, er, you know with our stuff in Britain, some of them are also outside Britain, some of them are also in Britain as well. What d'you call them again because N.'s son, no not son, his brother, he's one of these as well.

Individual with Primary Progressive Aphasia

Examiner: Could you tell me something about your holiday in Norway?

Patient: Er (holding up nine fingers) nides (= nine days) and an aeropload (= aeroplane) have flow and a mawnd bandelez and er the (unintelligible). When we came out a coach and took uz (= us) all round hoadle (= hotel) three days and er we a coach or two days and a splip ote and er ote five days it was all right. (Gives "thumbs up" sign)

From "Semantic Dementia: Implications for the Neural Basis of Language and Meaning," by P. Garrard & J. R. Hodges, in *Aphasiology*, *13*, 609–623. 1999. Reprinted by kind permission of Psychology Press.

Within the temporal and frontal lobes there is loss of the large pyramidal nerve cells. Medial temporal structures, such as the hippocampus and parahippocampal gyrus, typically are spared at least in the early stage of the disease (Mummery, Hodges, Patterson, & Price, 1999).

Differentiation of SD, Nonfluent PPA, and AD

Garrad and Hodges (1999) developed the following table (Table 10–4) in which comparison is made of the clinical features of SD, nonfluent PPA, and AD. Severe impairment of episodic memory is the key feature of AD. Nonfluency is the key feature of nonfluent PPA and individuals with SD are fluent but produce language that lacks content words.

Frontotemporal Dementia and Amyotrophic Lateral Sclerosis

Amyotrophic lateral sclerosis (ALS) is a progressive, adult-onset motor neuron disease characterized by loss of motor function and ultimately death. Amyotrophic refers to muscle atrophy, lateral refers to affected areas of the spinal cord, and sclerosis refers to thickening and hardening of motor neurons (Palmieri, 2005). Affected individuals experience weakness and progressive wasting of muscles that ultimately produces paralysis and the inability to speak and swallow. No diagnostic tests are definitive but electromyelogram and nerve conduction studies confirm lower motor neuron dysfunction and rule out other disorders. Diagnosis is based on history and signs of progressive dysfunction of lower motor neurons and upper motor neurons.

Table 10-4. Comparison of Clinical Features of Semantic Dementia, Progressive Nonfluent Aphasia and AD

	Semantic Dementia	Progressive Nonfluent Aphasia	Alzheimer-Type Dementia
Age at onset	Commonly <65	Commonly <65	Usually >65
Disease progression	Generally rapid	Slow	Variable
Spontaneous speech	Fluent and grammatically correct, but empty of content words	Labored, telegraphic with long word-finding pauses and frequent phonological and grammatical errors	Initially normal in most instances
Paraphasias	Semantic	Phonological	Semantic (early), phonological (late)
Comprehension:			
Single-words	Impaired	Intact	Initially intact
Syntax	Intact	Impaired	Initially intact
Repetition	Normal for single words	Phonemic errors	Generally intact
Episodic memory	Preserved for recent events	Intact	Severely impaired early in course
Frontal "executive" functions	Intact in early stages	Intact	May be impaired
Visuospatial and perceptual skills	Intact	Intact	Often impaired from early on; sometimes severely
Behavior	Appropriate initially but frontal features invariably appear later	Appropriate until very late	Normal in early stages, but commonly disturbed in later stages
General neurologic findings	Usually none	Buccofacial apraxia, and unilateral limb signs commonly seen	Usually normal until late stage
MRI findings	Focal polar and inferolateral temporal lobe atrophy, often worse on the left	Left perisylvian atrophy	Hippocampal ± medial temporal atrophy

From "Semantic Dementia: Implications for the Neural Basis of Language and Meaning," by P. Garrard and J. R. Hodges, in *Aphasiology, 13*, p. 609–623. 199. Reprinted with kind permission of Psychology Press.

The incidence rate is 1.0 to 1.8 in 100,000 and the average age of symptom onset is 59 years (SD = 10.8) (Strong, 1995). Disease duration averages 46 months from the time of the first symptom (Strong, Grace, Orange, & Leeper, 1996).

Historically, ALS was thought to spare cognitive functioning; however, research has shown that mild cognitive deficits are present in approximately 35% of ALS patients (Massman, Sims, Cooke, Haverkamp, & Appel, 1996) and frontotemporal dementia develops in 3 to 5% of patients (Abrahams et al., 2004). Of individuals who develop dementia (ALS-FTD), cognitive and behavioral changes often predate the development of motor signs by 6 to 12 months (Bak & Hodges, 2001). Patients with ALS-FTD have a rapid course and typically die from respiratory failure within three years of symptom onset.

Changes in personality, character, social conduct, and executive function are typical of ALS-FTD and reflect dysfunction of the anterior cerebral cortex (Neary, Snowden, & Mann, 2000). Although ALS-FTD patients are reported to have memory impairment, hippocampal structures are relatively spared, and memory impairment is secondary to executive function deficits (Neary et al., 2000). Today there is substantial evidence of frontal lobe pathology from neuropathologic (Nagy, Kato, & Kushner, 1994), neuroimaging (Abe et al., 1993; Abrahams, Goldstein, Al-Chalabi, Pickering, & Passingham, 1997; Frank, Haas, Heinze, Stark, & Munte, 1997), and electrophysiologic studies (Munte, Troger, Nusser, Wieringa, Johannes, et al., 1998; Munte, Troger, Nusser, Wieringa, Matke, et al., 1998).

Effects of ALS-FTD on Language

The most frequently reported change in language in individuals with ALS-FTD is progressive reduction in verbal output progressing to mutism (van Bogaert, 1925; Ziegler, 1930). Other reported changes include perseveration, echolalia, and use of stereotypic expressions (Constantinidis, 1987; Meyer, 1929). Several reports exist of aphasia (Caselli et al., 1993; Mitsuyama, 1984; Tsuchiya et al., 2000) that can present early. Caselli et al. (1993) described seven patients in whom progressive nonfluent aphasia was the first symptom. Five ALS patients reported by Doran, Xuereb, and Hodges (1995) had a similar clinical profile. Bak and Hodges (2001) documented language dysfunction in the seven ALS-FTD cases in the Cambridge series. In every case, language dysfunction preceded motor symptoms and both production and comprehension were compromised. Several of the patients in the Cambridge series used nonverbal means of communicating indicating that reduction in verbal output was not the result of apathy. Other interesting observations made by Bak and Hodges were that verbs were affected more than nouns in both language production and comprehension. This greater vulnerability of verbs has also been noted in individuals with nonfluent PPA (Cappa et al., 1998; Hillis, Tiffiash, & Caramazza, 2002) and those with progressive supranuclear palsy (Daniele, Giustolisi, Silveri, Colosimo, & Gainotti, 1994). The finding of selective vulnerability of action words in ALS-FTD patients, who have severe motor dysfunction, is intriguing given the finding of a relation between verb processing and motor function in healthy adults (Pülvermuller, Härle, & Hummel, 2000; Pülvermuller, Lutzenberger, & Preiss, 1999). As yet, neuroscientists do not understand this finding but the relation of movement, language, and cognition is likely to be the focus of much future research.

Summary of Important Points

- The term frontotemporal dementia describes a clinical syndrome associated with various degenerative conditions. Those of particular interest to speech-language pathologists are Pick disease, primary progressive aphasia, semantic dementia, and amyotrophic lateral sclerosis.
- Pick disease is a rare disorder affecting women more than men that results from lobar atrophy of the frontal and temporal lobes. The disease typically manifests when individuals are in their 50s and lasts from 3 to 17 years.
- The cognitive changes of individuals with Pick disease reflect frontal lobe pathology and include deficits in social judgment, attention, difficulty shifting mental sets, and executive dysfunction.
- The communication disorder associated with Pick disease is characterized by decreased verbal output, nonfluency, poor articulation, verbal stereotypies, and echolalia.
- Memory is better preserved in individuals with Pick disease than those with Alzheimer's disease.
- The diagnosis of primary progressive aphasia (PPA) is made when individuals present with progressive aphasia without other cognitive or behavioral problems.
- The features of PPA vary; some patients are fluent, others are not.
- Individuals with nonfluent PPA exhibit anomia and effortful agrammatic speech that lacks function words. Comprehension is typically good. Late in the disease, affected individuals may be mute.
- Individuals with fluent PPA exhibit anomia and often have language comprehension deficits but their articulation is relatively normal as are speech rate and phrase length. With disease progression, comprehension worsens as do other language functions.
- Semantic dementia is an uncommon but distinctive syndrome in which individuals progressively lose their semantic (conceptual) knowledge.
- The language disorder associated with semantic dementia includes empty spontaneous speech, loss of word meaning, impaired naming and comprehension, and semantic paraphasias, but with preserved word repetition and ability to read aloud and write orthographically regular words.
- Amytrophic lateral sclerosis (ALS) is a progressive, adult-onset motor neuron disease characterized by loss of motor function and untimely death.
- Historically, ALS was thought to spare cognitive functions; however, research has shown that mild cognitive deficits are present in approximately one-third of patients, and dementia develops in 3 to 5% of cases.
- Language dysfunction may precede motor symptoms in ALS.
- The most common change in language function in ALS is progressive reduction in verbal output progressing to mutism. Verbs appear to be affected more than nouns, and perseveration, echolalia, and use of stereotypic expressions may also be present.

References

Abe, K., Fujimura, H., Toyooka, K., Hazama, T., Hirono, N., Yorifuji, S., et al. (1993). Single-photon emission computed tomographic investigation of patients with motor neuron disease. *Neurology, 43,* 1569–1573.

Abe, K., Ukita, H., & Yanagihara, T. (1997). Imaging in primary progressive aphasia. *Neuroradiology, 39*, 556–559.

Abrahams, S., Goldstein, L. H., Al-Chalabi, A., Pickering, A., & Passingham, R. E. (1997). Relation between cognitive dysfunction and pseudo-bulbar palsy in amyotrophic lateral sclerosis. *Journal of Neurology, Neurosurgery, and Psychiatry, 62*, 464–472.

Abrahams, S., Goldstein, L. H., Simmons, A., Brammer, M., Williams, S. C. R., Giampietro, V., et al. (2004). Word retrieval in amyotrophic lateral sclerosis: A functional magnetic resonance imaging study. *Brain, 127*, 1507–1517.

Alzheimer, A. (1911). Uber eigenartige Krankheitsfalle des spateren Alters. *Zeitschrift für die Gesamte Neurologie und Psychiatrie, 4*, 356–385.

Ames, D., Cummings, J. L., Wirshing, W. C., Quinn, B., & Mahler, M. (1994). Repetitive and compulsive behavior in frontal lobe degenerations. *Journal of Neuropsychiatry and Clinical Neuroscience, 6*, 100–113.

Bak, T. H., & Hodges, J. R. (2001). Motor neurone disease, dementia and aphasia: Coincidence, co-occurrence or continuum? *Journal of Neurology, 248*, 260–270.

Cappa, S. F., Binetti, G., Pezzini, A., Padovani, A., Rozzini, L., & Trabucchi, M. (1998). Object and action naming in Alzheimer's disease and frontotemporal dementia. *Neurology, 50*, 351–355.

Caselli, R. J., Windebank, A. J., Petersen, R. C., Komori, T., Parisi, J. E., Okazaki, H., et al. (1993). Rapidly progressive aphasic dementia and motor neuron disease. *Annals of Neurology, 33*, 200–207.

Clark, D. G., Charuvastra, A., Miller, B. L., Shapira, J. S., & Mendez, M. F. (2005). Fluent versus nonfluent primary progressive aphasia: A comparison of clinical and functional neuroimaging features. *Brain and Language, 94*, 54–60.

Constantinidis, J. (1987). Syndrome familial: Association de Maladie de Pick at sclérose latérale amyotrophique. *Éncephale, 13*, 285–298.

Cummings, J. L., & Benson, D. R. (1983). *Dementia: A clinical approach*. Boston: Butterworth.

Daniele, A., Giustolisi, L., Silveri, M. C., Colosimo, C., & Gainotti, G. (1994). Evidence for a possible neuroanatomical basis for lexical processing of nouns and verbs. *Neuropsychologia, 32*, 1325–1341.

Doran, M., Xuereb, J., & Hodges, J. R. (1995). Rapidly progressive aphasia with bulbar motor neurone disease: A clinical and neuropsychological study. *Behavioural Neurology, 8*, 169–180.

Elfgren, C., Passant, U., & Risberg, J. (1993). Neuropsychological findings in frontal lobe dementia. *Dementia, 4*, 214–219

Frank, B., Haas, J., Heinze, H. J., Stark, E., & Munte, T. F. (1997). Relation of neuropsychological and magnetic resonance findings in amyotrophic lateral sclerosis: Evidence for subgroups. *Clinical Neurology and Neurosurgery, 99*, 79–86.

Gans, A. (1922). Pick Betrachtungen über Art und Ausbreitung des krankhaften Prozesses in einem Fall von Pickscher Atrophie des Stirnhirns. *Zeitschrift für die Gesamte Neurologie und Psychiatrie, 80*, 10–28.

Garrard, P., & Hodges, J. R. (1999). Semantic dementia: Implications for the neural basis of language and meaning. *Aphasiology, 13*, 609–623.

Graham, N. L., Patterson, K., & Hodges, J. R. (2000). The impact of semantic memory impairment on spelling: Evidence from semantic dementia. *Neuropsychologia, 38*, 143–163.

Gregory, C. A., Serra-Mestres, J., & Hodges, J. R. (1999). Early diagnosis of the frontal variant of frontotemporal dementia: How sensitive are standard neuroimaging and neuropsychologic tests? *Neuropsychiatry, Neuropsychology, and Behavioral Neurology, 12*, 128–135.

Grossman, M. (2002). Progressive aphasic syndromes: Clinical and theoretical advances. *Current Opinion in Neurology, 15*, 409–413.

Gustafson, L., Brun, A., & Risberg, J. (1990). Frontal lobe dementia of the non-Alzheimer type. In R. J. Wurtman, S. Corkin, J. H. Growdon, & E. Ritter-Walker (Eds.), *Advances in Neurology: Alzheimer's disease* (Vol. 51, pp. 65–71). New York: Raven Press.

Hillis, A. E., Tiffiash, E., & Caramazza, A. (2002). Modality-specific deterioration in naming verbs in nonfluent primary progressive aphasia. *Journal of Cognitive Neuroscience, 14,* 1099–1108.

Hodges, J. R. (2001). Frontotemporal dementia (Pick's disease): Clinical features and assessment. *Neurology, 56*(Suppl 4), S6–S10.

Hodges, J. R., Patterson, K., Oxbury, S., & Funnell, E. (1992). Semantic dementia. Progressive fluent aphasia with temporal lobe atrophy. *Brain, 115,* 1783–1806.

Hodges, J. R., Patterson, K., Ward, R., Garrard, P., Bak, T., Perry, R., et al. (1999). The differentiation of semantic dementia and frontal lobe dementia (temporal and frontal variants of frontotemporal dementia) from early Alzheimer's disease: A comparative neuropsychological study. *Neuropsychology, 13,* 31–40.

Holland, A. L., McBurney, D. H., Moossy, J., & Reinmuth, O. M. (1985). The dissolution of language in Pick's disease with neurofibrillary tangles: A case study. *Brain and Language, 24,* 36–58.

Howard, D., & Patterson, K. (1992). *Pyramids and Palm Trees: A test of semantic access from pictures and words.* Bury St. Edmunds, UK: Thames Valley.

Jeffries, E., Lambon Ralph, M. A., Jones, R., Bateman, D., & Patterson, K. (2004). Surface dyslexia in semantic dementia: A comparison of the influence of consistency and regularity. *Neurocase, 10,* 290–299.

Karbe, H., Kertesz, A., & Polk, M. (1993). Profiles of language impairment in primary progressive aphasia. *Archives of Neurology, 50,* 193–201.

Kertesz, A., Davidson, W., McCabe, P., Takagi, K., & Munoz, D. (2003). Primary progressive aphasia: Diagnosis, varieties, evolution. *Journal of the International Neuropsychological Society, 9,* 710–719.

Kirshner H. S., Tanridag, O., Thurman L., & Whetsell, W. O. Jr. (1987). Progressive aphasia without dementia: Two cases with focal spongiform degeneration. *Annals of Neurology, 22,* 527–532.

Lowenberg, K., Boyd, D. A., & Salon, D. D. (1939). Occurrence of Pick's disease in early adult years. *Archives of Neurology and Psychiatry, 41,* 1004–1020.

Macoir, J., & Bernier, J. (2002). Is surface dysgraphia tied to semantic impairment? Evidence from a case of semantic dementia. *Brain and Cognition, 48,* 452–457.

Massman, P. J., Sims, J., Cooke, N., Haverkamp, L. J., & Appel, V. (1996). Prevalence and correlates of neuropsychological deficits in amyotrophic lateral sclerosis. *Journal of Neurology, Neurosurgery and Psychiatry, 61,* 450–455.

McKhann, G. M., Albert, M. S., Grossman, M., Miller, B., Dickson, D., & Trojanowski, J. Q. (2001). Clinical and pathological diagnosis of frontotemporal dementia. *Archives of Neurology, 58,* 1803–1809.

Mendez, M. F., Selwood, A., Mastri, A. R., & Frey, W. H. (1993). Pick's disease versus Alzheimer's disease: A comparison of clinical characteristics. *Neurology, 43,* 280–292.

Mesulam, M. M. (1982). Slowly progressive aphasia without dementia. *Annals of Neurology, 11,* 592–598.

Mesulam, M. M. (1987). Primary progressive aphasia—differentiation from Alzheimer's disease. *Annals of Neurology, 22,* 522–524.

Mesulam, M. M. (2001). Primary progressive aphasia. *Annals of Neurology, 49,* 425–432.

Mesulam, M. M., Grossman, M., Hillis, A., Kertesz, A., & Weintraub, S. (2003). The core and halo of primary progressive aphasia and semantic dementia. *Annals of Neurology, 54*(Suppl 5), S11–S14.

Meyer, A. (1929). Uber eine der amyotrophischen Lateralsklerose nahestehende Erkrankung mit psychischen Storungen. Zugleich ein Beitrag zur Frage der spastischen pseudosklerose (A. Jakob). *Zeitschrift für die Gesamte Neurologie und Psychiatrie, 121,* 107–128.

Mitsuyama, Y. (1984). Presenile dementia with motor neuron disease in Japan: Clinico-pathological review of 26 cases. *Journal of Neurology, Neurosurgery & Psychiatry, 47,* 953–959.

Mummery, C. J., Hodges, J. R., Patterson, K., & Price, C. J. (1999). Functional neuroanatomy of the semantic system—divisible by what? *Journal of Cognitive Neuroscience, 10,* 766–777.

Munte, T. F., Troger, M., Nusser, I., Wieringa, B. M., Johannes, S., Matzke, M., et al. (1998). Alterations of early components of the visual evoked potential in amyotrophic lateral sclerosis. *Journal of Neurology, 245,* 206–210.

Munte, T. F., Troger, M., Nusser, I., Wieringa, B. M., Matzke, M., Johannes, S., et al. (1998). Recognition memory deficits in amyotrophic lateral sclerosis assessed with event-related brain potentials. *Acta Neurologica Scandinavia, 98,* 110–115.

Nagy, D., Kato, T., & Kushner, P. D. (1994). Reactive astrocytes are wide spread in the cortical gray matter of amyotrophic lateral sclerosis. *Journal of Neuroscience Research, 38,* 336–347.

Neary, D., Snowden, J. S., Gustafson, L., Passant, U., Stuss, D., Black, S., et al. (1998). Frontotemporal lobar degeneration: A consensus on clinical diagnostic criteria. *Neurology, 51,* 1546–1554.

Neary, D., Snowden, J. S., & Mann, D. M. A. (2000). Cognitive change in motor neurone disease/amyotrophic lateral sclerosis. *Journal of the Neurological Sciences, 180,* 15–20.

Palmieri, R. L. (2005). Take aim at amyotrophic lateral sclerosis. *Nursing, 35,* 32.

Pick, A. (1901). Senile hirnatrophie als grundlage für hernderscheinungen. *Wiener Klinische Wochenschrift, 14,* 403–404.

Pick, A. (1904). Zur symptomatologie der links-seitigen. Schlafenlappenatrophie. *Monatschrift für Psychiatrie und Neurologie, 16,* 378–388.

Pick, A. (1906). Uber einen weiteren symptomen-komplex in rahmen der dementia senilis, bedingt durch umschriebene starkere hirnatrophie (gemischte apraxie). *Monatsschrift für Psychiatrie und Neurologie, 19,* 97–108.

Pülvermuller, F., Härle, M. & Hummel, F. (2000). Neurophysiological distinction of verb categories. *NeuroReport, 11,* 2789–2793.

Pülvermuller, F., Lutzenberger, W., & Preiss, H. (1999). Nouns and verbs in the intact brain: Evidence from event-related potentials and high-frequency cortical responses. *Cerebral Cortex, 9,* 497–506.

Rahman, S., Sahakian, B. J., Hodges, J. R., Rogers, R. D., & Robbins, T. W. (1999). Specific cognitive deficits in mild frontal variant frontotemporal dementia. *Brain, 122,* 1469–1493.

Rascovsky, K., Salmon, D. P., Ho, G. J., Galasko, D., Peavy, G. M., Hansen, L. A., et al. (2002). Cognitive profiles differ in autopsy-confirmed

frontotemporal dementia and AD. *Neurology, 58,* 1801–1808.

Rosser, A., & Hodges, J. R. (1994). Initial letter and semantic category fluency in Alzheimer's disease, Huntington's disease, and progressive supranuclear palsy. *Journal of Neurology, Neurosurgery and Psychiatry, 57,* 1389–1394.

Siri, S., Benaglio, I., Frigerio, A., Binetti, G., & Cappa, S. F. (2001). A brief neuropsychological assessment for the differential diagnosis between frontotemporal dementia and Alzheimer's disease. *European Journal of Neurology, 8,* 125–132.

Snowden, J. S. (2005). Semantic dementia. In A. Burns, J. O'Brien & D. Ames (Eds.), *Dementia* (3rd ed., pp. 702–712). London: Hodder Arnold.

Snowden, J. S., Goulding, P. J., & Neary, D. (1989). Semantic dementia: A form of circumscribed cerebral atrophy. *Behavioural Neurology, 2,* 167–182.

Snowden, J. S., & Neary, D. (1993). Progressive language dysfunction and lobar atrophy. *Dementia, 4,* 226–231.

Strong, M. J. (1995, September). ALS: Update on a tragic illness. *Medicine in North America,* pp. 780–788.

Strong, M. J., Grace, G. M., Orange, J. B., & Leeper, H. A. (1996). Cognition, language, and speech in amyotrophic lateral sclerosis: A review. *Journal of Clinical and Experimental Neuropsychology, 18,* 291–303.

Tsuchiya, K., Ozawa, E., Fukushima, J., Yasui, H., Kondo, H., Nakano, I., et al. (2000). Rapidly progressive aphasia and motor neuron disease: A clinical, radiological and pathological study of an autopsy case with circumscribed lobar atrophy. *Acta Neuropathologica, 99,* 81–87.

Turner, R. S., Kenyon, L. C., Trojanowski, J. Q., Gonatas, N., & Grossman, M. (1996). Clinical, neuroimaging, and pathologic features of progressive nonfluent aphasia. *Annals of Neurology, 39,* 166–173.

van Bogaert, L. (1925). Les troubles mentaux dans la sclérose latérale amyotrophique. *Éncephale, 20,* 27.

Warren, J. D., Harvey, R. J., & Rossor, M. N. (2005). Progressive aphasia and other focal syndromes. In A. Burns, J. O'Brien, & D. Ames

(Eds.), *Dementia* (3rd ed., pp. 720–728). London: Hodder Arnold.

Warrington, E. K. (1975). Selective impairment of semantic memory. *Quarterly Journal of Experimental Psychology, 27,* 635–657.

Weintraub, S., & Mesulam, M. (1993). Four neuropsychological profiles in dementia. In F.

Boller & J. Grafman (Eds.), *Handbook of Neuropsychology* (Vol. 8, pp. 253–281). Amsterdam: Elsevier.

Ziegler, L. H. (1930). Psychotic and emotional phenomena associated with amyotrophic lateral sclerosis. *Archives of Neurology and Psychiatry, 24,* 930–936.

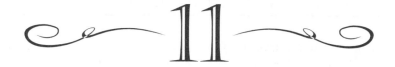

Assessment of Cognitive-Communication Disorders of Dementia

Assessment of cognitive function is critical to the diagnosis of dementia because *by definition*, dementia comprises multiple cognitive deficits. Early evaluation of individuals suspected of having dementia is important because 10 to 15% of cases are due to treatable causes (Clarfield, 1988; Larson, Reifler, Sumi, Canfield, & Chinn, 1986). Then, too, the advent of drugs that slow progression of some irreversible dementing diseases makes early detection vital. In this chapter three major topics are addressed: the process of assessment; tests for screening and comprehensive assessment of cognitive-communicative function; and differential diagnosis.

The Process of Assessment

Assessment of cognitive-communicative function serves many purposes (Tomoeda, 2001):

■ Detection of dementia
■ Identification of cognitive-communicative deficits
■ Identification of retained abilities

■ Establishment of a baseline of cognitive-communicative functioning for planning intervention and measuring response to treatment
■ Counseling caregivers
■ Predicting skills vulnerable to future decline

To ethically fulfill any of these purposes, clinicians must obtain valid and reliable information about the cognitive-communicative abilities of their clients. This is especially challenging in elders because normal nervous system aging and sensory losses affect cognition and communicative function. In addition to visual and auditory deficits, elders are slower at processing information. Thus, differentiating the older individual, who is highly intelligent, well-educated, and in the early stages of dementia, from a less intelligent, less-educated neurologically normal elder requires clinical expertise. Indeed, the presence of dementia cannot be determined by neuropsychological and cognitive communication testing alone, and laboratory tests should be administered to identify conditions that may account for a decline in cognitive function. By understanding the effects of the client's medical history, the skilled clinician contributes to the management of the client by providing appropriate assessment and interpretation of results that lead to the implementation of an effective care plan. The following principles will help clinicians control for sensory loss and other age-related conditions that can affect neuropsychological functioning and lead to inaccurate conclusions about mental status and functional abilities.

Prior to Testing

Review the Patient's Chart

Note whether the patient's medical history contains information about sensory impairment and other factors that can alter cognitive function (i.e., depression, drug effects). Is there evidence of more than one neurologic problem? Individuals with AD frequently have vascular disease and those with vascular disease often have AD. Are the symptoms variable? Variability in mental status is characteristic of individuals with Lewy body dementia.

If the client has previously been diagnosed with dementia, severity may be noted in the medical record. Clinicians should be familiar with the following commonly used rating scales for quantifying dementia severity.

Global Deterioration Scale (GDS) (Reisberg, Ferris, de Leon, & Crook, 1982). The GDS defines seven stages in the course of dementia with well-specified observational criteria. GDS stage 1 represents "normal" aging with no cognitive decline and GDS stage 7 represents "late dementia" and very severe cognitive decline.

Functional Assessment Stages (FAST) (Reisberg et al., 1984). The FAST is an exten-

sion of the GDS. It was developed to better elaborate functional changes in continence, affect, ambulation, and language in late-stage dementia (stages 6 and 7) in the order they typically appear.

Clinical Dementia Rating Scale (CDR) (Hughes et al., 1982). The CDR provides a rating of global cognitive function based on clinical information about: memory, orientation, judgment, problem-solving, community affairs, home and hobbies, and personal care. Impairment is rated as none (0), questionable (0.5), mild (1), moderate (2), or severe (3).

Dementia Rating Scale (DRS) (Mattis, 1976). The DRS is composed of items that evaluate five cognitive functions: attention, initiation and perseveration, construction, conceptualization, and memory. A maximum of 144 points can be awarded, and normal elders score 140 points or better.

Blessed Dementia Scale (BDS) (Blessed, Tomlinson, & Roth, 1968). The BDS is a short behavioral checklist that includes 22 items related to changes in cognitive function, everyday activities, habits, personality, interests, and drives. Items are rated from information provided by a caregiver. A score of 28 indicates extreme incapacity; scores of 4 or less indicate preserved capacity.

In Table 11–1 are scores associated with mild, moderate, and severe stages of dementia on three commonly used measures of dementia severity.

Arrange for a Good Test Environment

Testing should be conducted in a quiet room with adequate lighting. Be sure to light test materials in a way that prevents the presence of shadows, and remember that elders need two to three times more illumination than young adults. Avoid sitting with your

Table 11-1. Scores/Ratings on Three Commonly Used Measures of Dementia Severity Corresponding to Mild, Moderate, and Severe Dementia

	Mild	Moderate	Severe
Global Deterioration Scale Rating	3 or 4	5 or 6	7
Clinical Dementia Rating	CDR 1	CDR 2	CDR 3
Mattis Dementia Rating Scale	120–130	90–120	<90

back to a bright light or window which can make your facial features hard to perceive. Test stimuli should be printed in a font size that is readily perceptible. Black print on a white background is the easiest for elders to see.

During Testing

Check the Integrity of Vision

Most elders need glasses to read; be sure they are wearing them during assessment. When the patient's vision status is unknown, a standard eye chart can be used to screen for a visual deficit or you can ask the patient to read simple words or sentences in a print size smaller than test stimuli. If the patient can read text in the smaller print, the examiner can be assured that the patient has adequate visual acuity to see the printed test materials.

Check the Patient's Hearing

Hearing impairment is the most prevalent disability of older Americans (Ries, 1994). Check whether the examinee wears a hearing aid, and if so, make sure the aid is worn during testing. If a full audiometric evaluation cannot be obtained, a simple speech discrimination test can be given to ensure that the examinee can hear the clinician's voice in the test environment. Have the client repeat

words that sound similar (like "cake" and "take") to determine if they discriminate subtle differences. An example of this type of speech discrimination task can be found in the Arizona Battery for Communication Disorders of Dementia (ABCD) (Bayles & Tomoeda, 1993). Clients should be able to repeat words spoken by the examiner in the test environment with 85% or better accuracy.

Check Literacy

If a caregiver is unavailable to provide information about a patient's prior reading ability, check for literacy by having the examinee read two or three simple sentences. Generally, even individuals with moderately severe dementia are able to read aloud if they were literate prior to the onset of dementia.

Take Steps to Reduce Test-Taking Anxiety

Spend time at the beginning of the test session visiting with the examinee and describe what will occur during the session. Position score sheets so the client cannot see you record responses. When examinees ask about their performance, tell them the testing is going well. Do not tell examinees during testing if their responses are correct. Some patients become anxious about where their spouse or family member is during testing. Give assurance that the caregiver is nearby. If an examinee will not participate in the evaluation without the caregiver being in the room, advise the caregiver to offer encouragement but refrain from giving cues.

Be Alert to Depression

Depression is common in older adults and can negatively affect test performance. In fact, its effects can mimic dementia. Historically, the term "pseudodementia" was used to designate a dementia-like performance in a cognitively intact but depressed individual (Kiloh, 1961). However, in recent years the term has fallen out of favor (Alexopoulos, 2003; Dobie, 2002; Emery & Oxman, 2003) because research has shown that depression is a frequent early sign of dementing disease (Alexopoulos, Young, & Meyers, 1993; Kral & Emery, 1989; Shanmugham & Alexopoulos, 2005).

Individuals who are depressed generally convey a sense of distress or despair. Often they make self-deprecatory comments. Some are not interested in the testing and its outcome. A subsequent section of this chapter is devoted to differentiating mild AD from delirium and depression. Table 11–2 contains brief descriptions of tests that can be used to screen for depression in the elderly.

Be Alert to Drug Effects on Performance

Most elders take several medications to manage age-associated chronic disease (Lamy, 1986). In hospitals and long-term care settings, older patients average five to twelve daily medications (Kalchthaler, Coccaro, & Lichtige, 1977; Salzman, 1979). In Clarfield's (1988) review of 32 studies, in which the prevalence of different causes of dementia was examined, a common cause of reversible dementia was drug side effects. Many medications affect mental status or interact with other drugs to diminish cognitive function-

ing. Clinicians should check whether the examinee is taking medications and review their effects on cognitive and communicative functioning.

Orange (2001) listed classes of drugs that commonly interfere with speech, language, and cognition in persons with dementia. They include sedatives, antidepressants, anxiolytics (antianxiety drugs), antipsychotics, anticoagulants, antihypertensives, and narcotic-based analgesics. Massey (2005) cautioned that long-term use of benzodiazepines can interfere with the ability to learn, and long-term use of anticholinergic medications (Artane, Cogentin, atropine) and antihistamines (Benedryl, Dimetapp, Chlortrimeton) can contribute to confusion. Mental status changes also occur with medications for incontinence (Detrol, Ditropan), motility (Levsin, Bentyl), and pain.

Screening and Comprehensive Assessment

Clinicians should select assessment tools that have been normed on elders and individuals with dementia. If a test has been normed only on young adults, the performance of a normal elder may be mistaken for early dementia because of the effect of aging on cognition.

We have found, and others have confirmed (Locascio, Growdon, & Corkin, 1995), that measures suitable for early detection of dementia are generally ill-suited for documenting abilities over the course of the disease. By the moderate stage, patients struggle to perform these tests and floor effects develop in performance. Measures that are appropriate for characterizing cognition in the later stages of dementia are insensitive to the subtle early changes that characterize the preclinical or mild stages of cognitive decline.

Table 11–2. Tests That Can Be Used to Screen for Depression in the Elderly

Name of Measure	Citation	Description
Hamilton Rating Scale for Depression (HRS-D)	Hamilton, 1967; Hamilton, 1970	The HRS-D is one of the first developed and best known interview-based rating scales for depression. It is a 17-item inventory of symptoms that are rated for severity by an experienced clinician, based upon interview and other available data.
Beck Depression Inventory (BDI)	Beck et al., 1961	The BDI is a 21-item inventory of depressive symptoms and attitudes that are rated from 0 to 3 in terms of intensity. The BDI is commonly used as a self-administered measure, although it was originally designed to be administered by trained interviewers.
Zung Self-Rating Depression Scales (SDS)	Zung, 1965	The SDS comprises 20 items that evaluate four areas of disturbance: pervasive psychic, physiologic, psychomotor, and psychological. The patient rates the applicability, within the past week, of each item according to the following terms: "none or a little of the time," "some of the time," "good part of the time," and "most or all of the time."
Zung Depression Status Inventory (DSI)	Zung, 1972	The 20 items of the DSI correspond to the SDS, however, the interviewer rates the severity of symptoms or signs on a four-point scale from none to severe based on the results of a clinical interview.
Dementia Mood Assessment Scale	Sunderland et al., 1988	This two-part instrument is designed to measure the severity of mood disturbance of demented patients based on direct observation and a semistructured interview by health professionals. The first 17 items evaluate mood and are scaled from 0 (within normal limits) to 6 (most severe). The remaining seven items measure the patient's functional capacities.
Cornell Scale for Depression in Dementia	Alexopoulus, Abrams, Young, & Shamoian, 1988	The Cornell Scale is a 19-item clinician administered instrument that uses information obtained from interviews with the patient and a member of the nursing staff. This instrument was specifically designed for measuring depression in demented patients.

<table>
<tr><td>

Definitions

Ceiling effect—the failure of a test to identify the highest performance of the most competent because of a limited number of difficult test items.

Floor effect—the failure of a test to identify the lowest possible performance because of a limited number of easy or simple test items.

</td></tr>
</table>

That is, these tests are too easy for early stage patients, resulting in a ceiling effect. It is the clinician's responsibility to have measures in their clinical armamentarium that are sensitive to early dementia and others that will characterize changes in function across the disease course.

Screening for Dementia

The purpose of screening is the identification of individuals with cognitive deficits greater than those associated with normal aging in a time-efficient way. Individuals who fail the screening test should be given in-depth evaluation. SLPs are not qualified to diagnose dementia and should refer individuals who fail a screening test to a physician for further evaluation. Two kinds of measures are routinely used to screen for dementia: mental status and episodic memory tests.

Mental Status Tests

Mini-Mental State Examination (MMSE) (Folstein, Folstein, & McHugh, 1975). The MMSE is popular worldwide and evaluates orientation to person, place, and time, general knowledge, memory, communication, and copying. The MMSE requires 5 to 10 minutes to administer. The total possible score is 30. Most clinicians consider a score less than 24 as indicative of dementia (Desmond, 2002); however, based on results of our longitudinal studies, we suspect early dementia in literate people with scores of 25 to 26 (Bayles, Tomoeda, Montgomery, Cruz, & Azuma, 2000). Similarly, Monsch et al. (1995) recommended that an MMSE score of less than 26 be used to indicate impairment. Comprehensive reviews of the psychometric properties and uses of the MMSE can be found in Tombaugh and McIntyre (1992) and Lezak, Howieson, and Loring (2004).

Short Portable Mental Status Questionnaire (SPMQ) (Pfeiffer, 1975). This 10-item measure assesses a patient's knowledge of personal and general information including orientation to time and place, age, date of birth, mother's maiden name, telephone number, address, current and previous U.S. Presidents, and serial subtraction ability. Pfeiffer (1975) provided the following scoring criteria:

0 to 2 errors—intact intellectual functioning

3 to 4 errors—mild intellectual impairment

5 to 7 errors—moderate intellectual impairment

8 to 10 errors—severe intellectual impairment.

The SPMQ has been widely used in epidemiologic studies, and a cutoff score of three errors provided high sensitivity and specificity in screening for moderate to severe dementia in community- and hospital-based populations (Erkinjuntti, Sulkava, Wikström, & Autio, 1987).

> ### Definitions
>
> **Test sensitivity**—the ability of the test to identify people with a certain trait
>
> **Test specificity**—the ability of the test to identify people without the trait

Alzheimer Disease Assessment Scale (ADAS) (Rosen, Moh, & Davis, 1984, 1986). The ADAS is primarily used by researchers for detecting small cognitive and behavioral changes in AD patients (Weiner, 2003). It is a 21-item scale that combines a mental status or cognitive portion (items 1–11) with a behavior rating or noncognitive portion (items 12–21). The cognitive portion, sometimes referred to as the ADAS-COG, consists of measures of:

word recall

spoken language

language comprehension

test instruction recall

word finding

following commands

naming

figure construction

ideational praxis

orientation

word recognition

Examples of noncognitive behaviors are tremor, tearfulness, depressed mood, and hallucinations. Most items are rated on a scale of 0 to 5, with higher scores indicating greater severity of dysfunction. The test takes approximately 45 minutes to administer and must be given by a professional trained in its administration (Weiner, 2003). Information about the psychometric properties of the ADAS and ADAS-COG can be found in Lezak et al. (2004).

Mental Status Subtest of the ABCD (Bayles & Tomoeda, 1993). The simple and reliable mental status subtest of the ABCD is increasingly being used, especially by speech-language pathologists. The subtest's 13 items evaluate orientation to time, place, person, and general knowledge. It takes less than 5 minutes to give and requires no special training. The maximum score possible is 13. In the ABCD standardization study only 5% of the normal elderly had a score below 11.5; mild AD patients averaged 9.9 and moderate AD patients averaged 4.5.

Episodic Memory Tests

Measures of Learning and Delayed Recall. Because the primary feature of Alzheimer's dementia is memory impairment, it is unsurprising that the best measures for screening for Alzheimer's dementia are tests of episodic memory (Rentz & Weintraub, 2000). Reports from studies involving individuals in the preclinical phase of AD indicate that *initial learning of information and loss of information over a delay* interval are the key characteristics that discriminate between nondemented elders and those with the earliest signs of AD (Grober & Kawas, 1996; Locascio et al., 1995; Robinson-Whelen & Storandt, 1992; Rubin et al., 1998; Welsh, Buttters, Hughes, Mohs, & Heyman, 1991). Examples of tests routinely used to measure a patient's ability to learn and recall information after a delay include: the Logical Memory subtest (basically a story recall task) of the Wechsler Memory Scale—Third Edition (Wechsler, 1999) and the Buschke Selective Reminding

Test (Buschke & Fuld, 1974) which requires learning, storing, and retrieving information after a delay via free- and cued-recall and recognition. Measures similar to these can be found in the Arizona Battery for Communication Disorders of Dementia (ABCD) (Bayles & Tomoeda, 1993), specifically, the Story Retelling (Immediate and Delayed) and Word Learning subtests. Only one of these measures need be used for screening and the shorter test is Story-Retelling (Immediate and Delayed).

The 7-Minute Screen. Solomon and colleagues (1998) selected four tests with previously demonstrated sensitivity to AD and called the measure "The 7-Minute Screen" because it reportedly took research subjects an average of 7 minutes to complete it. Additional criteria for selecting these tests were that they are easy to administer and score. The 7-Minute Screen consists of (1) Enhanced Cued Recall, (2) Category Fluency, (3) Benton Temporal Orientation Test (Benton, 1983), and (4) Clock Drawing. It had high sensitivity (92%) and specificity (96%) for identifying individuals with AD in a population of patients referred to a memory disorders clinic and community-dwelling volunteer controls (Solomon et al., 1998).

Comprehensive Evaluation of Cognitive-Communicative Functioning

The comprehensive evaluation of cognitive-communicative functioning is an essential part of the information gathering process that is requisite to good patient care. Comprehensive evaluation of individuals with dementia should provide information about the patient's mental status, verbal memory, and basic skills of language comprehension and production.

Tests used to measure these constructs should be standardized on individuals with dementia for whom etiology and severity are specified and controlled. The Arizona Battery for Communication Disorders of Dementia (ABCD) (Bayles & Tomoeda, 1993) designed for mild and moderate patients, and the Functional Linguistic Communication Inventory (FLCI) (Bayles & Tomoeda, 1994), designed for severely demented patients, are standardized batteries that provide information about cognitive-communicative functioning. However, many other tests are available from which a clinician can fashion a test battery. The Wechsler Memory Scale—Third Edition (WMS-III) (Wechsler, 1999) is widely used to evaluate memory as is the Rivermead Behavioral Memory Test—Second Edition (Wilson, Cockburn, & Baddeley, 1991). The Block Design and Similarities subtests from the Wechsler Adult Intelligence Scale—Revised (WAIS-R; Wechsler, 1981) have been shown to be sensitive to early dementia and are measures of visual spatial processing and verbal associative reasoning, respectively.

As described in earlier chapters, individuals with different dementia etiologies may present with impairment in executive functioning making it important to be familiar with neuropsychological tests of executive functions (see Tingus, McPherson, & Cummings [2002] for an overview of assessment of executive function). The Wisconsin Card Sorting Test (Heaton, 1981; Heaton, Chelune, Talley, Kay, & Curtiss, 1993) is a widely used nonverbal test of attention and set shifting that has been administered to individuals with dementia. Other tests of executive function that an SLP might administer include the Controlled Oral Word Association Test (Benton & Hamsher, 1989) in which patients generate as many words as possible within a minute that begin with the letters F, A, and S; the Digit Span subtest of the Wechsler Adult Intelligence Scale—Third Edition

(WAIS-III) (Wechsler, 1997) and WMS-III (Wechsler, 1999) in which individuals must recall number strings of increasing length; and the California Verbal Learning Test (CLVT) (Delis, Kramer, Kaplan, & Ober, 2000). The CVLT is a standardized memory test that assesses rate of word learning, retention after short- and long-delay intervals, semantic encoding ability, recognition memory, intrusion and perseverative errors, and response biases.

Whereas many fine aphasia test batteries exist, they were not designed for individuals with dementia. Most are too easy for mildly and moderately demented Alzheimer's and Parkinson's patients and lack subtests of verbal episodic memory and mental status, important in differential diagnosis. For individuals with frontotemporal and vascular disease, aphasia batteries can be appropriate but still need to be paired with tests of memory, mental status, and executive function to track the emergence and course of dementia. Further, Kertesz, Davidson, McCabe, and Munoz (2003) report that behavioral quantitation is particularly sensitive to frontotemporal dementia.

Arizona Battery for Communication Disorders of Dementia (ABCD)

The ABCD (Bayles & Tomoeda, 1993) consists of 14 subtests (Table 11–3) that evaluate mental status, verbal memory, and the basic skills of language comprehension and production in addition to visuospatial skill. The ABCD also contains four screening measures to help clinicians identify problems that can invalidate test results including: Speech Discrimination, Visual Perception and Literacy, Visual Field, and Visual Agnosia.

Standardization of the ABCD. The ABCD was standardized on individuals with AD, Parkinson's disease, and young and older

Table 11–3. The Constructs and Subtests of the Arizona Battery for Communication Disorders of Dementia (Bayles & Tomoeda, 1993)

CONSTRUCT 1: LINGUISTIC COMPREHENSION
Subtests:
Following Commands
Comparative Questions
Repetition
Reading Comprehension

CONSTRUCT 2: LINGUISTIC EXPRESSION
Subtests:
Object Description
Generative Naming
Confrontation Naming
Concept Definition

CONSTRUCT 3: VERBAL MEMORY
Subtests:
Story Retelling—Immediate
Story Retelling—Delayed
Word Learning

CONSTRUCT 4: VISUOSPATIAL SKILL
Subtests:
Generative Drawing
Figure Copying

CONSTRUCT 5: MENTAL STATUS
Subtest:
Mental Status

nondemented community-dwelling individuals. It has also been given to individuals with multiple sclerosis (Wallace & Holmes, 1993) and to individuals with Down syndrome with and without dementia (Moss, Tomoeda, &

Bayles, 2000). The ABCD was modified for individuals in the United Kingdom (Armstrong, Borthwick, Bayles, & Tomoeda, 1996), Australia (Moorhouse, Douglas, Panaccio, & Steel, 1999), and The Netherlands.

ABCD subtests can be used individually or the full battery can be given. When all 14 subtests are administered, four types of scores are obtained: raw, summary, construct, and a total overall (Table 11–4). The full ABCD typically requires 60 to 90 minutes to complete.

Reliability of the ABCD. In the ABCD manual are data demonstrating high test-retest reliability of the battery and good internal consistency of subtests. Reliability of subtest scoring (interrater agreement) was also high and ranged from 93 to 100%.

Validity of the ABCD. Criterion validity was determined in the standardization study through correlation with three well-known measures of dementia severity: the Global Deterioration Scale (Reisberg et al., 1982), the Mini-Mental State Examination (Folstein et al., 1975), and the Block Design subtest

Table 11–4. Four Types of Scores Available from the ABCD and Their Uses

RAW:	Scores on the individual subtests.
SUMMARY:	Standardized scores that permit performance comparisons between subtests.
CONSTRUCT:	Standardized scores that permit interconstruct performance comparisons.
TOTAL:	One score that represents performance on the whole test.

of the Wechsler Adult Intelligence Scale-Revised (WAIS-R; Wechsler, 1981). Correlations between these three measures and ABCD subtests were high, ranging from .62 to .85 (Bayles & Tomoeda, 1993).

In a later, post-standardization study, Bayles, Tomoeda, Wood, Cruz, and McGeagh (1996) compared the ABCD to five measures known to be sensitive to dementia to determine which was the best for discriminating individuals with early AD from normal elders: the Block Design subtest of the WAIS-R (Wechsler, 1981), the Modified Wisconsin Card Sorting Test (Hart, Kwentus, Wade, & Taylor, 1988; Jenkins & Parsons, 1978), a test of verbal fluency (Bayles, Trosset, Tomoeda, Montgomery, & Wilson, 1993), a verbal picture description test (Tomoeda & Bayles, 1993), and the MMSE (Folstein et al., 1975). The ABCD was the best measure for discriminating early dementia and for distinguishing mild from moderate Alzheimer's dementia.

ABCD Subtests Most Sensitive to AD. Of the 14 ABCD subtests, Story Retelling—Delayed and Word Learning were those most sensitive to AD and thus are the best for screening individuals at risk for dementing diseases. As can be seen by comparing scores in Table 11–5, the disparity in performance between normal elders and AD patients is greatest on these measures. The shorter of these subtests is Story Retelling making it more appropriate for screening. Individuals are told a short story and asked to retell it immediately after hearing it and again after a short delay. It is quick to administer and score.

Performance of *Mild* AD Patients on ABCD. The average performance of mild AD patients (mean age = 76.74) on ABCD subtests is charted in Table 11–5 and can be compared to the performance of normal elders (mean age = 70.44) and young normals (mean age = 20.29).

Table 11–5. Means (M) for RAW, SUMMARY, CONSTRUCT, and TOTAL OVERALL Scores of Young and Old Normal Control (NC) and Mild and Moderate (Mod) Alzheimer's Disease (AD) Subjects

	Sign. Diff. p<.05	Young NC *M*	Old NC *M*	Mild AD *M*	Mod AD *M*
Raw Scores					
Mental Status	2, 3	12.9	12.8	9.9	4.5
Story Retelling—Immediate	2, 3	14.9	14.0	7.3	2.6
Following Commands	1, 2, 3	9.0	8.8	8.3	6.1
Comparative Questions	3	5.9	5.9	5.7	4.6
Word Learning—Free Recall	1, 2, 3	10.4	7.6	2.3	0.8
Word Learning—Total Recall	1, 2, 3	15.7	15.1	7.7	3.3
Word Learning—Recognition	1, 2, 3	47.8	46.6	36.3	30.0
Repetition	1, 2, 3	73.7	67.9	59.2	36.8
Object Description	1, 2, 3	10.9	9.1	6.6	3.4
Reading Comp.—Word	3	8.0	7.9	7.7	5.6
Reading Comp.—Sentences	1, 2, 3	6.9	6.4	6.0	3.6
Generative Naming	1, 2, 3	13.4	11.4	7.1	3.1
Confrontation Naming	2, 3	18.6	18.1	15.5	8.8
Concept Definition	2, 3	57.8	56.60	41.20	10.00
Generative Drawing	1, 2, 3	13.9	12.4	10.7	5.2
Figure Copying	1, 3	11.8	11.4	11.1	6.7
Story Retelling—Delayed	1, 2, 3	14.9	12.4	1.0	0.0
Summary Scores					
Mental Status	2, 3	4.93	4.80	3.36	2.15
Story Retelling—Immediate	1, 2, 3	4.73	4.50	3.32	2.22
Following Commands	1, 2, 3	5.00	4.84	4.32	2.96
Comparative Questions	2, 3	4.73	4.84	4.44	3.00
Word Learning—Free Recall	1, 2, 3	4.97	4.41	2.98	2.42
Word Learning—Total Recall	1, 2, 3	4.77	4.42	2.98	2.24
Word Learning—Recognition	1, 2, 3	4.93	4.65	3.10	2.73
Repetition	1, 2, 3	4.93	4.50	3.80	2.55
Object Description	1, 2, 3	4.90	4.50	3.76	2.53
Reading Comp.—Word	1, 2, 3	5.00	4.84	4.51	2.86
Reading Comp.—Sentences	1, 2, 3	4.90	4.45	4.02	2.62
Generative Naming	1, 2, 3	4.83	4.42	3.54	2.27

continues

Table 11–5. *continued*

	Sign. Diff. p<.05	Young NC M	Old NC M	Mild AD M	Mod AD M
Confrontation Naming	2, 3	4.60	4.48	3.76	2.40
Concept Definition	2, 3	4.60	4.48	3.35	1.83
Generative Drawing	1, 2, 3	4.97	4.55	4.02	2.44
Figure Copying	1, 3	4.87	4.55	4.46	2.89
Story Retelling—Delayed	1, 2, 3	4.83	4.46	3.17	3.00
Construct Scores					
Mental Status	2, 3	4.93	4.80	3.36	2.15
Episodic Memory	1, 2, 3	4.85	4.48	3.11	2.52
Linguistic Expression	2, 3	4.73	4.66	3.48	1.88
Linguistic Comprehension	1, 2, 3	4.91	4.69	4.22	2.84
Visuospatial Construction	1, 2, 3	4.92	4.55	4.24	2.67
Total Overall					
Total	1, 2, 3	24.34	23.58	18.12	10.15

1 = Old NC vs. Young NC, 2 = Old NC vs. Mild AD, 3 = Mild AD vs. Mod. AD.
Adapted from Bayles, K. A., & Tomoeda, C. K. (1993). *Arizona Battery for Communication Disorders of Dementia—manual.* Austin, TX: Pro-Ed. Used with permission.

Mild AD patients were significantly inferior to normal elders on all subtests except Comparative Questions, Word Reading Comprehension, and Figure Copying. However, when construct scores (composite scores) were considered, the mild AD group was, in all cases, significantly inferior in performance to normal elders. Finally, the average total overall score for individuals with mild AD was significantly lower than that for normal elders.

Performance of *Moderate* AD Patients on ABCD. Moderate AD patients in the standardization study performed significantly more poorly than mild AD patients and normal elders on every ABCD subtest. Their poorest performance was on the Story Retelling task in the delayed condition.

Performance of *Severe* AD Patients on ABCD. The ABCD was designed to differentiate normal elders from persons with early dementia and to track functional abilities until advanced dementia. Individuals who are severely demented find the ABCD too difficult. The Functional Linguistic Communication Inventory (FLCI) (Bayles & Tomoeda, 1994) was developed to document their functional communication abilities.

Functional Linguistic Communication Inventory (FLCI)

The FLCI (Bayles & Tomoeda, 1994) characterizes the functional linguistic communication of moderately and severely demented individuals. It takes approximately 30 minutes to test the following skills:

- naming and greeting
- answering questions
- participating in a conversation
- comprehending signs and matching objects to pictures
- reading and comprehending words
- reminiscing
- following commands
- pantomiming
- gesturing
- writing

The FLCI score sheet enables clinicians to compare the performance of the examinee to that of AD patients in the standardization study. Also, the examinee's intact communicative functions can be charted (see Chapter 14, Figure 14–2 for typical FLCI profiles of individuals in the mild, moderate, moderately severe, and very severe stages of dementia) and predictions made of skills vulnerable as AD progresses. Test results are useful in the preparation of functional maintenance programs and caregiver counseling.

The FLCI evolved from longitudinal studies of individuals with AD. It was standardized on 40 individuals with AD whose dementia severity was staged with a modified version of the Functional Assessment Stages (Reisberg, Ferris, & Franssen, 1985). Twenty individuals were tested twice with a one-week interval between administrations and high test-retest correlations were obtained for all FLCI subtests.

Differential Diagnosis

Normal Aging from Mild AD

Humans do not suffer a gradual year-by-year decline in their knowledge of language nor the ability to use language. The reported effects of age on communicative function are modest as can be seen by comparing the performance of young and older normals on ABCD subtests (see Table 11–5). Effects are most commonly reported in individuals who are in advanced old age (75+ years) and on tasks requiring speed or a directed search of memory. Results of the literature on aging and language effects are summarized in Table 11–6.

Table 11–6. Summary of Normal Aging Effects on Language

Form:	In general, no loss of phonologic or syntactic knowledge. May simplify grammar.
Content:	Vocabulary grows throughout life. Reduced information in verbal descriptions of individuals older than 70. Individuals older than 70 may be less concise in verbal description (fewer information units per words uttered). No across-the-decades decline in the content of language.
Use:	Slower to process complex language. Less efficient in deducing implied information. Less efficient in confrontation naming. Reading speed slows. Name fewer exemplars in generative naming.

The primary differences in communicative functioning of normal elders and individuals with mild AD are that the mild AD patients have:

1. Diminished quality in the content of language.
2. Reduction in total verbal output.
3. Difficulty processing complex speech acts.
4. Frequent repetitions.
5. Greater difficulty with word finding.

Example of the Use of ABCD Performance to Differentiate Normal Aging from Mild AD

Table 11–7 compares the performance on the ABCD of an individual suspected of having early AD, Mr. Lee, and a healthy age-mate, Mr. Smith. Mr. Lee, is 79 years of age and has been referred for evaluation because he is verbally repetitious. Mr. Smith is a neurologically normal 78-year-old man. Note that their performances differ most on

Table 11–7. Performance of Mr. Lee (individual with AD) and Mr. Smith (nondemented elder) on the ABCD

ABCD Subtests	Mr. Lee Raw Scores	Mr. Smith Raw Scores
Mental Status	11	12
Story Retelling — Immediate	10	14
Following Commands	9	9
Comparative Questions	6	6
Word Learning Free Recall	2	7
Word Learning Cued Recall	8	9
Word Learning Total Recall	10	16
Word Learning Recognition	39	47
Repetition	75	73
Object Description	4	6
Reading Comprehension—Words	8	8
Reading Comprehension—Sentences	7	7
Generative Naming	11	13
Confrontation Naming	18	20
Concept Definition	54	56
Generative Drawing	14	12
Figure Copying	12	12
Story Retelling—Delayed	0	13

the tests of verbal episodic memory (Story Retelling and Word Learning). Mr. Lee's scores on Story Retelling are inferior to those of Mr. Smith in both the immediate and delayed conditions. Whereas Mr. Smith gave approximately 90% of the information in the delayed condition that he told in the immediate condition, Mr. Lee could recall nothing of the story. On the Word Learning test, Mr. Lee had serious difficulty in the free recall segment recalling only 2 of 16 items. His Word Learning - Total Recall score, with the benefit of cues, is improved but not as much as Mr. Smith's score. On the Word Learning—Recognition subtest, Mr. Lee performed slightly better than most mild AD patients, but not as well as Mr. Smith and elders in the normal control group.

Both Mr. Lee and Mr. Smith received the maximum scores allowable for the following ABCD subtests: Following Commands, Comparative Questions, Reading Comprehension of Words and Sentences, and Figure Copying. With the exception of the Reading Comprehension of Sentences subtest, these tasks are relatively simple and most mild AD patients perform well on them. Mr. Lee and Mr. Smith also performed well on the Concept Definition task, and Mr. Lee actually received higher scores on the Generative Drawing and Repetition subtests.

Differentiating Mild AD from Delirium and Depression

Delirium

As described in Chapter 1, the DSM-IV-TR of the American Psychiatric Association (2000) defines dementia as a syndrome with multiple cognitive deficits that results in significant problems with employment and social functioning *in the absence of delirium*. To detect dementia, it is important for SLPs to know how to distinguish it from delirium.

Delirium is a confusional state that develops over a short period of time in which an individual experiences disturbances of consciousness, attention, cognition, and perception (American Psychiatric Association, 1999). Although cognitive deficits are omnipresent in dementia and common in delirium, patients with dementia are typically alert and do not have the disturbances of consciousness that characterize delirium.

Depression

Depression is a disorder of mood in which an individual is preoccupied with negative thoughts. Although depressed individuals experience moments of happiness and laughter, overall their perspective is pessimistic. As previously mentioned, depression is particularly common in the elderly and associated with the following signs and somatic complaints:

- Poor appetite
- Loss of weight
- Constipation
- Fatigue
- Sleep problems
- Agitation
- Flat affect
- Irritability

In addition certain behaviors are common in depressed individuals and include:

- Self-deprecatory comments
- Statements about feeling sad or helpless
- Failure to try
- Inattentiveness
- Indecisiveness
- Inconsistency in performance (better performance on some hard tasks than would be expected and poorer performance on some easy tasks than would be expected)
- Worse performance in the morning
- Slow speaking rate

■ Monotonous voice
■ Low volume

Popplewell and Phillips (2002) provide guidelines for distinguishing between dementia, delirium, and depression (Table 11–8). The features best for identifying depression include the onset of the condition, the patient's conscious state, and mood.

Of course, depression can co-occur with dementia. In fact, it is not unusual for *mild* AD patients, who realize that their memory and cognitive abilities are deteriorating, to become depressed. Similarly, delirium can complicate dementia, but it is typically triggered by another medical condition (e.g., high fever, bacterial infection, toxicity). If delirium is suspected, medical professionals should be alerted.

Differentiating Mild AD from Frontotemporal Dementia (FTD) Presenting with Progressive Changes in *Behavior*

As described in Chapter 10, the consensus criteria for FTD describe two forms: (1) a *behavioral variant* in which early and progressive changes in personality and frontal executive functions are prominent (includes Pick disease), and (2) a *language variant* in which early and progressive changes in language function dominate the clinical picture (includes semantic dementia and primary progressive aphasia). The following differences in clinical presentation can help distinguish individuals with mild AD from those with the behavioral variant of FTD (Table 11–9).

Table 11–8. Differentiating Dementia from Delirium and Depression

	Dementia	Delirium	Depression
Onset	Insidious	Acute	Acute
Conscious state	Impaired very late	Highly variable	Unusual
Mood	Stable	Variable consciousness	Depressed with diurnal variation
Duration	Long term	Short (days)	Short (weeks)
Cognitive features	Reduced short-term Reduced long-term memory	Short attention span	Reduced short- and long-term memory
Sleep/Wake cycle	Day/night reversal	Hour to hour variation	Hypersomnia, insomnia
Psychomotor changes	Late	Marked	—
Associated features	—	Medical conditions	Past history

From Popplewell, P., & Phillips, P. (2002). Is it dementia?—Which one? *Australian Family Physician, 31,* 319–322. Copyright 2006 Australian Family Physician. Reproduced with permission from The Royal Australian College of General Practitioners.

Table 11–9. Comparison of Clinical Features in FTD-Behavioral Variant and AD

Features	FTD-Behavioral Variant	AD
Onset	Typically early (age 45–65)	Typically late (after age 65)
Personality changes	Appears early	Appears later
Affect	Blunted; unconcerned indifferent	Concerned; may be anxious
Eating and oral behaviors	Disturbances appear early; overeating common; hyperoral	Preserved until later
Speech/language	Reduced output; more perseverations and stereotypes; may become mute	Output remains steady until late

Assessment Instruments for the Behavioral Variant of FTD

Individuals with the behavioral variant of FTD often have relatively preserved memory, visuo-spatial skills, and orientation in the early stage, making traditional dementia screening measures, such as the MMSE, insensitive to the condition (Gregory & Hodges, 1993). Gregory and Hodges (1996) recommend the use of the FAS test (also called the Controlled Oral Word Association Test) to detect FTD. In this verbal fluency measure the examinee is asked to generate as many words as possible within a minute that begin with the letters F, A, and S.

Caregiver questionnaires have also been developed for differentiating AD and the behavioral variant of FTD. These include the Neuropsychiatric Inventory (NPI) (Cummings, 1997; Cummings et al., 1994), the Frontal Behavioral Inventory (FBI) (Kertesz, Davidson, & Fox, 1997), and a 39-item questionnaire developed by Bozeat, Gregory, Lamdon Ralph, and Hodges (2000).

Neuropsychiatric Inventory (NPI) (Cummings, 1997; Cummings et al., 1994). The NPI was

developed to assess psychopathology in individuals with dementia. It evaluates the frequency and severity of 12 behavioral disturbances common in patients with dementia:

Delusions

Dysphoria

Agitation

Disinhibition

Hallucinations

Anxiety

Euphoria

Irritability

Apathy

Aberrant motor activity

Nighttime behavior disturbances

Appetite/eating abnormalities

The NPI also evaluates the amount of caregiver distress generated by these behavioral disturbances. Cummings et al. (1994) demonstrated the content and concurrent validity, interrater reliability, test-retest reliability, and internal consistency of the NPI. Levy, Miller, Cummings, Fairbanks, and Craig (1997) reported that the NPI behavioral profiles are capable of differentiating patients with FTD from those with AD.

Frontal Behavioral Inventory (FBI) (Kertesz et al., 1997). The FBI is a 24-item questionnaire administered to caregivers. Half the items address *deficit* behaviors:

Apathy

Indifference

Disorganization

Verbal apraxia

Aspontaneity

Inflexibility

Personal neglect

Alien hand

Inattention

Concreteness

Loss of insight

Logopenia (paucity of speech)

The other half address *excess* behaviors:

Perseveration

Inappropriateness

Restlessness

Hypersexuality

Irritability

Impulsivity

Aggression

Incontinence

Irresponsibility

Excessive or childish jocularity

Hyperorality

Utilization behavior (need to touch objects)

Each item is scored on a 4-point scale (none, mild, moderate, and severe). A cutoff score of 30 differentiates individuals with FTD from individuals with AD or depressive dementia (who typically score below 24) (Kertesz et al., 1997). The FBI has been found to be better than the Mini-Mental State Examination (Folstein et al., 1975) and the Mattis Dementia Rating Scale (Mattis, 1976) for differentiating FTD and AD patients (Kertesz et al., 2003). Kertesz, Nadkarni, Davidson, and Thomas (2000) report that FBI items also discriminate between individuals with the behavioral and language variants of FTD.

Caregiver Questionnaire (Bozeat et al., 2000). Bozeat and colleagues (2000) developed a 39-item questionnaire to assess the following:

Elation

Aggression

Risk taking

Disinhibition

Hallucinations

Social withdrawal

Irritability

Distractibility

Empathy

Depression

Personal care

Sleep patterns

Anxiety

Executive functioning

Apathy

Aberrant motor behavior

Ritualistic/stereotypic behavior

Changes in food preferences

Caregivers rate the frequency of these behaviors on a 4-point scale. Bozeat et al. (2000) reported that responses to the questionnaire distinguished between the FTD and AD groups, but that individuals with the behavioral and language variants of FTD had similar profiles.

Differentiating Mild AD from FTD Presenting with Progressive Changes in *Language* (Primary Progressive Aphasia and Semantic Dementia)

AD and FTD-Primary Progressive Aphasia

Primary progressive aphasia (PPA) is a slowly developing language disorder associated with relative sparing of nonverbal cognitive functions until late in the disease (Warren, Harvey, & Rossor, 2005). As described in Chapter 10, individuals with PPA have been characterized as having fluent or nonfluent aphasia (Mesulam et al., 2003) although this distinction is controversial. The SLP is often the first rehabilitation professional to see an individual with PPA because aphasia is the presenting symptom in the form of anomia, spelling difficulty (Warren et al., 2005), and semantic or phonemic paraphasias (Mesulam, 2001). In many PPA patients, language comprehension is spared until late in the disease course. To differentiate AD and PPA, SLPs must consider the clinical features of the two conditions (Table 11–10). Then, too, careful assessment of communicative skills and memory function is required.

AD and FTD—Semantic Dementia

Another type of FTD is semantic dementia, "a disorder characterized by a progressive loss of semantic (conceptual) knowledge about the world" (Snowden, 2005, p. 702). The clinical features that distinguish semantic dementia from AD can be found in Table 11–11. Snowden (2005) reports that semantic dementia is most commonly misdiagnosed as AD and urges the use of tests of word naming and comprehension, and face and object recognition to aid in their differentiation.

Table 11–10. Comparison of Clinical Features in FTD-PPA and AD

Features	FTD-PPA	AD
Onset	Age 50–80	After age 65
Speech/language Expression	Presenting problems include dysnomia; paraphasias; empty speech	Naming problems also occur but expressive problems are not as pronounced early
Speech/language Comprehension	Generally spared	Early difficulty with episodic and working memory can affect encoding and comprehension
Memory	Spared until later	Affected early

Table 11–11. Comparison of Clinical Features in FTD-Semantic Dementia and AD

Features	FTD-Semantic Dementia	AD
Onset	Age 50 to 65	Over age 65
Speech/language Expression	Selective semantic disorder appears early	No selective semantic disorder
Speech/language Comprehension	Impaired single word comprehension	Impaired sentence comprehension
Memory	Spared until late	Affected early

Assessment Instruments for the Language Variant of FTD. As previously noted, Kertesz and colleagues (2000) have administered the FBI to individuals with various forms of dementia including those with FTD-behavioral variant, PPA, and AD. They observed that verbal apraxia was a predominant characteristic of patients with PPA. Furthermore, PPA patients had significantly higher logopenia (decrease in amount of speech associated with word finding difficulty) scores than individuals with AD. It should be reiterated that whereas speech and language impairments are early features of the language variant of FTD, memory appears relatively unaffected early and memory measures should distinguish between AD and the FTD-language variant. Snowden (2005) suggests careful testing of memory. In early semantic dementia, autobiographical (episodic) memory should be relatively preserved; in early AD, it will be impaired. Le Rhun, Richard, and Pasquier (2006) reported that an analysis of responses on MMSE items also can aid differentiation of early PPA from AD. In their study, patients with PPA were significantly better on MMSE items related to word recall and constructional praxis whereas AD patients were better on items related to word registration,

object naming, sentence repetition, and following verbal instructions.

Differentiating AD from Vascular Dementia

Researchers have documented that vascular pathology and AD often co-occur; therefore, it is helpful to know the medical/clinical features of both diseases. Tables 11–12 and 11–13 provide general summary information that can be useful in distinguishing the two patient populations and recognizing their co-occurrence.

Assessment Instruments for VaD

Neuropsychological assessment and rating scales have been used to determine the presence of VaD. The most widely used instrument is the Hachinski Ischemic Scale (HIS) (Hachinski et al., 1975).

Hachinski Ischemic Scale (HIS) (Hachinski et al., 1975). The HIS comprises 13 items that are considered typical of the dementia associated with multiple infarctions. Moroney and colleagues (1997) administered the HIS to a large number of neuropathologically

Table 11–12. Comparison of Clinical Features in Vascular Dementia (VaD) and AD

	VaD	AD
History of hypertension	Usually present	Not necessarily present
Focal neurologic signs	Present	Generally absent
Brain areas involved	Cortical or subcortical dysfunction	Cortical dysfunction
Disease progression	Usually abrupt or stepwise deterioration, but may also be gradual	Gradual decline over time
Gait disturbance	Present early	May appear late
Illness duration	Usually short (3 years)	Usually longer (8 years)

Table 11–13. Differences in Cognitive Profiles Between VaD and AD

Feature	Difference Between VaD and AD
Cognitive impairment	May be greater overall in VaD
Executive function impairment	Prominent in VaD
	Often early feature in VaD
	Manifests as relatively greater degree of impairment in frontal lobe functions in VaD, such as:
	attention
	working memory
	planning
	sequencing
	abstraction
	speed of mental processing
Perseveration	More prominent in VaD

Modified from Ferris, S., & Gauthier, S. (2002). Cognitive outcome measures in vascular dementia. In T. Erkinjuntti & S. Gauthier (Eds.), *Vascular cognitive impairment* (pp. 395–400). London: Martin Dunitz.

confirmed patients with AD, VaD, and mixed dementia (AD and VaD) and reported that a score of 4 or less was typical of individuals with AD and a score of 7 or more was typical of those with VaD. Items that distinguished *MID from AD* included:

Stepwise deterioration

Fluctuating course

Focal neurologic symptoms

Hypertension

History of stroke

The two items that differentiated *mixed dementia from VaD* were stepwise deterioration and emotional incontinence and the two that *differentiated mixed dementia from AD* were fluctuating course and history of stroke.

Results of a Critical Analysis of the Published Literature. Sachdev and Looi (2003) conducted a systematic computerized literature search of several bibliographic databases for articles published between January 1966 and December 2000 that reported a comparison of patients with VaD and AD on neuropsychological tests. The studies were scrutinized to determine if they met strict criteria for inclusion in their analysis, resulting in 32 studies being selected for the final review. Studies were grouped by the broad cognitive domain(s) that were assessed (e.g., intelligence, language, nonverbal memory, etc.). Sachdev and Looi reported that despite the relative heterogeneity of VaD pathology and diagnostic criteria used, group differences were found in neuropsychological profiles of the two groups based on the overall analysis. Individuals with VaD are likely to have relatively preserved long-term memory, greater impairment in frontal-executive function, and greater motor dysfunction than AD. No clear differences could be determined on tests of language, constructional abilities, memory registration, conceptual function, visual perception, and attention and tracking. Based on these findings, Sachdev and Looi recommend tests of verbal long-term memory, such as the California Verbal Learning Test (Delis et al., 2000).

Differentiating Mild AD from Lewy Body Dementia (LBD)

As described in Chapter 8, LBD is associated with the presence of Lewy bodies in cortical and subcortical structures and neuronal loss. Also, Hansen and colleagues (1990) found that 75% of individuals with LBD have the characteristic neuropathologic features of AD, particularly neuritic plaques. Both LBD and AD patients exhibit progressive decline in cognitive functioning; however, the other characteristic features of LBD distinguish it from AD as can be seen in Table 11–14.

Assessment Instruments for LBD

Evidence is accumulating that patients with LBD can be distinguished from individuals with AD using certain standardized neuropsychological measures. Hamilton and colleagues (2004) used the CVLT and the Logical Memory Test of the WMS-R (Wechsler, 1987) and reported unique patterns of performance. Whereas LBD and AD groups were equally impaired in learning new verbal information, the LBD patients exhibited better retention and recognition memory than AD patients.

Hansen and colleagues (1990) compared the neuropsychological profiles of autopsy-proven LBD and AD patients and found that the groups had equivalent performance on tests of episodic memory, confrontation naming (Boston Naming Test), and arithmetic, but the LBD group was significantly worse than the AD group on a test of attention (WAIS-R Digit Span subtest) and on tests of visuospatial and construction ability. Interestingly, LBD and AD groups performed differently on tests of verbal fluency. The AD patients were better than LBD patients on the letter fluency test (i.e., generating words that begin with a certain letter),

Table 11–14. Comparison of Clinical Features of LBD and AD

Clinically, LBD patients are more likely than AD patients to have the following:

1. **Fluctuating cognitive impairment**—Fluctuation in cognitive function is common and apparent in the early stages of LBD (McKeith et al., 1996). The degree and frequency of fluctuation can vary between individuals and within the same individual.

2. **Visual and/or auditory hallucinations**—The visual hallucinations of LBD patients are typically detailed, well-formed, and recurrent (McKeith et al., 1996) and occur in 93% of cases whereas auditory hallucinations are less common, occurring in approximately 50% of cases (Bolla, Filley, & Palmer, 2000). Hallucinations appear early in the disease course (Luis et al., 1999).

3. **Confusional state and clouding of consciousness**—The fluctuation in cognitive status can be the result of transient confusion and variability in attention and alertness (McKeith et al, 1996).

4. **Symptoms of parkinsonism**—Parkinsonian features that can appear early in LBD include rigidity and bradykinesia, hypophonia, stooped posture, problems with balance, and a slow shuffling gait. In AD, parkinsonian features appear late in the disease.

5. **Shorter duration of illness**—Patients with LBD experience a shorter illness duration that is about half as long as that for patients with AD (McKeith, Fairbairn, Perry, & Thompson, 1994).

6. **Sensitivity to neuroleptics**—LBD patients are extremely sensitive to neuroleptic drugs such as risperidone or haloperidol, to the degree that the reaction can be life-threatening (Bolla et al., 2000).

but the two groups performed similarly on a semantic category fluency test (i.e., generating words in a particular category such as "animals").

Summary of Important Points

- Assessment of cognitive function is critical to the diagnosis of dementia because by definition, dementia comprises multiple cognitive deficits.
- Early identification of dementia is important because some cases are treatable and

others will benefit from drugs that slow disease progression.

- Prior to testing: review the medical history; check hearing, vision, and literacy; and build rapport to reduce test anxiety.
- Be alert to possible depression and drug effects that can affect test performance.
- Clinicians have a role in screening for dementia and in comprehensive evaluation. However, diagnosis of dementia is the province of the physician.
- To obtain valid and reliable information about a client's cognitive-communicative abilities, use tests that have been standardized on individuals with dementia

(for whom etiology was specified) and healthy elders.

- The best behavioral measures for screening for dementia are mental status and episodic memory tests.
- Comprehensive evaluation should include measures of language comprehension and production, verbal memory, executive function, and mental status.
- The Arizona Battery of Communication Disorders of Dementia (ABCD) is a standardized battery designed to comprehensively evaluate individuals with mild and moderate dementia.
- The Story-Retelling subtest of the ABCD is a time-efficient, sensitive instrument for screening for Alzheimer's dementia.
- The Functional Linguistic Communication Inventory is a standardized battery for evaluating individuals with moderately-severe and severe dementia.
- The primary differences in communicative functioning between healthy elders and individuals with mild AD are: diminished quality of the content of language, reduced verbal output; repetitiveness; difficulty processing complex speech acts; and greater dysnomia.
- Depressed individuals typically have many somatic complaints and communicate a sense of helplessness and despair. Inconsistency of performance is a red flag for depression.
- Individuals with delirium typically have an acute medical condition that causes variability in their conscious state.
- Individuals with FTD-behavioral variant present with early changes in personality and executive functioning and relatively preserved memory and visuospatial skills.
- Individuals with FTD-language variant (PPA) present with early changes in language with relative sparing of nonverbal cognitive functions.

- Individuals with FTD-language variant (SD) present with progressive loss of conceptual knowledge with relative sparing of memory.
- Individuals with VaD typically have: history of hypertension, focal neurologic signs, abrupt or stepwise deterioration, and impairment in executive function.
- Individuals with LBD often have: fluctuating cognitive impairment, visual and auditory hallucinations, and parkinsonian features.

References

Alexopoulos, G. S. (2003). Depressive dementia. In V. O. B. Emery & T. E. Oxman (Eds.). *Dementia: Presentation, differential diagnosis, and nosology* (pp. 398–416). Baltimore: The Johns Hopkins University Press.

Alexopoulos, G. S., Abrams, R. C., Young, R. C., & Shamoian, C. A. (1988). Cornell scale for depression in dementia. *Biological Psychiatry, 23*, 271–284.

Alexopoulos, G., Young, R., & Meyers, B. (1993). Geriatric depression: Age of onset and dementia. *Biological Psychiatry, 34*, 141–145.

American Psychiatric Association (2000). *Diagnostic and statistical manual of mental disorders DSM-IV-TR*. Washington, DC: Author.

American Psychiatric Association, Work Group on Delirium. (1999). Practice guideline for the treatment of patients with delirium. *The American Journal of Psychiatry, 156*(Suppl.), 1–20.

Armstrong, L., Borthwick, S. E., Bayles, K. A., & Tomoeda C. K. (1996). Use of the Arizona Battery for Communication Disorders of Dementia in the UK. *European Journal of Disorders of Communication. 31*, 171–180.

Bayles, K. A., & Tomoeda, C. K. (1993). *Arizona Battery for Communication Disorders of Dementia*. Austin, TX: Pro-Ed.

Bayles, K. A., & Tomoeda, C. K. (1994). *Functional Linguistic Communication Inventory*. Austin, TX: Pro-Ed.

Bayles, K. A., Tomoeda, C. K., Montgomery, E. B., Cruz, R. F., & Azuma, T. (2000). The relationship of mental status to performance on lexical-semantic tasks in Parkinson's disease. *Advances in Speech-Language Pathology, 2,* 67–75.

Bayles, K. A., Tomoeda, C. K., Wood, J. A., Cruz, R. F., & McGeagh, A. (1996). Comparison of the sensitivity of the ABCD and other measures of Alzheimer's dementia. *Journal of Medical Speech-Language Pathology, 4,* 183–194.

Bayles, K. A., Trosset, M. W., Tomoeda, C. K., Montgomery, E. B., & Wilson, J. (1993). Generative naming in Parkinson's disease patients. *Journal of Clinical and Experimental Neuropsychology, 15,* 547–562.

Beck, A. T., Ward, C. H., Mendelson, M., Mock, J., & Erbaugh, J. (1961). An inventory for measuring depression. *Archives of General Psychiatry, 4,* 561–571.

Benton, A. L. (1983). *Contributions to neuropsychological assessment.* New York: Oxford University Press.

Benton, A. L., & Hamsher, K. deS. (1989). *Multilingual Aphasia Examination.* Iowa City, IA: AJA Associates.

Blessed, G., Tomlinson, B. E., & Roth, M. (1968). The association between quantitative measures of dementia and of senile changes in the cerebral grey matter of elderly subjects. *British Journal of Psychiatry, 114,* 797–811.

Bolla, L. R., Filley, C. M., & Palmer, R. M. (2000). Dementia DDx: Office diagnosis of the four major types of dementia. *Geriatrics, 55,* 34–46.

Bozeat, S., Gregory, C. A., Lambon Ralph, M. A., & Hodges, J. R. (2000). Which neuropsychiatric and behavioural features distinguish frontal and temporal variants of frontotemporal dementia from Alzheimer's disease? *Journal of Neurology, Neurosurgery, and Psychiatry, 69,* 178–186.

Buschke, H. & Fuld, P. A. (1984). Evaluating storage, retention, and retrieval in disordered memory and learning. *Neurology, 24,* 1019–1025.

Clarfield, A. M. (1988). The reversible dementias: Do they reverse? *Annals of Internal Medicine, 109,* 476–486.

Cummings, J. L. (1997). The Neuropsychiatric Inventory: Assessing psychopathology in dementia patients. *Neurology, 48*(Suppl. 6), S10–S16.

Cummings, J. L., Mega, M., Gray, K., Rosenberg-Thompson, S., Carusi, D. A., & Gornbein, J. (1994). The Neuropsychiatric Inventory: Comprehensive assessment of psychopathology in dementia. *Neurology, 44,* 2308–2314.

Delis, D. C., Kramer, J. H., Kaplan, E., & Ober, B. A. (2000). *California Verbal Learning Test®—Second Edition* (CVLT®—II). San Antonio, TX: Harcourt Assessment.

Desmond, D. W. (2002). General approaches to neuropsychological assessment. In T. Erkinjuntti & S. Gauther (Eds.), *Vascular cognitive impairment* (pp. 323–338). London: Martin Dunitz.

Dobie, D. J. (2002). Depression, dementia and pseudodementia. *Seminars in Clinical Neuropsychiatry, 7,* 170–186.

Emery, V. O. B., & Oxman, T. E. (2003). Depressive dementia. In V. O. B. Emery & T. E. Oxman (Eds.), *Dementia: Presentation, differential diagnosis, and nosology* (pp. 361–397). Baltimore: The Johns Hopkins University Press.

Erkinjuntti, T., Sulkava, R., Wikström, J., & Autio, L. (1987). Short portable mental status questionnaire as a screening test for dementia and delirium among the elderly. *Journal of the American Geriatrics Society, 35,* 412–416.

Ferris, S., & Gauthier, S. (2002). Cognitive status measures in vascular dementia. In T. Erkinjuntti & S. Gauthier (Eds.), *Vascular cognitive impairment* (pp. 395–400). London: Martin Dunitz.

Folstein, M. F., Folstein, S. E., & McHugh, P. R. (1975). "Mini-mental state": A practical method for grading the mental state of patients for the clinician. *Journal of Psychiatric Research, 12,* 189–198.

Gregory, C. A., & Hodges, J. R. (1993). Dementia of frontal type and the focal lobar atrophies. *International Review of Psychiatry, 5,* 397–406.

Gregory, C. A., & Hodges, J. R. (1996). Frontotemporal dementia: Use of consensus criteria and prevalence of psychiatric features. *Neuropsychiatry, Neuropsychology, and Behavioral Neurology, 9,* 145–153.

Grober, E., & Kawas, C. (1997). Learning and retention in preclinical and early Alzheimer's disease. *Psychology and Aging, 12,* 183–188.

Hachinski, V. C., Iliff, L. D., Zilhka, E., duBoulay, G. H. D., McAllister, V. L., Marshall, J., et al. (1975). Cerebral blood flow in dementia. *Archives of Neurology, 32,* 632–637.

Hamilton, J. M., Salmon, D. P., Galasko, D., & Hansen, L. A. (2004). Distinct memory deficits in dementia with Lewy bodies and Alzheimer's disease. *Journal of the International Neuropsychological Society, 10,* 689–697.

Hamilton, M. (1967). A rating scale for depression. *Journal of Neurology, Neurosurgery, and Psychiatry, 23,* 56–62.

Hamilton, M. (1970). Development of a rating scale for primary depressive illness. *British Journal of Social & Clinical Psychology, 6,* 278–296.

Hansen, L., Salmon, D., Galasko, D., Masliah, E., Katzman, R., DeTeresa, R., et al. (1990). The Lewy body variant of Alzheimer's disease: A clinical and pathological entity. *Neurology, 40,* 1–8.

Hart, R. P., Kwentus, J. A., Wade, J. B., & Taylor, J. R. (1988). Modified Wisconsin Card Sorting Test in elderly normal, depressed, and demented patients. *Clinical Neuropsychologist, 2,* 49–52.

Heaton, R. K. (1981). *Wisconsin Card Sorting Test manual.* Odessa, FL: Psychological Assessment Resources.

Heaton, R. K., Chelune, G. J., Talley, J. L., Kay, G. G., & Curtiss, G. (1993). *Wisconsin Card Sorting Test manual: Revised and expanded.* Odessa, FL: Psychological Assessment Resources.

Hughes, C. P., Berg, L., Danziger, W. L., Coben, L. A., & Mastin, R. L. (1982). A new clinical scale for the stageing of dementia. *British Journal of Psychiatry, 140,* 566–572.

Jenkins, R. L. & Parsons, O. A. (1978). Cognitive deficits in male alcoholics as measured by a modified Wisconsin Card Sorting Test. *Alcohol Technical Reports, 7,* 76–83.

Kalchthaler, T., Coccaro, E., & Lichtiger, S. (1977). Incidence of polypharmacy in a long-term care facility. *Journal of the American Geriatrics Society, 25,* 308–313.

Kertesz, A., Davidson, W., & Fox, H. (1997). Frontal behavioral inventory: Diagnostic criteria for frontal lobe dementia. *Canadian Journal of Neurological Sciences, 24,* 29–36.

Kertesz, A., Davidson, W., McCabe, P., & Munoz, D. (2003). Behavioral quantitation is more sensitive than cognitive testing in frontotemporal dementia. *Alzheimer Disease and Associated Disorders, 17,* 223–229.

Kertesz, A., Nadkarni, N., Davidson, W., & Thomas, A. W. (2000). The Frontal Behavioral Inventory in the differential diagnosis of frontotemporal dementia. *Journal of the International Neuropsychological Society, 6,* 460–468.

Kiloh, L.G. (1961). Pseudo-dementia. *Acta Psychiatrica Scandinavica, 37,* 336–351.

Kral, V. A., & Emery, O. B. (1989). Long-term follow up of depressive pseudodementia of the aged. *Canadian Journal of Psychiatry, 34,* 445–446.

Lamy, P. P. (1986). The elderly and drug interactions. *Journal of the American Geriatric Society, 34,* 586–592.

Larson, E. B., Reifler, B. V., Sumi, S. M., Canfield, C. G., & Chinn, N. M. (1986). Diagnostic tests in the evaluation of dementia: A prospective study of 200 elderly outpatients. *Archives of Internal Medicine, 146,* 1917–1922.

Le Rhun, E., Richard, F., & Pasquier, F. (2006). Different patterns of Mini Mental Status Examination responses in primary progressive aphasia and Alzheimer's disease. *European Journal of Neurology, 13,* 1124–1127.

Levy, M. L., Miller, B. L., Cummings, J. L., Fairbanks, L. A., & Craig, A. (1997). Alzheimer disease and frontotemporal dementias: Behavioral distinctions. *Archives of Neurology, 53,* 687–690.

Lezak, M. D., Howieson, D. B., Loring, D. W., with Hannay, H. J., & Fischer, J. S. (2004). *Neuropsychological assessment* (4th ed.). New York: Oxford University Press.

Locascio, J. J., Growden, J. H., & Corkin, S. (1995). Cognitive test performance in detecting, staging and tracking Alzheimer's disease. *Archives of Neurology, 52,* 1087–1099.

Luis, C. A., Barker, W .W., Gajaraj, K., Harwood, D., Petersen, R., Kashuba, A., et al. (1999). Sensitivity and specificity of three clinical criteria for dementia with Lewy bodies in an autopsy-verified sample. *International Journal of Geriatric Psychiatry, 14,* 526–533.

Massey, A. J. (November 8, 2005). Medication-related issues associated with the management of dementia. *The ASHA Leader, 10,* 12–13.

Mattis, S. (1976). Mental status examination for organic mental syndrome in the elderly patient. In L. Bellak & T. B. Karasu (Eds.), *Geriatric psychiatry* (pp. 77–121). New York: Grune & Stratton.

McKeith, I. G., Fairbairn, A.F., Perry, R. H., & Tompson, P. (1994). The clinical diagnosis and misdiagnosis of senile dementia of Lewy body type (SDLT). *British Journal of Psychiatry, 165,* 324–332.

McKeith, I. G., Galasko, D., Kosaka, K., Perry, E. K., Dickson, D. W., Hansen, L. A., et al. (1996). Consensus guidelines for the clinical and pathologic diagnosis of dementia with Lewy bodies (DLB). *Neurology, 47,* 1113–1124.

Mesulam, M. M. (2001). Primary progressive aphasia. *Annals of Neurology, 49,* 425–432.

Mesulam, M. M., Grossman, M., Hillis, A., Kertesz, A., & Weintraub, S. (2003). The core and halo of primary progressive aphasia and semantic dementia. *Annals of Neurology, 54*(Suppl 5), S11–S14.

Monsch, A. U., Foldi, N. S., Ermini-Fünfschilling, Berres, M., Taylor, K. I., Seifritz, E., et al. (1995). Improving the diagnostic accuracy of the Mini-Mental State Examination. *Acta Neurologica Scandinavica, 92,* 145–150.

Moorhouse, B., Douglas, J., Panaccio, J., & Steel, G. (1999). Use of the Arizona Battery for Communication Disorders of Dementia in an Australian context. *Asia Pacific Journal of Speech, Language and Hearing, 4,* 93–107.

Moroney, J. T., Bagiella, E., Desmond, D. W., Hachinski, V. C., Molsa, P. K., Gustafson, L., et al. (1997). Meta-analysis of the Hachinski Ischemic Score in pathologically verified dementias. *Neurology, 49,* 1096–1105.

Moss, S. E., Tomoeda, C. K., & Bayles, K. A. (2000). Comparison of the cognitive-linguistic profiles of Down syndrome adults with and without dementia to individuals with Alzheimer's disease. *Journal of Medical Speech-Language Pathology, 8,* 69–81.

Neary, D. (2005). Frontotemporal dementia. In A. Burns, J. O'Brien, & D. Ames (Eds.), *Dementia* (3rd ed., pp. 667–677). London: Hodder Arnold.

Orange, J. B. (2001). Family caregivers, communication, and Alzheimer's disease. In M. L. Hummert & J. F. Nussbaum (Eds.), *Aging, communication, and health: Linking research and practice for successful aging* (pp. 225–248). Mahwah, NJ: Lawrence Earlbaum Associates.

Pfeiffer, E. (1975). A Short Portable Mental Status Questionnaire for the assessment of organic brain deficit in elderly patients. *Journal of the American Geriatrics Society, 23,* 433–441.

Popplewell, P., & Phillips, R. (2002). Is it dementia?—Which one? *Australian Family Physician, 31,* 319–322.

Reisberg, B., Ferris, S. H., Anand, R., de Leon, M. J., Schneck, M. K., Buttinger, C., et al. (1984). Functional staging of dementia of the Alzheimer type. *Annals of the New York Academy of Sciences, 435,* 481–483.

Reisberg, B., Ferris, S. H., de Leon, M. J., & Crook, T. (1982). The global deterioration scale (GDS): An instrument for the assessment of primary degenerative dementia (PDD). *American Journal of Psychiatry, 139,* 1136–1139.

Reisberg, B., Ferris, S. H., & Franssen, E. (1985). An ordinal functional assessment tool for Alzheimer's type dementia. *Hospital and Community Psychiatry, 36,* 593–595.

Rentz, D. M. & Weintraub, S. (2000). Neuropsychological detection of early probable Alzheimer's disease. In L. F. M. Scinto & K. R. Daffner (Eds.), *Early diagnosis of Alzheimer's disease* (pp. 169–189). Totowa, NJ: Humana Press.

Ries, P. W. (1994). Prevalence and characteristics of persons with hearing trouble: United States, 1990–1991: National Center for Health Statistics. *Vital Health Statistics, 193,* 1–75.

Robinson-Whelen, S., & Storandt, M. (1992). Immediate and delayed prose recall among normal and demented adults. *Archives of Neurology, 49,* 32–34.

Rosen, W. G., Mohs, R. C., & Davis, K. L. (1984). A new rating scale for Alzheimer's disease. *American Journal of Psychiatry, 141,* 1356–1364.

Rosen, W. G., Mohs, R. C., & Davis, K. L. (1986). Longitudinal changes: Cognitive, behavioral, and affective patterns in Alzheimer's disease. In L. W. Poon (Ed.), *Handbook for clinical memory assessment of older adults* (pp. 294–301). Washington, DC: American Psychological Association.

Rubin, E. H., Storandt, M., Miller, J. P., Kinscherf, D. A., Grant, E. A., Morris, J. C., et al. (1998). A prospective study of cognitive function and onset of dementia in cognitively healthy elders. *Archives of Neurology, 55,* 395–401.

Sachdev, P. S., & Looi, J. C. L. (2003). Neuropsychological differentiation of Alzheimer's disease and vascular dementia. In J. V. Bowler & V. Hachinski (Eds.), *Vascular cognitive impairment* (pp. 153–175). New York: Oxford University Press.

Salzman, C. (1979). Update on geriatric psychopharmacology. *Geriatrics, 34,* 87–90.

Shanmugham, B., & Alexopoulos, G. (2005). Depression with cognitive impairment. In A. Burns, J. O'Brien, & D. Ames (Eds.), *Dementia* (3rd ed., pp. 731–737). London: Hodder Arnold.

Snowden, J. S. (2005). Semantic dementia. In A. Burns, J. O'Brien, & D. Ames (Eds.), *Dementia* (3rd, ed., pp. 702–712). London: Hodder Arnold.

Solomon, P. R., Hirschoff, A., Kelly, B., Relin, M., Brush, M., DeVeaux, R. D., et al. (1998). A 7 minute neurocognitive screening battery highly sensitive to Alzheimer's disease. *Archives of Neurology, 55,* 349–355.

Sunderland, T., Alterman, I. S., Yount, D., Hill, J. L., Tariot, P. N., Newhouse, P. A., et al. (1988). A new scale for the assessment of depressed mood in demented patients. *American Journal of Psychiatry, 145,* 955–959.

Tingus, K., McPherson, S., & Cummings, J. L. (2002). Neuropsychological examination of executive functions. In T. Erkinjuntti & S. Gauthier (Eds.), *Vascular cognitive impairment* (pp. 339–363). London: Martin Dunitz.

Tombaugh, T., & McIntyre, N. (1992). The Mini-Mental State Examination: A comprehensive review. *Journal of the American Geriatrics Society, 40,* 922–935.

Tomoeda, C. K. (2001). Comprehensive assessment for dementia: A necessity for differential diagnosis and management. *Seminars in Speech and Language, 22,* 275 – 289.

Tomoeda, C. K. & Bayles, K. A. (1993). Longitudinal effects of Alzheimer's disease on discourse production. *Alzheimer's Disease and Associated Disorders, 7,* 223–236.

Wallace, G. L. & Holmes, S. (1993). Cognitive-linguistic assessment of individuals with multiple sclerosis. *Archives of Physical Medical Rehabilitation, 74,* 637–643.

Warren, J. D., Harvey, R. J., & Rossor, M. N. (2005). Progressive aphasia and other focal syndromes. In A. Burns, J. O'Brien, & D. Ames (Eds.), *Dementia* (3rd ed., pp. 720–728). London: Hodder Arnold.

Wechsler, D. (1981). *Wechsler Adult Intelligence Scale—Revised manual.* New York: Harcourt Brace & Jovanovich.

Wechsler, D. (1987). *Wechsler Memory Scale—Revised.* New York: The Psychological Corporation.

Wechsler, D. (1997). *Wechsler Adult Intelligence Scale—Third Edition.* San Antonio, TX: Harcourt Assessment.

Wechsler, D. (1999). *Wechsler Memory Scale—Third Edition.* San Antonio, TX: Harcourt Assessment.

Weiner, M. F. (2003). Clinical diagnosis of cognitive dysfunction and dementing illness. In M. F. Weiner & A. M. Lipton (Eds.), *The dementias: Diagnosis, treatment, and research* (pp. 1–48). Washington, DC: American Psychiatric Publishing.

Welsh, K., Butters, N., Hughes, J., Mohs, R., & Heyman, A. (1991). Detection of abnormal memory decline in mild cases of Alzheimer's disease using CERAD neuropsychological measures. *Archives of Neurology, 48,* 278–281.

Wilson, B., Cockburn, J., & Baddeley, A. (1991). *Rivermeade Behavioral Memory Test* (2nd ed.). Reading, England: Thames Valley Test Co.

Zung, W. W. K. (1965). A self-rating depression scale. *Archives of General Psychiatry, 1,* 63–70.

Zung, W. W. K. (1972). The Depression Status Inventory: An adjunct to the Self-Rating Depression Scale. *Journal of Clinical Psychology, 28,* 539–543.

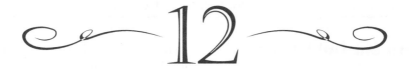

Treating Cognitive-Communicative Disorders of Dementia: Direct Interventions

The cognitive-communicative dysfunction of individuals with dementia can be improved with direct and indirect interventions. *Direct* interventions are those in which the SLP provides individual or group therapy. *Indirect* interventions are those in which the physical and/or linguistic environments are modified to support communication as a result of training of professional or personal caregivers. The focus of this chapter is on direct interventions. Indirect interventions are the focus of Chapter 13.

Historically, the value of therapy for dementia patients with irreversible conditions, such as AD, was questioned likely because the term "therapy" implies a reduction in or elimination of the cause of the problem. In recent years, however, therapy has been interpreted to mean ensuring that patients function maximally. Indeed, federal legislation in the form of the Omnibus Budget Reconciliation Act of 1987 (OBRA, 1987), that governs accreditation of long-term care facilities, requires that residents be comprehensively evaluated and care plans developed that will enable them to function at their highest level of ability.

Today, SLPs routinely receive reimbursement for assessing the patient's ability to improve in a reasonable period of time. If improvement is expected and the special skills of the SLP are needed, claims reviewers will approve "restorative therapy" and the clinician will be reimbursed (ASHA, 2004). When a patient's restoration potential is judged insignificant after a trial of restorative therapy, the clinician can develop a functional maintenance plan (FMP). The time involved in plan development, the time needed to instruct supportive personnel in carrying it out and periodic oversight are reimbursable services if the FMP is created during the period of diagnostic or restorative therapy.

Definitions

Restorative therapy—therapy in which clients are brought to a functional level they are capable of but have not been achieving.

Functional Maintenance Plan—a plan of care designed to maintain clients at a level of functioning.

Treatment Guidelines

Regardless of the cause of dementia, clinicians will find the following guidelines helpful in designing a care plan for maximizing function (Bayles & Tomoeda, 1997).

1. Strengthen the knowledge and processes that have the potential to improve.
2. Reduce demands on impaired cognitive systems.
3. Increase reliance on spared cognitive systems.
4. Provide stimuli that evoke positive fact memory, action, and emotion.

Etiologically different dementia patients have different profiles of spared and impaired cognitive abilities. Identifying the profile of preserved abilities and knowledge is as important to good therapy planning as identifying deficits because spared systems can be used to compensate for those impaired. For example, individuals with AD have poor episodic memory but relatively preserved procedural learning ability (Salmon, Heindel, & Butters, 1992) and other types of nondeclarative memory (see De Vreese, Neri, Fioravanti, Belloi, & Zanetti, 2001 for a review). The spared nondeclarative systems can be used to teach new behaviors. Indeed, many investigators have reported improved skill learning in AD patients through repetition priming (Deweer, Pillon, Michon, & Dubois, 1993; Dick, Hsieh, Bricker, & Dick-Muehlke, 2003; Dick et al., 1996; Grober, Ausubel, Sliwinski, & Gordon, 1992; Keane, Gabrieli, Fennema, Groudon, & Corkin, 1991; Verfaellie, Keane, & Johnson, 2000).

In planning therapy care should be taken to use stimuli that evoke positive emotion and action. Neither individuals with dementia nor their caregivers benefit from the creation of a negative emotion in the patient. Negative moods and behavior often persist long after the provoking stimulus is forgotten increasing caregiver stress, staff time, and diminishing the quality of life of the patient.

Techniques That Facilitate Learning

Many variables have been empirically demonstrated to influence learning in healthy adults and individuals with dementia, (Table 12–1). Taking them into account when planning intervention will produce greater learning.

Facilitate Perception

Aging significantly affects human sensory systems and perception. Diminished perception impedes learning because perception is

Table 12–1. Variables That Influence Learning

Perceptibility of stimuli
Task complexity
Number of tasks
Working memory span
Level of learner engagement
Self-generation of response
Multimodal stimulation
Personal relevancy of task and stimuli
Emotion
Minimization of error responses
Repetition of desired response
Elaborateness of encoding

the first step in information processing. An awareness of how aging affects sensory systems is needed to help elders compensate. The sensory systems most influential in information processing are the visual and auditory systems.

Vision and Aging

The best known age-related change in vision is loss of focusing power, a condition known as *presbyopia* (National Institute on Aging, 1995). Although the eye stops growing in adolescence, the lens continues to grow in adulthood, becoming denser and less elastic. The result is that elders are less able to focus and need two to three times more light than a person 20 years of age (Clark, 1975). Aging also affects the ability to adjust to changes in levels of illumination. In youth, one can go from a sunny afternoon to a darkened movie theatre and quickly accommodate the change in illumination. With age, this adjustment is slower and less efficient leaving individuals temporarily blind. Finally, age-related changes in vision affect the ability to perceive patterns and increase the need for contrast to aid perception (Brawley, 1997).

Many elders develop cataracts, glaucoma, and macular degeneration (Schieber, 2006). With cataracts, vision becomes blurred. People who have cataracts say it is like looking at the world through a cloud or thick haze. Glaucoma also causes blurred vision and loss of peripheral perception. Macular degeneration is the condition in which degeneration occurs in the center of the retina. The result is a blind spot in the center of the visual field. Macular degeneration is also associated with increased sensitivity to light and altered color vision (Fangmeier, 1994).

Individuals with AD experience these age-related changes in vision plus others that are disease related, specifically, deficits in color discrimination and contrast sensi-

tivity (Cronin-Golomb, Corkin, & Growdon, 1991; Cronin-Golomb, Sugiura, Corkin, & Growdon, 1993). Of clinical significance is how sensory loss can negatively affect the ability to communicate, perform tests, and carry out daily activities. Consider that vision is needed to read lips, recognize facial expressions, interpret contexts, follow directions, and read. People with impaired depth perception, a decreased ability to focus, and reduced sensitivity to contrast may appear more demented than they really are because sensory losses diminish performance on tests and ADLs. Even young adults who wear glasses often remark that they have trouble hearing and thinking without their glasses on. Unfortunately, the need for accommodations that will enhance vision is underappreciated by many professional and personal caregivers. In short, impaired vision reduces patients' quality of life, increases dependency, and makes them appear more intellectually impaired than they are by virtue of neuropathology.

Managing Problems with Vision to Facilitate Learning

First and foremost, clinicians need to screen for vision problems. A simple screening technique is included in the Arizona Battery of Communication Disorders of Dementia (Bayles & Tomoeda, 1993). However, clinicians without access to the ABCD can easily create a similar one. Type a variety of letters on a page of paper turned horizontally. Repeat one letter, like "A," several times in each quadrant of the page. Have the examinee identify all the "As" in each quadrant. Note whether the target letter is unnoticed in an area of the page. Also note whether the individual has to move the paper to find the "As." If so, a visual field defect may be present and the patient should be referred for neurologic evaluation.

Before neuropsychological testing, ensure that patients who need glasses wear them. Use printed materials that are in large font size and colors that provide strong contrast (black on white or vice versa) to make print perceptible. Because of the frequency of vision problems, clinicians should introduce themselves when greeting a client. Although elders may be able to see them, they may be unable to discern their facial features sufficiently to recognize them. Finally, do not stand in front of a window or bright light when talking to an elder as glare can reduce perception of your face.

It is important for individuals with dementia to have adequate light throughout the day. "Sunlight starvation" negatively impacts the health and quality of life of many elders (Campbell, Kripke, Gillin, & Hrubovcak, 1988; Clark, 1975). Lack of sunlight disturbs circadian rhythms that regulate a host of biological processes (Brawley, 1997), among them body temperature, hormone release, heart rate, blood pressure, and the sleep-wake cycle. Sunlight also benefits the body's immune system. In addition to the negative effects of sunlight deprivation on bioregulatory processes, victims of sunlight starvation are at greater risk for depression and sleep disorders that can diminish cognitive functioning. Increased agitation is also a byproduct of light deprivation (Satlin, Volicer, Ross, Herz, & Campbell, 1992), and investigators have demonstrated that exposure to bright light can reduce agitation and improve sleep-wake cycles even in late-stage dementia patients (Ancoli-Israel et al., 2003; Singer & Hughes, 1995).

Brawley (1997, p. 87) recommended the following guide for lighting in long-term care facilities. Her recommendations are of value to SLPs and other personnel responsible for the care of elders.

- Raise the level of illumination
- Provide consistent, even light levels
- Eliminate glare
- Provide access to natural daylight
- Provide gradual changes in light levels in transition spaces
- Provide focused task lighting
- Improve color rendition from lamps or light sources so that colors of the environment and people in the environment are not distorted

Color and Vision

Not only does the lens of the eye thicken with age, it yellows, filtering out the short wavelengths. The consequence is distortion of color perception, particularly after age 60 (Cooper, Ward, Gowland, & McIntosh, 1991). Discriminating along the blue-yellow axis is particularly affected as is discriminating among light colors. AD patients are less able to distinguish between blue and green hues and between blue and violet hues. Most resistant to age effects are the ability to discriminate the red hue and the brightness of color (Cooper, 1993). By providing high contrast, clinicians can increase function (Figures 12–1 and 12–2). For example, table tops and countertops should contrast strongly with the color of the floor. Dishes that contrast with the color of the table facilitate eating. The best contrast is provided by using a dark color against a light background or vice-versa (e.g., black against white, light yellow against dark blue). Poor contrasts result from dark green against bright red, yellow against white, blue against green, and lavender against pink.

Hearing and Aging

Hearing loss is the most prevalent disability of elderly Americans (Adams & Marano, 1995; Jerger, Chmiel, Wilson, & Luchi, 1995; Ries, 1994). Cruickshanks et al. (1998) conducted a population-based study of 4,541 people aged 48 to 92 and reported the preva-

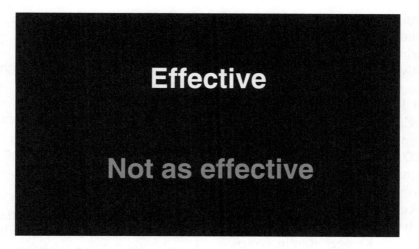

Figure 12–1. Example of high and low letter contrasts.

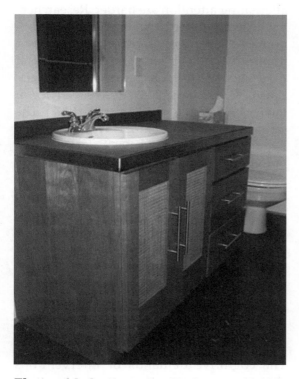

Figure 12–2. Example of bathroom with high contrast between sink and countertop and between toilet and floor.

lence of all degrees of hearing loss to be 45.9% among those 65 years and older. Among nursing home residents, the percent-age appears to be even higher approaching 90% (Hull, 1995). In addition, adults with hearing loss often experience further deterioration of hearing ability with advancing age (Cruickshanks et al., 2003).

Hearing loss in persons with AD is not less prevalent than in nondemented elders (Hodkinson, 1974) and some researchers suggest that it may be more prevalent (Herbst & Humphrey, 1980; Uhlmann, Larson, Rees, Koepsell, & Duckert, 1989). Indeed, Uhlmann et al. (1989) found that the risk of dementia increased with progressively greater amounts of hearing loss. It has been reported that between 70 to 80% of nursing home residents have hearing loss (Schow & Nerbonne, 1980; Voeks, Gallager, Langer, & Drinka, 1990; Weinstein & Amsel, 1986). Gold, Lightfoot, and Hnath-Chisolm (1996) documented the prevalence of hearing loss in 94% of a sample of individuals with AD.

Just as a deficit in vision can make individuals with dementia seem more intellectually and functionally impaired than they are, so can a deficit in hearing (Gates et al., 1996; Ohta, Carlin, & Harmon, 1981; Uhlmann et al., 1989; Weinstein & Amsel, 1986). Yet, it is shocking how few investigators have controlled for the hearing abilities of individuals with dementia in neuropsychological and treatment studies. Additionally, without correction, hearing loss can contribute to more rapid cognitive decline. Using longitudinal data from individuals with AD, Uhlmann, Larson, and Koepsell (1986) observed that cognitive decline over a one-year period was almost twice as great in the group of hearing impaired AD than in the nonhearing impaired AD group.

Furthermore, when individuals with dementia receive amplification, their cognitive and behavioral functioning improves (Allen et al., 2003; Kreeger, Raulin, Grace, & Priest, 1995; Palmer, Adams, Bourgeois, Durrant, & Rossi, 1999; Palmer, Adams, Durrant, Bourgeois, & Rossi, 1998; Weinstein & Amsel, 1986). Palmer and colleagues (1999) documented reduction in problem behaviors reported by caregivers for all eight AD subjects in their study after hearing aid use. Allen and associates (2003) reported improvement on measures of hearing handicap over 24 months of hearing aid use in their study of 31 individuals with dementia.

Before making a judgment about the existence and severity of dementia in any individual, hearing should be tested. If comprehensive assessment of hearing is possible, clinicians may wish to follow the procedures described by Mahendra, Bayles, and Harris (2005) in which otoscopy, pure-tone threshold testing, word recognition testing, and the Hearing Handicap Inventory for the Elderly —Screening Version (Ventry & Weinstein, 1983) were used. If comprehensive hearing assessment is unavailable, clinicians can screen hearing by simply administering a speech discrimination test (repeating spoken words or judging whether two spoken words are the same) in the environment in which the testing will occur. Regardless of dementia severity, most individuals with AD can complete a simple speech discrimination test (Bayles & Tomoeda, 1993).

To facilitate hearing, clinicians should do the following:

- Have clients who need hearing aids wear them
- Eliminate noise
- Ensure that clients can see their face
- Amplify their voice

Focus on Single Tasks

Most individuals with dementia have attention deficits (Duchek, Hunt, Ball, Buckles, & Morris, 1997; Perry, Watson, & Hodges, 2000). As we know from personal experience, tasks requiring division of attention or alternating attention are harder. Researchers have demonstrated that the neural activation associated with a given task decreases in healthy adults if a second task is done at the same time (Just, Carpenter, Keller, Emery, Zajac, & Thulborn, 2001; Rees, Frith, & Lavie, 1997; Vandenberghe et al., 1997). The same is true for individuals with dementia. Filoteo and colleagues (1992) reported that individuals with AD were better at focusing attention on a single aspect of a stimulus than dividing attention between two aspects of the same stimulus. Camicioli, Howieson, Lehman, and Kay (1997) observed that AD patients slowed their walking speed when asked to perform a verbal fluency task (reciting male names) while walking.

Control Task Complexity

The cognitive demands of interventions should be considered when planning therapy. What makes a task harder or easier? The number and type of mental operations differentiate tasks as does the complexity of stimuli. Bayles, Tomoeda, Kaszniak, and Trosset (1991) documented that those tasks requiring multiple cognitive processes and more cognitive effort were those on which the performance of healthy elders and Alzheimer dementia patients were the worst. In the Bayles et al. study, 11 different tasks were given to AD patients in the order shown in Table 12–2. All tasks used the same 13 conceptual stimuli (Table 12–2) thereby enabling the investigators to make intertask comparisons of difficulty. The most difficult tasks were superordinate and coordinate naming that required recall of conceptual information.

Recall tasks, in which learners have to search memory for answers, are widely recognized as more difficult than tasks in which learners have only to recognize the answer (Anderson & Bower, 1972; Hasher & Zacks, 1979; Kintsch, 1970). In superordinate naming, study subjects had to grasp the relation between the stimulus concept and the larger category of things to which the stimulus concept belonged, retrieve the superordinate, and express it orally. This task placed demands on working memory span, attention, and

Table 12–2. Tasks and Concepts Used in the Bayles et al. (1991) Study

11 Tasks	13 Concepts
Confrontation naming	Pencil
Auditory comprehension	Comb
Dictation	Hanger
Oral reading	Mask
Definition	Racquet
Reading comprehension	Dart
Coordinate naming	Harmonica
Superordinate naming	Domino
Superordinate identification	Knocker
Pantomime expression	Stethoscope
Pantomime recognition	Compass
	Tongs
	Abacus

decision-making as well as semantic memory. In coordinate naming, study subjects had to grasp the relation between the stimulus concept and other objects in the same category and provide the names of coordinates. Like superordinate naming, this task taxed working and semantic memory systems.

The least difficult tasks were oral reading of words, auditory comprehension, and reading comprehension, the latter two being multiple-choice tasks that required recognition of the answer rather than recall. Oral reading of words is a mechanical task that does not require comprehension of the word to be read or manipulation of information.

Bayles et al. (1991) also observed that concept difficulty affected performance. Less common concepts were those most likely to produce an error. The concepts of compass, stethoscope, and abacus accounted for most errors. The concepts of pencil and comb elicited the fewest errors.

In sum, remember that recognition is easier than recall, comparing features of items is harder than item recognition, and expressing relationships is harder than confirming relationships. Also, remember that complexity of stimuli interacts with task complexity. Performing multiple cognitive operations on complex information is more difficult than performing multiple cognitive operations on simple information. Tasks that require few cognitive manipulations of simple information are easier yet. Finally, dementia patients are often unable to remember task instructions. By making task instructions simple and visible throughout the intervention, performance will be enhanced.

Work Within Memory Span

Working memory span capacity, or the ability to hold incoming information in consciousness, attenuates slightly with age and markedly in individuals with dementia (Belleville, Peretz, & Malenfant, 1996; Cherry, Buckwalter, & Henderson, 1996). Reduction in span capacity can affect an individual's ability to comprehend task instructions. Daneman and Carpenter (1980) documented that a large span capacity for auditory-verbal information is associated with better language comprehension than a small span capacity. Having knowledge of a patient's span capacity for verbal and visual information is important in designing tasks that will not be overwhelming and discourage participation. Often, when dementia patients are given more information than they can process, they withdraw and refuse to participate in the activity. Span capacity for verbal and visual information can be tested with the Digit Span and Spatial Span subtests of the Wechsler Memory Scale-Third Edition (Wechsler, 1997). The Digit Span subtest involves having patients repeat strings of numbers that increase in length in the same order (forward) and in reverse order (backward). In the Spatial Span subtest, span capacity for visual information is tested by having patients touch a sequence of blocks of increasing length in the same order as presented by the examiner and in reverse order.

Active Engagement Facilitates Learning

For healthy individuals and dementia patients, learning is both faster and better when the individual is actively engaged in the learning process (Engelkamp & Zimmer, 1989; Karlsson et al., 1989). Active engagement in its fullest form is learning by doing. Action-oriented learning involves the non-declarative procedural memory system that enables us to develop skills and habits. This

system is generally preserved in individuals with AD (Deweer et al., 1993; Dick, 1992). If individuals are provided the opportunity to practice new procedures, such as making transfers from a wheel chair, they become habitual and increase independence. Further, by providing opportunities for the execution of previously learned procedures, this knowledge can be sustained (Zanetti et al., 1997; Zanetti et al., 2001).

Self-Generation of a Response

One technique for actively involving dementia patients is to have them generate a response during learning rather than just watching and listening. This "generation effect" was first described by Slamecka and Graf (1978) who observed that young adults had better memory for words they generated, in response to cues, than for words they simply heard. Mitchell, Hunt, and Schmitt (1986) reported the same effect in old and young adults and individuals with AD. Study participants read 30 sentences of subject-verb-object (SVO) form and generated the object in another 30 SVO sentences (for example, "The gentleman opened the _____."). Later they were presented with the verbs from the 60 sentences and asked to supply the objects associated with them. Study results showed that individuals with AD, like healthy young and older adults, better remembered self-generated objects than those already present in the stimulus sentences they read.

Lipinska, Bäckman, Mäntylä, and Viitanen (1994) conducted a study in which they provided a 20-page booklet to individuals with AD. On each page was the name of a concrete noun. Patients had to generate "general properties" of 10 of the nouns. For the other 10, they had to make yes/no judgments about whether the item was a member of the category provided by the experimenter. At recall, the AD patients were provided their own self-generated cues for 10 of the words and the experimenter provided cues for the remainder. Recall was best when subjects were provided their self-generated cues.

Multimodal Stimulation Strengthens Learning

Learning is advantaged when the learner has the opportunity to see, hear, feel, smell, and actively engage with the concept to be learned. For example, an individual is more likely to learn how to safely transfer from a bed to a wheelchair if they are told how to do it, shown how to do it, and can practice making the transfer. Similarly, learning the name of a new acquaintance is facilitated by seeing and hearing the name, writing the name, and pairing the name with attributes of the person.

Montessori methods are gaining prominence in rehabilitation settings because they actively engage clients and involve multimodality stimulation (Camp, 1999; Camp & Brush, 1999; Mahendra, 2001). The defining principles of the Montessori method are: having choices, purposeful activities, multisensory experience, action-oriented, and incremental learning. Several investigators recommend Montessori methods for engaging individuals with Alzheimer's dementia (Dreher, 1997; Vance, Camp, Kabacoff, & Greenwalk, 1996; Vance & Porter, 2000). Orsulic-Jeras, Judge, and Camp (2000) reported that AD patients who participated in Montessori-based activities (such as category sorting using pictures or words and memory bingo) were more attentive than when they participated in regular, more passive activities like watching an event.

Personal Relevancy Makes a Difference

Perlmuter and Monty (1989) observed that personalizing a task, by permitting the patient to make choices, increased their engagement, motivation, and performance. Clinicians should interview patients about the activities they enjoyed premorbidly or goals they would like to achieve. Then, by offering a choice of activities or a choice of goals to focus on, clinicians give patients a sense of control over their learning.

Many nursing homes allow residents to bring personal items from home, such as a favorite chair and bedspread, to create a sense of familiarity. Familiarity promotes a feeling of security. Unfamiliar environments can create insecurity that heightens anxiety and negatively affects learning. Our experience is that many dementia patients are best treated in their home environments.

Emotion

Emotional memory enables humans, and other organisms to recognize and avoid danger (Darwin, 1872; Damasio, 1999; Emery, 2003). Events, people, and objects with emotional significance are more memorable and produce changes in brain chemistry that facilitate learning. LaBar, Mesulam, Gitelman, and Weintraub (2000) demonstrated that emotionally charged information captures the attention of dementia patients better than neutral information. Individuals with AD and normal controls were shown pairs of visual scenes, some emotionally charged and some neutral. Recordings of eye movements revealed that AD patients, like normal controls, were more attentive to the emotionally charged scenes. Moayeri, Cahill, Jin, and Potkin (2000) presented AD subjects with stories accompanied by slides containing either emotionally charged or neutral elements. Although AD patients were inferior to normal controls at recalling both types of story elements, emotional passages were better remembered than neutral ones.

Minimize Error Responses

Dementia patients with episodic memory deficits typically do not remember their error responses. Consequently, they don't self-correct as neurologically normal adults do in trial and error learning (Baddeley & Wilson, 1994). When an error response is repeatedly given, its engram is strengthened making it more accessible in the future. To reduce the probability of error response, the clinician can manipulate stimulus characteristics and response contingencies. The technique of vanishing cues has frequently been used to reduce the production of errors in amnesic individuals (Baddeley & Wilson, 1994; Clare et al., 2000; Wilson, Baddeley, Evans, & Shiel, 1994; Winter & Hunkin, 1999). In the vanishing cues technique learners are given strong cues at first. Gradually, cue strength is reduced until the target response is given in the absence of cues. For example, if you wanted to teach the patient that the name of the night nurse was Janet, you could present the name in its full form on a card and ask the learner to read the card to answer the question, "What is the name of your night nurse?" On subsequent learning trials, the patient would read a card with the name in a reduced form (Jane, Jan _, Ja _ _,). The vanishing cues method has been used successfully in nondemented amnesic patients (Glisky, Schacter, & Tulving, 1986; Leng, Copello, & Sayegh, 1991; Van der Linden & Coyette, 1995) and two studies report its effectiveness in teaching new facts to AD patients (Fontaine, 1995; Wilson & Moffat, 1992).

Repetition Is Key to Learning

When individuals repeatedly access information and bring it to conscious awareness for manipulation, the engram for the information is strengthened making it more accessible for future recall (Green, 1992). All of us learned the importance of this fact as students. The more frequently we thought about the information presented in lectures and class exercises, the more likely we were to recall it on a test. Just as repetition helps healthy individuals learn information and skills, it also helps memory-impaired individuals learn (Glisky, 1997). Many researchers have demonstrated that repetition facilitates learning in dementia patients (Heun, Burkart, & Benkert, 1997; Little, Volans, Hemsley, & Levy, 1986; Mahendra, 2001; Small, Kemper, & Lyons, 1997). If the information to be learned is new information, as opposed to previously known information, learning will be slower and forgotten more quickly by individuals with dementia. For some dementia patients, new fact learning is impossible. When this is the case, the clinical focus will be on maintaining preserved knowledge (e.g., names of grandchildren, how to make a 911 call) through repeated opportunities to use it.

Spaced Retrieval Training (SRT)

Spaced retrieval training (SRT) is a shaping procedure in which an individual is asked to recall information (e.g., a name, procedure, location) over increasingly longer intervals of time (Brush & Camp, 1998a). It is a simple procedure requiring little cognitive effort from the patient (Schacter, Rich, & Stampp, 1985). SRT can be nested in other activities such as conversation, physical therapy, or doing a craft project and used by both personal and professional caregivers (Brush & Camp, 1998a).

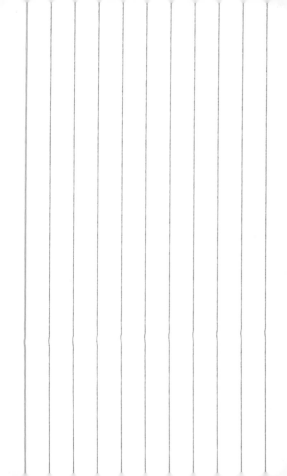

Clinicians control the type of target response, duration of the intervals between retention probes, and the number of learning trials. The first intervals between recall probes are very short and gradually extended. When an incorrect response is given, the clinician returns to the length of interval that last produced a correct response. Activities during the intervals between retention probes can be related to the desired response or unrelated.

Originally described by Landauer and Bjork in 1978, SRT was not used with a dementia patient until 1985. Since then, its efficacy has been explored by many investigators who report success in teaching face-name associations (Abrahams & Camp, 1993; Camp 1989; Camp & Schaller, 1989; Moffat, 1989; Vanhalle, Van der Linden, Belleville, & Gilbert, 1998), object location (Camp, 1989), object names (Abrahams & Camp, 1993; Jacquemin, Van der Linden, & Feyereisen, 1993; McKitrick & Camp, 1993; Moffat, 1992) and various verbal and motor responses (Bird, 2000; Camp, Bird, & Cherry, 2000; McKitrick & Camp, 1993). Brush and Camp (1998b) used SRT to teach seven dementia patients and two memory-impaired stroke patients three pieces of information: the therapist's name, a fact important to the person (e.g., room number, spouse's birthday), and a compensatory technique for improving communication. Five participants with dementia completed the study and all learned the three pieces of information as did the two stroke patients. However, participants had varying levels of recall a month later. Davis, Massman, and Doody (2001) tested the efficacy of using spaced retrieval to teach previously known but forgotten personal information in a randomized placebo-controlled study of 37 AD patients. Cognitive stimulation served as the placebo and consisted of home-administered attention exercises. AD patients in the intervention group improved in the recall of personal information during the 5-week intervention whereas the performance of patients in the placebo group remained constant.

The efficacy of spaced retrieval with dementia patients is thought to result from spared nondeclarative memory processes that enable individuals to learn associations even though they cannot remember the event of learning. A common question is how long does a dementia patient remember what is learned through SRT? Researchers have reported retention of information for many months in some individuals with dementia. In these cases, the individuals had frequent occasions to use the learned information. If the information to be learned is not needed, and therefore never accessed, it will not be retained long.

Examples of Uses for SRT

Both fact knowledge and procedures can be taught with SRT. Examples of useful facts are: previously known but forgotten personal information; name-face associations of caregivers and family members; location of important objects; 911 as an emergency number. Examples of useful procedures are: making a phone call for help; making a safe transfer; finding an important location (e.g., bathroom, bedroom, nurses' station, dining room); increasing volume of voice; operating a faucet; and inserting a hearing aid.

Elaborate Encoding Builds Stronger Engrams

Healthy elders show improved memory when strategies such as visual imagery or organization of information to be learned are provided during encoding (Kliegl, Smith, & Baltes, 1989; Verhaeghen, Marcoen,

& Goossens, 1992; Yesavage, Rose, & Bower, 1983). Such strategies promote a greater depth of processing that may result in better learning. The greater the depth of processing of the to-be-retained information, the greater the learning. Good teachers know the truth of this principle.

The depth-of-processing principle also applies to individuals with AD (see Bäckman & Small, 1998 for a review). Bird and Luszcz (1991) observed that AD patients learned better when they were engaged in tasks like thinking of attributes of the to-be-remembered information or its category membership compared to trying to recall pictures in the absence of any type of cue. Similarly, Herlitz and Viitanen (1991) noted improved learning when material to be remembered had a logical structure. Arkin, Rose, and Hopper (2000) found that working within a semantic schema by linking a target to its superordinate category facilitated learning.

Glasgow, Zeiss, Barrera, and Lewinshon (1977) developed a technique, known as The PQRST method (Preview, Question, Read, State, Test), for increasing the depth of processing of information. The PQRST method is a systematic way of involving the learner actively at encoding. First, the information is previewed. Next, the learner is asked to answer questions about it. Thereafter, the learner reads the information, summarizes it, and is subsequently tested. A similar technique is having learners listen to text, identify key propositions, and later use them in a story they create (Van der Linden & Van der Kaa, 1989).

Another technique for learning text is to divide it into segments and have the learner summarize each before proceeding to the next segment. Stevens, King, and Camp (1993) used question asking and reading (QAR) to increase memory for the content of stories. The reading of the text was distributed among group members and scripted to include text-based questions that group members had to answer. The QAR technique increased the learning of text and the frequency of verbal interactions among group members.

A three-step strategy for making face-name associations was described by McCarthy (1980). First the learner identifies a prominent facial feature, then transforms the name into a concrete image, and finally formulates an interactive visual image of the two elements (feature and image of name).

Techniques That Facilitate Retrieval of Information

Many techniques have been empirically demonstrated to facilitate recall of information in healthy adults and individuals with dementia, Table 12–3. Like the variables that facilitate learning, the techniques that facilitate recall of information should be incorporated in therapy programs.

Table 12–3. Variables that Facilitate Retrieval of Information

Recognition paradigm
Priming
Reminiscence
Use of retrieval cues that reflect support given at encoding
Cognitive stimulation
Avoid multitasking
Allow more time to respond

Recognition Is Easier Than Recall

Free recall of information is harder than recognizing information. All students know the truth of this statement. A multiple-choice test is easier than an essay test because it contains the correct answers that have only to be recognized. Answering an essay question requires an effortful search of memory and formulation and generation of a coherent, correct response. The same is true for dementia patients. Table 12–4 shows the performance of mild and moderate Alzheimer's patients and young and older normal individuals on tests of free recall, cued recall, and recognition. As the data show, the ability to freely recall information diminishes with age and the performances of healthy adults and those with dementia were better in the cued recall and recognition conditions. *Note:* To determine the effect of cued recall, subtract the free recall score from the total recall score.

When individuals with episodic memory deficits are asked to recall information, they are set up to fail. A simple technique for preserving their dignity is avoidance of free recall questions, such as "What's new?" or "What have you been doing?" or "What did you have for dinner?" Questions like these require the recall of recent events. Recogni-tion questions that require yes/no answers are easier, for example asking "Did you go to the store today?" "Is that a new dress?" or "Does dinner with the Smith's sound like fun?" Choice questions such as "Would you like fish or chicken for dinner?" "Shall we watch television or go for a walk?" have the answer in the question making them easier (Bayles & Tomoeda, 1994).

Another type of question that can pose difficulty for dementia patients is one that asks for a listing of things, for example, "What are your favorite TV shows?" or "Where have you traveled?" These require a search of memory while holding the question in mind.

Priming Facilitates Recall

Recent exposure to a word, concept, or proposition makes the word, concept, or proposition more likely to come to mind. For example, if you have recently seen the word "desert," you will recognize it more quickly on tasks requiring you to make judgments about it (for example whether it is a real word). You will also make faster judgments about the words "hot" and "dry" because they are associated with the concept of desert. The prior exposure to the word "desert" heightened the level of activation

Table 12–4. Mean Raw Scores and Standard Deviations of Young and Old Normal Control and Individuals with Mild and Moderate Alzheimer's Disease (AD) on the Word Learning Subtest of the ABCD

	Young Normal	Old Normal	Mild AD	Moderate AD
Word Learning—Free Recall	10.4	7.6	2.3	0.8
Word Learning—Total Recall	15.7	15.1	7.7	3.3
Word Learning—Recognition	47.8	46.6	36.3	30.0

of the concept "desert" and its lexical representation. It also heightened the level of activation of related concepts and their lexical representations. The heightened activation of "desert," "hot," and "dry" occurred without your awareness and is the result of the spreading activation of energy within semantic and lexical memory. The phenomenon of advantaging a response, by virtue of prior exposure to the target or a related item, is called *priming*. Priming is demonstrated empirically by an increase in the frequency, speed, or accuracy of a response as a consequence of prior exposure to a particular stimulus (Ochsner, Chiu, & Schacter, 1994; Tulving & Schacter, 1990).

Storms (1958) conducted one of the early studies that fueled interest in the phenomenon of priming. Storms asked students to study a list of words, List A, all of which elicit high-frequency associations. For example, the word "eagle" typically elicits the word "bird." Then Storms presented the students with a second list of words, List B, which were high-frequency responses to the words on List A, but which do not usually elicit words on the A list. For example, the List A word "eagle" elicits "bird," but the word "bird" (List B) does not usually elicit the word "eagle." However, Storms observed that the production of words on the A list, as responses to the words on the B list, was significantly higher when the A list was previously seen. Cofer (1960) subsequently labeled this phenomenon as "priming of associations." Over the decades, the term "priming" has been extended to refer to a variety of events, or paradigms, that facilitate the production of target information.

Repetition or Direct Priming

Repetition or direct priming refers to the paradigm in which an item presented in the training (or study phase) of an experiment, is identical to, or composed of fragments of the target item to be produced. For example, exposure to the word "boat" in the training phase will result in faster judgments about the word "boat" when it is seen again. Or, prior exposure to the word "boat" will result in individuals saying "boat" when later shown the fragment "bo_ _." Repetition, or direct priming, is perceptual, that is, it is modality specific and independent of the meaning of the item. Commonly used repetition priming tasks require subjects to complete a word, make a decision about a word, or identify previously seen words.

Associative or Indirect Priming

Associative or indirect priming refers to the paradigm in which the item presented in the training phase is associated with the item to be produced. Associative/indirect priming is conceptual or semantic. Commonly used indirect, associative priming tasks are word associations, category production, and general knowledge tests. In word association tasks, a word presented in the training phase produces a preference for an associated word. For example, the word "snow" produces a preference for "cold."

In category production tasks the subject is presented with items from a particular category, for example, fruits, and later asked to generate as many exemplars of fruit as possible. The prior exposure to items from the category increases the likelihood that they will be produced later in the category production task.

In a general knowledge task, the prior presentation of a word increases the probability of it being given as the answer to questions related to the word. For example, prior exposure to the word "saguaro" will increase the probability that saguaro will be given as an answer to the question, "What is a large cactus that grows in southern Arizona?"

Using Priming Clinically

Many SLPs are unfamiliar with the term "priming" but routinely use priming to facilitate the performance of clients through cuing. Clinicians often give an associate of a word to facilitate its recall ("use it to cut through wood" for "saw"). Often they provide the name of the larger category of things the target word belongs to ("it's a form of transportation" for "car"). Sometimes they provide the opposite of a word to stimulate the target ("up" for "down").

Clinicians use more than words to prime desired behavior, among them routines, memory books, music, and contexts. A routine is a behavioral chain in which each behavior functions as a discriminative stimulus for the next behavior and a conditioned reinforcer for the previous link (Halle & Spradlin, 1993). Ylvisaker and Feeney (2002) described routines as concrete structured event complexes that become organized mental representations that cue behavior.

Wallets and memory books with photographs of past events and loved ones, together with text, have been demonstrated to improve the meaningfulness of verbiage produced by dementia patients in conversation (Bourgeois, 1990, 1991, 1992). The photographs and text in the memory wallets and books activate memories and prime associations with the pictured events and people.

All of us have memories and emotions associated with music. Often a song transports us to a past event. If the event is positive, our mood may improve. Music is a tool clinicians can use to stimulate memory. Foster and Valentine (2001) used music to facilitate autobiographical recall in individuals with dementia. They observed increased arousal and interest when background music was played during recall. Mahendra (1999, 2001) used music to stimulate the recall of autobiographical events with individuals

with dementia and observed greater animation, increased verbal output, and greater physical action (imitating drum playing, toe tapping, and in one case, dancing).

Context can also cue behavior. Recognition of this fact has led clinicians to train individuals in the contexts in which the desired behavior is needed. This is important because skills acquired in a clinical context often do not transfer to real world contexts (Martin & Pear, 1996).

Reminiscence

Reminiscence therapy stimulates recall (Thornton & Brotchie, 1987). When individuals with dementia and healthy adults are presented with pictures, newspaper articles, video clips, clothes, and props associated with a theme, their personal experiences related to the theme come to mind (Hellen, 1992). Sheridan (1995) recommends using a variety of materials to trigger all the senses. A synergy can develop in reminiscence sessions in which group members aid each other in the recall of past events. When one member of the group shares a memory, it stimulates memories in other group members.

Good reminiscence sessions require planning (Gillies & James, 1994). In addition to selecting a theme and obtaining related tangibles, the clinician should develop a list of questions that probe for the obvious and less obvious recollections individuals are likely to have. Plan how to include all group participants. For example, have some individuals describe a tangible item, then ask other members what they think about the tangible. Group members can share the responsibility for reading newspaper articles or article headlines. Finally, reminiscence can be a stimulus for physical activity such as dancing, food preparation (Boczko, 1994), or exercise.

> ### Good Themes for Reminiscence Sessions
>
> ■ culturally appropriate holidays
> ■ personal milestone events (getting married, graduation)
> ■ notable world events
> ■ weather events
> ■ national traditions
> ■ geography

Use Retrieval Cues That Reflect Support Given at Encoding

The amount of informational overlap between a retrieval cue and the memory engram established at the time of encoding is vital to memory proficiency. This is known as the *encoding specificity principle* (Tulving & Thomson, 1973). A substantial literature exists demonstrating that recall is improved when retrieval cues reflect support given at encoding (Diesfeldt, 1984; Herlitz & Viitanen, 1991; Karlsson et al., 1989). All of us are familiar with detectives having witnesses return to the scene of a crime as a memory trigger. Many of us have experienced the same phenomenon at high school and college reunions. Back at our alma maters, surrounded by old friends, we recall events we likely would never have thought of again had we not returned to the setting in which they occurred. Most of us are familiar with the phenomenon of being at a loss for the correct answer to a test question when the question is worded differently from how the information was presented in class. To facilitate recall, use retrieval cues that reflect support given at the time of encoding.

Cognitive Stimulation

Some researchers report success in improving recall, learning new information, and sustaining cognitive status through cognitive stimulation and practice. Arkin (1992) developed memory training interventions that resulted in the learning of new factual information and its retention two weeks later by subjects presumed to have AD whose MMSE scores ranged from 13 to 26. The primary method of cognitive stimulation was having subjects listen to audiotapes. Some heard the tapes twice, others heard them once and then were quizzed about the contents. Learning occurred in both conditions but was better in the tape plus quiz format. Arkin developed the procedure based on reports that normal subjects learn better when they are actively involved with the to-be-learned material and when they have to answer questions about it. Although Arkin's subjects did not have confirmed AD and the sample size was modest, the results inspire us to consider that training may be beneficial in individuals who retain semantic and some episodic memory function.

Quayhagen and Quayhagen (1989) assessed the value of a home program in which dementia patients had 6 hours per week of memory-provoking and problem-solving exercises. Although caregivers did not report gains in patients' cognitive function, they reported positive emotional outcomes, notably greater interaction, less depression, and increased confidence.

Avoid Having Client Multitask

Multitasking is more cognitively effortful than doing a single task. Recent research suggests that the "timesaving" technique of multitasking makes healthy adults less efficient (Newman, Keller, & Just, 2007) and consumes more time. The process of switching back and forth between tasks can take longer than doing one task to completion and then doing the next task. The brain has to overcome "inhibitions" imposed to stop the first task to do the second task. Newman and colleagues had subjects listen to sentences while comparing rotating objects. When done together, the resources available for processing visual input dropped 29%. Brain activation for listening dropped 53%. Too much multitasking can cause attention gaps, stress, trouble concentrating, and problems with recent memory. Because of their deficits in attention and memory, dementia patients have much greater difficulty with multitasking than healthy adults.

Allow More Time to Respond

As previously mentioned in Chapter 3, information processing slows with age. Birren, Woods, and Williams (1980) demonstrated that between the ages of 65 and 91, slowing in psychomotor speed occurs even in healthy elders and adversely affects performance on neuropsychological tests. However, when healthy elders are given sufficient time to respond, they often perform like young adults and the age effect disappears. Dementia patients are slower in processing as a function of age and as a function of pathology that has disrupted their neurochemistry and interfered with intercellular communication. Particularly slow are individuals with Parkinson's dementia. Allow more time for responding and counsel others to do the same.

Rehabilitation of Dementia: The Future

Before ending this chapter, it is important to note that behavioral therapy as a means of habilitating and rehabilitating individuals with brain damage as a function of disease and injury looks brighter than ever before because of advances in our understanding of neural plasticity. Over the last decade, neuroscientists have demonstrated that the central nervous system has remarkable adaptive capacity. We now know that the human brain continuously remodels its neural circuitry as a function of experience (Kleim & Jones, in press). Said another way, neural plasticity is experience-dependent. There is a burgeoning body of evidence, primarily from animal research, that indicates that behavioral training is key to promoting reorganization of brain tissue after brain damage (Johansson, 2000, 2003; Jones et al., 2003; Jones, Hawrylak, Klintsova, & Greenough, 1998; Monfils, Plautz, & Kleim, 2005). Kleim and Jones have specified the empirically-derived principles of experience-dependent plasticity that are of importance to rehabilitation professionals.

- Neural circuits not actively engaged in task performance for an extended period of time begin to degrade.
- Plasticity can be induced within specific brain regions through extended training.
- Learning or skill acquisition, rather than mere use, seem to be required to produce significant changes in patterns of neural connectivity.
- Repetition matters and may be essential for inducing lasting neuronal changes.
- Intensity matters—too little can induce a weakening of synaptic responses but higher intensity can induce long-term potentiation and learning.
- Timing matters—there appear to be time windows in which behavioral treatments are particularly effective in inducing plasticity.
- Salience matters and it has long been known that emotion modulates the strength of memory consolidation.
- Age matters—synaptic potentiation synaptogenesis and cortical map regoranization are reduced with aging.

- Plasticity in response to one training experience can enhance the acquisition of similar behaviors.
- Plasticity in response to one experience can interfere with the acquisition of other behaviors.

Kleim and Jones acknowledge that a better understanding is needed of when and how much training should be given for optimal response and how training interacts with neural reactions to brain damage, aging, and self-derived compensatory behaviors. Nonetheless, the fundamental fact that the brain appears to need training to maximize appropriate functional reorganization remains, a fact that will ultimately influence the delivery of services by rehabilitation personnel.

Treating the dementia patient poses a greater challenge than treating an individual with a traumatic brain injury or stroke because dementia-producing diseases are usually progressive. However, as has been pointed out in earlier chapters, the human brain has more than one memory or learning system and research has already shown that individuals with dementia can use these to compensate for those that are damaged from disease. What is now a modest literature on the benefit of cognitive training for individuals with dementia can be expected to dramatically expand as more is learned about experience-dependent neural plasticity.

Summary of Important Points

- Direct interventions are those in which SLPs provide individual or group therapy.
- Federal legislation requires that residents of long-term care facilities have a care plan that will enable them to function at their highest level of ability.

- SLPs routinely receive reimbursement for providing direct interventions that improve the communicative functioning of individuals with dementia.
- Four guidelines are helpful in designing a care plan for maximizing patient function:
  - Strengthen the knowledge and processes that have the potential to improve.
  - Reduce demands on impaired cognitive systems.
  - Increase reliance on spared cognitive systems.
  - Provide stimuli that evoke positive fact memory, action, and emotion.
- To improve learning, take the following into account when planning intervention:
  - Facilitate perception.
  - Focus on single tasks.
  - Control task complexity.
  - Work within memory span.
  - Actively engage the patient in learning.
  - Use multimodal stimulation.
  - Make therapy personally relevant.
  - Use emotion to capture attention.
  - Minimize error responses.
  - Provide opportunity for repetition of information to be learned or strengthened.
  - Provide opportunity for elaborate encoding to build strong engrams.
- To facilitate the retrieval of information, take the following into account:
  - Recognition of information is easier than free recall of information.
  - Priming facilitates recall.
  - Use retrieval cues that reflect support given at encoding.
  - Provide cognitive stimulation.
  - Avoid having individuals with dementia multitask
  - Allow more time for responding.
- The human brain continuously remodels its neural circuitry as a function of experience. Neural circuits not actively engaged will ultimately degrade.

- With greater understanding and awareness of this fact, the demand for cognitive stimulation to facilitate the remodeling of neural circuitry will dramatically increase.

References

Abrahams, J. P., & Camp, C. J. (1993). Maintenance and generalization of object naming training in anomia associated with degenerative dementia. *Clinical Gerontology, 12,* 57–72.

Adams, P. F., & Marano, M. A. (1995). Current estimates from the National Health Interview Survey, 1994: National Center for Health Statistics. *Vital Health Statistics 10, 193,* 83–84.

Allen, N. H., Burns, A., Newton, V., Hickson, F., Ramsden, R., Rogers, J., Butler, et al. (2003). The effects of improving hearing in dementia. *Age and Ageing, 32,* 189–193.

Ancoli-Israel, S., Martin, J., Gehrman, P., Shochat, T., Corey-Bloom, J., Marler, M., et al. (2003). Effect of light on agitation in institutionalized patients with severe Alzheimer disease. *American Journal of Geriatric Psychiatry, 11,* 194–203.

American Speech-Language-Hearing Association. (2004). *ASHA's Medicare handbook for speechlanguage pathologists.* Rockville, MD: Author.

Anderson, J. R. & Bower, G. H. (1972). *Human associative memory.* Washington, DC: Winston.

Arkin, S. M. (1992). Audio-assisted memory training with early Alzheimer's patients. *Clinical Gerontologist, 12,* 77–96.

Arkin, S. M., Rose, C., & Hopper, T. (2000). Implicit and explicit learning gains in Alzheimer's patients: Effects of naming and information retrieval training. *Aphasiology, 14,* 723–742.

Bäckman, L., & Small, B. (1998). Influences of cognitive support on episodic remembering: Tracing the process of loss from normal aging to Alzheimer's disease. *Psychology and Aging, 13,* 267–276.

Baddeley, A. D., & Wilson, B.A. (1994). When implicit learning fails: Amnesia and the problem of error elimination. *Neuropsychologia, 32,* 53–68.

Bayles, K. A., & Tomoeda, C. K. (1993). *Arizona Battery for Communication Disorders in Dementia.* Austin, TX: Pro-Ed.

Bayles, K. A., & Tomoeda, C. K. (1994). *Functional Linguistic Communication Inventory.* Austin, TX: Pro-Ed.

Bayles, K. A., & Tomoeda, C. K. (1997). *Improving function in dementia and other cognitive-linguistic disorders.* Austin, TX: Pro-Ed.

Bayles, K. A., Tomoeda, C. K., Kaszniak, A. W., & Trosset, M. W. (1991). Alzheimer's disease effects on semantic memory: Loss of structure or function. *Journal of Cognitive Neuroscience, 3,* 166–182.

Belleville, S., Peretz, I., & Malenfant, D. (1996). Examination of the working memory components in normal aging and in dementia of the Alzheimer type. *Neuropsychologia, 34,* 195–207.

Bird, M. J. (2000). Psychosocial rehabilitation for problems arising from cognitive deficits in dementia. In R. D. Hill, L. Bäckman, & A. Stigsdotter-Neely, (Eds.), *Cognitive rehabilitation in old age* (pp. 249–267). New York: Oxford University Press.

Bird, M., & Luszcz, M. (1991). Encoding specificity, depth of processing, and cued recall in Alzheimer's disease. *Journal of Clinical and Experimental Neuropsychology, 13,* 508–520.

Birren, J. E., Woods, A., & Williams, M. V. (1980). Behavioral slowing with age: Causes, organization, and consequences. In L. Poon (Ed.), *Aging in the 1980s* (pp. 293–308). Washington, DC: American Psychological Association.

Boczko, F. (1994). The Breakfast Club: A multimodal language stimulation program for nursing home residents with Alzheimer's disease. *American Journal of Alzheimer's Care and Related Disorders and Research, 9,* 35–38.

Bourgeois, M. S. (1990). Enhancing conversation skills in patients with Alzheimer's disease using a prosthetic memory aid. *Journal of Applied Behavior Analysis, 23,* 29–42.

Bourgeois, M. S. (1991). Communication treatment for adults with dementia. *Journal of Speech and Hearing Research, 34,* 831–844.

Bourgeois, M. S. (1992). Evaluating memory wallets in conversations with persons with dementia. *Journal of Speech and Hearing Research, 35,* 1344–1357.

Brawley, E. (1997). *Designing for Alzheimer's disease*. New York: John Wiley & Sons.

Brush, J. A., & Camp, C. J. (1998a). *A therapy technique for improving memory: Spaced retrieval*. Beachwood, OH: Authors.

Brush, J. A., & Camp, C. J. (1998b). Using spaced-retrieval as an intervention during speech-language therapy. *Clinical Gerontologist, 19*, 51–64.

Camicioli, R., Howieson, D., Lehman, S., & Kaye, J. (1997). Talking while walking: The effect of a dual task in aging and Alzheimer's disease. *Neurology, 48*, 955–958.

Camp, C. J. (1989). Facilitation of new learning in Alzheimer's disease. In G. C. Gilmore, P. J. Whitehouse, & M. L. Wykle (Eds.), *Memory, aging and dementia* (pp. 212–225). New York: Springer.

Camp, C. J. (1999). *Montessori-based activities for persons with dementia, Vol. 1*. Beachwood, OH: Meyers Research Institute.

Camp, C. J., Bird, M. J, & Cherry, K. E. (2000). Retrieval strategies as a rehabilitation aid for cognitive loss in pathological aging. In R.D. Hill, L. Bäckman, & A. Stigsdotter-Neely (Eds.), *Cognitive rehabilitation in old age* (pp. 224–248). New York: Oxford University Press.

Camp, C. J., & Brush, J. A. (1999). *Montessori-based interventions for persons with dementia*. University of Arizona, National Center for Neurogenic Communication Disorders Telerounds No. 46: National Videoconference Series. Tucson, AZ: Arizona Board of Regents.

Camp, C. J., & Schaller, J. R. (1989). Epilogue: Spaced-retrieval memory training in an adult day-center. *Educational Gerontology, 15*, 641–648.

Campbell, S. S., Kripke, D. F., Gillin, J. C., & Hrubovcak, J. C. (1988). Exposure to light in healthy elderly subjects and Alzheimer's patients. *Physiological Behavior, 42*, 141-144.

Cherry, B. J., Buckwalter, J. G., & Henderson, V. W. (1996). Memory span procedures in Alzheimer's disease. *Neuropsychology, 10*, 286–293.

Clare, L., Wilson, B. A., Carter, G., Breen, K., Gosses, A., & Hodges, J. R. (2000). Intervening with everyday memory problems in dementia of Alzheimer type: An errorless learning approach. *Journal of Clinical and Experimental Neuropsychology, 22*, 132–146.

Clark, L. (1975). *The ancient art of color therapy*. New York: Pocket Books.

Cofer, C. N. (1960). Experimental studies of the role of verbal processes in concept formation and problem solving. *Annals of the New York Academy of Sciences, 91*, 94–107.

Cooper, B. (1993). Long-term care design: Current research on the use of color. *The Journal of Healthcare Design, 6*, 61–67.

Cooper, B., Ward, M., Gowland, C., & McIntosh, J. (1991). The use of the Lanthony New Color Test in determining the effects of aging on color vision. *Journal of Gerontology, 46*, 320–324.

Cronin-Golomb, A., Corkin, S., & Growdon, J. H. (1991). Visual dysfunction in Alzheimer's disease: Relation to normal aging. *Annals of Neurology, 29*, 41–52.

Cronin-Golomb, A., Sugiura, R., Corkin, S., & Growdon, J. H. (1993). Incomplete achromatopsia in Alzheimer's disease. *Neurobiology of Aging, 14*, 471–477.

Cruickshanks, K. J., Tweed, T. S., Wiley, T. L., Klein, B. E. K., Klein, R., Chappell, R., et al. (2003). The 5-year incidence and progression of hearing loss: The epidemiology of hearing loss study. *Archives of Otolaryngology–Head and Neck Surgery, 129*, 1041–1046.

Cruickshanks, K. J., Wiley, T. L., Tweed, T. S., Klein, B. E. K., Klein, R., Mares-Perlman, J. A., et al. (1998). Prevalence of hearing loss in older adults in Beaver Dam, Wisconsin. *American Journal of Epidemiology, 148*, 879–886.

Damasio, A.R. (1999). *The feeling of what happens: Body and emotion in the making of consciousness*. New York: Harcourt, Brace.

Daneman, M., & Carpenter, P. A. (1980). Individual differences in working memory and reading. *Journal of Verbal Learning and Verbal Behavior, 19*, 450–466.

Darwin, C. (1872). *The expression of the emotions in man and animals*. London: Murray.

Davis, R. N., Massman, P. J., & Doody, R. S. (2001). Cognitive intervention in Alzheimer's disease: A randomized placebo-controlled study. *Alzheimer Disease and Associated Disorders, 15*, 1–9.

De Vreese, L. P., Neri, M., Fioravanti, M., Belloi, L. & Zanetti, O. (2001). Memory rehabilitation in Alzheimer's disease. *International Journal of Geriatric Psychiatry, 16*, 794–809.

Deweer, B., Pillon, B., Michon, A., & Dubois, F. (1993). Mirror reading in Alzheimer's disease: Normal skill learning and acquisition of item-specific information. *Journal of Clinical and Experimental Neuropsychology, 15*, 789–804.

Dick, M. B. (1992). Motor and procedural memory in Alzheimer's disease. In L. Bäckman (Ed.), *Memory functioning in dementia* (pp. 135–150). Amsterdam: North-Holland.

Dick, M. B., Hsieh, S., Bricker, J., & Dick-Muehlke, C. (2003). Facilitating acquisition and transfer of a continuous motor task in healthy older adults and patients with Alzheimer's disease. *Neuropsychology, 17*, 202–212.

Dick, M. B., Shankel, R. W., Beth, R. E., Dick-Muehlke, C., Cotman, C. W., & Kean, M. L. (1996). Acquisition and long-term retention of a fine motor skill in Alzheimer's disease. *Brain and Cognition, 29*, 294–306.

Diesfeldt, H. F. A. (1984). The importance of encoding instructions and retrieval cues in the assessment of memory in senile dementia. *Archives of Gerontology and Geriatrics, 3*, 51–57.

Duchek, J. M., Hunt, L., Ball, K., Buckles, V., & Morris, J. C. (1997). The role of selective attention in driving and dementia of the Alzheimer type. *Alzheimer Disease and Associated Disorders, 11*(Suppl. 1), 48–56.

Dreher, B. B. (1997). Montessori and Alzheimer's: A partnership that works. *American Journal of Alzheimer's Disease, 12*, 138–140.

Emery, V. O. B. (2003). Retrophylogenesis. In V. O. B. Emery & T. E. Oxman (Eds.), *Dementia* (pp. 177–236). Baltimore: The Johns Hopkins University Press.

Engelkamp, J., & Zimmer, H. D. (1989). Memory for action events: A new field of research. *Psychological Research, 51*, 153–157.

Fangmeier, R. (1994). *The world through their eyes: Understanding vision loss.* New York: The Lighthouse.

Filoteo, J. V., Delis, D. C., Massman, P. J., Demadura, T., Butters, N. & Salmon, D. P. (1992). Directed and divided attention in Alzheimer's disease: Impairment in shifting attention to global and local stimuli. *Journal of Clinical and Experimental Neuropsychology, 14*, 871–883.

Fontaine, F. (1995). *Apprentissage de nouvelles connaissances chez les patients Alzheimer* [Acquisition of new knowledge in Alzheimer patients]. Unpublished doctoral dissertation, Université de Montreal.

Foster, N. A., & Valentine, E. R. (2001). The effect of auditory stimulation on autobiographical recall in dementia. *Experimental Aging Research, 27*, 215–228.

Gates, G. A., Cobb, J. L., Linn, R. T., Rees, T., Wolf, P. A., & D'Agostino, R. B. (1996). Central auditory dysfunction, cognitive dysfunction, and dementia in older people. *Archives of Otolaryngology–Head and Neck Surgery, 122*, 161–167.

Gillies, C., & James, A. (1994). *Reminiscence work with old people.* London: Chapman & Hall.

Glasgow, R. E., Zeiss, R. A., Barrera, M., & Lewinshon, P. M. (1977). Case studies on remediating memory deficits in brain-injured patients. *Journal of Clinical Psychology, 33*, 1049–1054.

Glisky, E. L. (1997). Rehabilitation and memory disorders: Tapping into preserved mechanisms. *Brain and Cognition, 35*, 291–292.

Glisky, E. L., Schacter, D. L., & Tulving, E. (1986). Learning and retention of computer-related vocabulary in memory-impaired patients: Method of vanishing cues. *Journal of Clinical and Experimental Neuropsychology, 8*, 292–312.

Gold, M., Lightfoot, L. A., & Hnath-Chisolm, T. (1996). Hearing loss in a memory disorders clinic: An especially vulnerable population. *Archives of Neurology, 53*, 922–928.

Green, R. L. (1992). *Human memory: Paradigms and paradoxes.* Hillsdale, NJ: Lawrence Erlbaum Associates.

Grober, E., Ausubel, R., Sliwinski, M., & Gordon, B. (1992). Skill learning and repetition priming in Alzheimer's disease. *Neuropsychologia, 30*, 849–858.

Halle, J. W., & Spradlin, J. E. (1993). Identifying stimulus control of challenging behavior. In J. Reichle & D. W. Wacker (Eds.), *Communicative alternatives to challenging behavior: Integrating functional assessment and intervention strategies* (pp. 83–109). Baltimore: Paul H. Brookes.

Hasher, L. & Zacks, R. T. (1979) Automatic and effortful processes in memory. *Journal of Experimental Psychology: General, 108*, 356–388.

Hellen, C. R. (1992). *Alzheimer's disease: Activity-focused care.* Newton, MA: Butterworth-Heinemann.

Herbst, K. G., & Humphrey, C. (1980). Hearing impairment and mental state in the elderly living at home. *British Medical Journal, 281,* 903–905.

Herlitz, A., & Viitanen, M. (1991). Semantic organisation and verbal episodic memory in patients with mild and moderate Alzheimer's disease. *Journal of Clinical and Experimental Neuropsychology, 13,* 559–574.

Heun, R., Burkart, M., & Benkert, O. (1997). Improvement of picture recall by repetition in patients with dementia of the Alzheimer type. *International Journal of Geriatric Psychiatry, 12,* 85–92.

Hodkinson, H. (1973). Mental impairment in the elderly. *Journal of the Royal College of Physicians London, 7,* 305.

Hull, R. H. (1995). *Hearing in aging.* San Diego, CA: Singular.

Jacquemin, A., Van der Linden, M., & Feyereisen, P. (1993). Thérapie du manque du mot chez un patient bilingue présentant une maladie d'Alzheimer probable. *Questions de Logopédie, 27,* 91–96.

Jerger, J., Chmiel, R., Wilson, N., & Luchi, R. (1995). Hearing impairment in older adults: New concepts. *Journal of the American Geriatrics Society, 43,* 928–935.

Johansson B. B. (2000). Brain plasticity and stroke rehabilitation. The Willis lecture. *Stroke, 31,* 223–230.

Johansson B. B. (2003). Environmental influence on recovery after brain lesions—experimental and clinical data. *Journal of Rehabilitation Medicine, 41*(Suppl.), 11–16.

Jones T. A., Bury, S. D., Adkins-Muir, D. L., Luke, L. M., Allred, R. P., & Sakata, J. T. (2003). Importance of behavioral manipulations and measures in rat models of brain damage and brain repair. *ILAR Journal, 44,* 144–152.

Jones, T. A., Hawrylak, N., Klintsova, A. Y., & Greenough W. T. (1998). Brain damage, behavior, rehabilitation, recovery, and brain plasticity. *Mental Retardation and Developmental Disabilities Research Reviews, 4,* 231–237.

Just, M. A., Carpenter, P. A., Keller, T. A., Emery, L., Zajac, H., & Thulborn, K. R. (2001). Interdependence of nonoverlapping cortical systems in dual cognitive tasks. *NeuroImage, 14,* 417–426.

Karlsson, T., Bäckman, L., Herlitz, A., Nilsson, L.-G., Winblad, B., & Österlind, P.-O. (1989). Memory improvement at different stages of Alzheimer's disease. *Neuropsychologia, 27,* 737–742.

Keane, M. M., Gabrieli, J. D. E., Fennema, A. C., Growdon, J. H., & Corkin, S. (1991). Evidence for a dissociation between perceptual and conceptual priming in Alzheimer's disease. *Behavioral Neuroscience, 105,* 326–342.

Kintsch, W. (1970). Models for free recall and recognition. In D. A. Norman (Ed.), *Models of human memory* (pp. 333–374). New York: Academic Press.

Kleim J. A., & Jones, T. A. (in press). Principles of experience-dependent neural plasticity: Implications for rehabilitation after brain damage. *Journal of Speech, Language, Hearing Research.*

Kliegl, R., Smith, J., & Baltes, P. B. (1989). Testing-the-limits of the study of adult age differences in cognitive plasticity of a mnemonic skill. *Developmental Psychology, 25,* 247–256.

Kreeger, J. L., Raulin, M. L., Grace, J., & Priest, B. L. (1995). Effect of hearing enhancement on mental status ratings in geriatric psychiatric patients. *American Journal of Psychiatry, 152,* 629–631.

LaBar, K. S., Mesulam, M. M., Gitelman, D. R., & Weintraub, S. (2000). Emotional curiosity: Modulation of visuospatial attention by arousal is preserved in aging and early-stage Alzheimer's disease. *Neuropsychologia, 38,* 1734–1740.

Landauer, T. K., & Bjork, R. A. (1978). Optimum rehearsal patterns and name learning. In M. M. Gruneberg, P. E. Morriss, & R. N. Sykes (Eds.), *Practical aspects of memory* (pp. 625–632). New York: Academic Press.

Leng, N. R. C., Copello, A. G., & Sayegh, A. (1991). Learning after brain injury by the method of vanishing cues: A case study. *Behavioural Psychotherapy, 19,* 173–181.

Lipinska, B., Bäckman, L., Mäntylä, T., & Viitanen, M. (1994). Effectiveness of self-generated cues in early Alzheimer's disease. *Journal of Clinical and Experimental Neuropsychology, 16,* 809–816.

Little, A. G., Volans, P. J., Hemsley, D. R., & Levy, R. (1986). The retention of new information in senile dementia. *British Journal of Clinical Psychology, 25,* 71–72.

Mahendra, N. (November, 1999). Manipulation of working memory through sensory stimulation. In Bayles, K. A., Hopper, T, Mahendra, N., Cleary, S., & Tomoeda, C. K., *What works with dementia patients and why.* Short course presented at the American Speech-Language-Hearing Association Convention, San Francisco, CA.

Mahendra, N. (2001). Direct interventions for improving the performance of individuals with Alzheimer's disease. *Seminars in Speech and Language, 22,* 291–304.

Mahendra, N., Bayles, K. A., & Harris, F. P. (2005). Effect of presentation modality on immediate and delayed recall in individuals with Alzheimer's disease. *American Journal of Speech-Language Pathology, 14,* 144–155.

Martin, G., & Pear, J. (1996). *Behavior modification. What it is and how to do it.* Upper Saddle River, NJ: Prentice-Hall.

McCarthy, D. L. (1980). Investigation of a visual imagery mnemonic device for acquiring name-face associations. *Journal of Experimental Psychology: Human Learning and Memory, 6,* 145–155.

McKitrick, L. A., & Camp, C. J. (1993). Relearning the names of things: The spaced retrieval intervention implemented by caregivers. *Clinical Gerontology, 14,* 60–62.

Mitchell, D. B., Hunt, R. R., & Schmitt, F. A. (1986). The generation effect and reality monitoring: Evidence from dementia and normal aging. *Journal of Gerontology, 41,* 79–84.

Moayeri, S. E., Cahill, L., Jin, Y., & Potkin, S. G. (2000). Relative sparing of emotionally influenced memory in Alzheimer's disease. *NeuroReport, 11,* 643–645.

Moffat, N. J. (1989). Home-based cognitive rehabilitation with the elderly. In L. Poon, D. C. Rubin, & B.A. Wilson (Eds.), *Everyday cognition in adulthood and late life* (pp. 659–690). Cambridge: Cambridge University Press.

Moffat, N. (1992). Strategies of memory therapy. In B. A. Wilson & N. Moffat (Eds.), *Clinical management of memory problems* (2nd ed., pp. 86–119). London: Chapman & Hall.

Monfils M. H., Plautz, E. J., & Kleim J. A. (2005). In search of the motor engram: Motor map plasticity as a mechanism for encoding motor experience. *Neuroscientist, 11,* 471–483.

National Institute on Aging. (1995). *Aging and your eyes.* AgePages. Bethesda, MD: Author (http://www.healthandage.com/html/min/nih/content/eyes.htm)

Newman, S. D., Keller, T. A., & Just, M. A. (2007). Volitional control of attention and brain activation in dual task performance. *Human Brain Mapping, 28,* 109-117.

Ochsner, K. N, Chiu, C- Y. P., & Schacter, D. L. (1994). Varieties of priming. *Current Biology, 4,* 189–194.

Ohta, R. J., Carlin, M. R., & Harmon, B. M. (1981). Auditory acuity and performance on the mental status questionnaire in the elderly. *Journal of the American Geriatrics Society, 27,* 476–478.

Omnibus Budget Reconciliation Act of 1987. (1987). Public Law No. 100–203, 483.15.

Orsulic-Jeras, S., Judge, K. S., & Camp, C. J. (2000). Use of Montessori-based activities for clients with dementia in adult day care: Effects on engagement and affect. *Gerontologist, 40,* 107–111.

Palmer, C. V., Adams, S. W., Bourgeois, M., Durrant, J., & Rossi, M. (1999). Reduction in caregiver-identified problem behaviors in patients with Alzheimer disease post-hearing-aid fitting. *Journal of Speech, Language, and Hearing Research, 42,* 312–328.

Palmer, C. V., Adams, S. W., Durrant, J. D., Bourgeois, M., & Rossi, M. (1998). Managing hearing loss in a patient with Alzheimer's disease. *Journal of the American Academy of Audiology, 9,* 275–284.

Perlmuter, L. C., & Monty, R. A. (1989). Motivation and aging. In L. Poon, D. C. Rubin, & B. A. Wilson (Eds.), *Everyday cognition in adulthood and late life* (pp. 373–393). Cambridge: Cambridge University Press.

Perry, R. J., Watson, P. & Hodges, J. R. (2000). The nature and staging of attention dysfunction in early (minimal and mild) Alzheimer's disease: Relationship to episodic and semantic memory impairment. *Neuropsychologia, 38,* 252–271.

Quayhagen, M. P., & Quayhagen, M. (1989). Differential effects of family based strategies on Alzheimer's disease. *The Gerontologist, 29,* 150–155.

Rees, G., Frith, C. D., & Lavie, N. (1997). Modulating irrelevant motion perception by varying attentional load in an unrelated task. *Science, 278,* 1616–1619.

Ries, P. W. (1994). Prevalence and characteristics of persons with hearing trouble: United States, 1990-1991. National Center for Health Statistics. *Vital Health Statistics 10, 188,* 1–75.

Salmon, D. P., Heindel, W. C., & Butters, N. (1992). Semantic memory, priming and skill learning in Alzheimer's disease. *Advances in Psychology, 89,* 99–118.

Satlin, A., Volicer, L., Ross, V., Herz, L., & Campbell, S. (1992). Bright light treatment of behavioral and sleep disturbances in patients with Alzheimer's disease. *American Journal of Psychiatry, 149,* 1028–1032.

Schacter, D. L., Rich, S. A., & Stampp, M. S. (1985). Remediation of memory disorders: An experimental evaluation of the spaced retrieval technique. *Journal of Clinical and Experimental Neuropsychology, 7,* 79–96.

Schieber, F. (2006). Vision and aging. In J. E. Birren & K. W. Schaie (Eds.), *Handbook of the psychology of aging* (6th ed., pp. 129–161). Burlington, MA: Elsevier.

Schow, R., & Nerbonne, M. (1980). Hearing levels among elderly nursing home residents. *Journal of Speech and Hearing Disorders, 45,* 124–132.

Sheridan, C. (1995). Reminiscence. In Alzheimer's Association, *Activity programming for persons with dementia: A sourcebook.* Chicago: The Alzheimer's Association.

Singer, C., & Hughes, R. (1995, March). Clinical use of bright light in geriatric neuropsychiatry. *Lighting for Aging Vision and Health,* (LRI-1995), pp. 143–146. (http://www.epri.com/LRO/publication.html)

Slamecka, N. J., & Graf, P. (1978). The generation effect: Delineation of a phenomenon. *Human Learning and Memory, 4,* 592–604.

Small, J. A., Kemper, S., & Lyons, K. (1997). Sentence comprehension in Alzheimer's disease: Effects of grammatical complexity, speech rate, and repetition. *Psychology and Aging, 12,* 3–11.

Stevens, A., King, C. A., & Camp, C. J. (1993). Improving prose memory and social interaction using question asking reading with adult day care clients. *Educational Gerontology, 19,* 651–662.

Storms, L. H. (1958). Apparent backward association: A situational effect. *Journal of Experimental Psychology, 55,* 390–395.

Thornton, S., & Brotchie, J. (1987). Reminiscence: A critical review of the empirical literature. *British Journal of Clinical Psychology, 26,* 93–111.

Tulving, E., & Schacter, D. L. (1990). Priming and human memory systems. *Science, 247,* 301–306.

Tulving, E., & Thomson, D. M. (1973). Encoding specificity and retrieval processes in episodic memory. *Psychological Review, 80,* 352–373.

Uhlmann, R. F., Larson, E. B., & Koepsell, T. D. (1986). Hearing impairment and cognitive decline in senile dementia of the Alzheimer's type. *Journal of the American Geriatrics Society, 34,* 207–210.

Uhlmann, R. F., Larson, E. B., Rees, T. S., Koepsell, T. D., & Duckert, L.G. (1989). Relationship of hearing impairment to dementia and cognitive dysfunction in older adults. *Journal of the American Medical Association, 261,* 1916–1919.

Van der Linden, M., & Coyette. F. (1995). Acquisition of word processing knowledge in an amnesic patient: Implications for theory and rehabilitation. In R. Campbell & M. Conway (Eds.), *Broken memories: Neuropsychological case studies* (pp. 54–80). Oxford: Blackwell.

Van der Linden, M., & Van der Kaa, M. M. (1989). Reorganization therapy for memory impairments. In X. Seron & G. Deloche (Eds.), *Cognitive approaches in neuropsychological rehabilitation* (pp. 105–158). Hillsdale, NJ: Lawrence Erlbaum Associates.

Vance, D., Camp, C. J., Kabacoff, M., & Greenwalk, L. (1996). Montessori methods: Innovative interventions for adults with Alzheimer's disease. *Montessori Life, 8,* 10–12.

Vance, D. E., & Porter, R. J. (2000). Montessori methods yield cognitive gains in Alzheimer's day cares. *Activities, Adaptation and Aging, 24,* 1–21.

Vandenberghe, R., Duncan, J., Dupont, P., Ward, R., Pline, J.-B, Bormans, G., et al. (1997). Attention to one or two features in left or right visual field: A positron emission tomography study. *Journal of Cognitive Neuroscience, 9,* 419–432.

Vanhalle, C., Van der Linden, M., Belleville, S., & Gilbert, B. (1998). Putting names on faces: Use of spaced retrieval strategy in a patient with dementia of Alzheimer type. American Speech Language & Hearing Association, Special Interest Division 2 Newsletter. *Neurophysiology and Neurogenic Speech and Language Disorders, 8,* 17–21.

Ventry, I. M., & Weinstein, B. E. (1983). Identification of elderly people with hearing problems. *ASHA, 25,* 37–42.

Verfaellie, M., Keane, M. M., & Johnson, G. (2000). Preserved priming in auditory perceptual identification in Alzheimer's disease. *Neuropsychologia, 38,* 1581–1792.

Verhaeghen, P., Marcoen, A., & Goossens, L. (1992). Improving memory performance in the aged through mnemonic training: A meta-analytic study. *Psychology and Aging, 7,* 242–251.

Voeks, S., Gallager, C., Langer, E., & Drinka, P. (1990). Hearing loss in the nursing home: An institutional issue. *Journal of the American Geriatrics Society, 38,* 141–145.

Wechsler, D. (1999). *Wechsler Memory Scale-Third Edition.* San Antonio, TX: Harcourt Assessment.

Weinstein, B. E., & Amsel, L. (1986). Hearing loss and senile dementia in the institutionalized elderly. *Clinical Gerontologist, 4,* 3–15.

Wilson, B. A., Baddeley, A., Evans, J., & Shiel, A. (1994). Errorless learning in the rehabilitation of memory impaired people. *Neuropsychological Rehabilitation, 4,* 307–326.

Wilson, B. A., & Moffat, N. (1992). The development of group memory therapy. In B. A. Wilson & N. Moffat (Eds.), *Clinical management of memory problems* (2nd ed., pp. 243–273). London: Chapman & Hall.

Winter, J., & Hunkin, N. M. (1999). Re-learning in Alzheimer's disease. *International Journal of Geriatric Psychiatry, 14,* 988–990.

Yesavage, J. A., Rose, T. L., & Bower, G. H. (1983). Interactive imagery and affective judgments improve face-name learning in the elderly. *Journal of Gerontology, 38,* 197–203.

Ylvisaker, M. & Feeney, T. (2002). Executive functions, self-regulation, and learned optimism in pediatric rehabilitation: A review and implications for intervention. *Pediatric Rehabilitation, 5,* 51–70.

Zanetti, O., Binetti, G., Magni, E., Rozzini, L., Bianchetti, A., & Trabucchi, M. (1997). Procedural memory stimulation in Alzheimer's disease: Impact of a training program. *Acta Neurologica Scandinavia, 95,* 152–157.

Zanetti, O., Zanieri, G., Di Giovanni, G., De Vreese, L. P., Pezzini, A., Metitieri, T., et al. (2001). Effectiveness of procedural memory stimulation in mild Alzheimer's disease patients. A controlled study. *Neuropsychological Rehabilitation, 11,* 263–272.

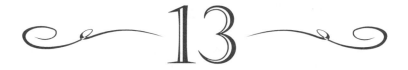

Treating Cognitive-Communicative Disorders of Dementia: Indirect Interventions

Whereas direct interventions were the focus of Chapter 12, indirect interventions are the focus of this chapter. Indirect interventions involve modifying the linguistic and physical environments of individuals with dementia to improve cognitive-communicative functioning and quality of life. SLPs do not carry out indirect interventions but recommend them in care plans, teach them to caregivers, and oversee their implementation. Medicare will pay for the development of functional maintenance plans, caregiver training, and the oversight of implementation of indirect interventions.

interventions are extrinsic environmental supports for orientation, prospective memory, communication, executive functioning, and ADLs. They can provide reminders, cue and monitor performance, alert caregivers to problems, expose patients to virtual environments, stimulate communication, and help people compensate for sensory loss. Although the application of ATC to the treatment of individuals with progressive dementia is still in its infancy, reports to date are encouraging especially regarding prospective memory aids (see LoPresti, Mihailidis, & Kirsch, 2004, for a review)

Computer Technology: An Indirect Intervention

Advances in computer technology are increasingly being used to support the functioning of cognitively and communicatively impaired individuals. "Cognitive prostheses" or "cognitive orthoses" are collectively known as ATC, or assistive technology for cognition (LoPresti, Mihailidis, & Kirsch, 2004). ATC

Prospective Memory Aids

Many prospective memory aids are commercially available. Most are pocket-sized devices that can record and play back verbal messages. They contain software that stores a schedule (and in some cases, other information) and sophisticated models can send and receive information. These aids can signal users to do scheduled things through auditory and/or visual cues.

Zanetti, Zanieri, Vreese, Frisoni, and Binetti (2000) studied the ability of mild and moderate AD patients to use a prospective memory aid, specifically an electronic agenda. Five subjects were given seven memory tasks to complete at fixed times over the course of a day. Task completion with and without the device was compared. When the electronic agenda was available, task completion significantly improved and two of the subjects had perfect scores.

Mihailidis, Fernie, and Barbenel (2001) used artificial intelligence to develop COACH (Cognitive Orthosis for Assisting aCtivities in the Home), a device to help individuals with dementia complete the task of handwashing. COACH uses artificial intelligence algorithms and a video camera connected to a computer to monitor handwashing and provides prerecorded verbal prompts. It was tested for 60 days with 10 individuals with moderate to severe dementia. Results showed that the number of handwashing steps completed without caregiver assistance increased by 25% when group data were analyzed. Systems like COACH could be used to support myriad other activities.

Augmenting Short-Term Memory to Support Conversation

A multidisciplinary team in Scotland designed a conversation support and prompting system for people with dementia (Alm, Astell, Ellis, Dye, Gowans, & Campbell, 2004). The system uses touch screen technology to access a multimedia reminiscence presentation that prompts conversation. The rationale for the system's development is the difficulty that dementia patients have conversing because of deficits in the ability to freely recall information and events. The conversation support system compensates for that difficulty. It provides information that dementia patients have difficulty recalling but

retain in long-term memory thereby stimulating reminiscence. Results of a pilot study show that the reminiscence presentation system maintains the interest of individuals with dementia, is easy to use, and gives the patient control over the communication interaction. Staff and family members also responded positively to the system and modifications are underway to increase the quantity and quality of the communication the systems prompts.

Life-History Videos

Multimedia systems can be used to make life-history videos of people with dementia (Cohen, 2000). If available, they could serve many purposes: acquainting staff with patients, helping patients maintain memory of life events, stimulating conversation, and providing comfort to agitated patients.

Robots

Even robots are being developed to assist elders. They can be programmed with information about the elder's daily activities and have the capacity to provide needed reminders (Ramakrishnan & Pollack, 2000). Also their sensing systems can detect problems and alert caregivers.

A House as a Cognitive Orthotic

Mynatt, Essa, and Rogers (2000) have described their concept of an "instrumented environment" or house. It will have information about the inhabitants' activities and life style and contain sensors that detect task disruptions. Various auditory and visual cuing systems throughout the house will assist inhabitants in the completion of multistep activities (e.g., washing clothes, making breakfast, emptying the trash). Finally, the sensors will be used to detect the need for emergency assistance.

Virtual Reality Technology

Virtual reality (VR) technology is designed to simulate natural environments and its potential for assessment and rehabilitation of cognitively impaired individuals is mind-boggling. As Rizzo, Schultheis, Kerns, and Mateer (2004) point out, within virtual environments (VEs), researchers and clinicians can present ecologically relevant stimuli with exquisite control to teach desired behaviors and foster their generalization to real world contexts. VR also has potential for nurturing and entertaining people with dementia. Gaming activities can be integrated into VR-based rehabilitation systems to increase client motivation. As Rizzo et al. (2004) wrote, "More believable virtual humans inhabiting VEs would open up possibilities for assessment and rehabilitation scenarios that target social interaction, naturalistic communication and awareness of social cues" (p. 207).

The challenge of providing quality care for people with dementia is to engage them in enjoyable activities *all day every day*. Through advances in computer technology, clinicians and caregivers will have more tools for meeting this challenge. One can imagine that prospective memory aids, robotics, "instrumented" environments, multimedia, and virtual environments will support independence and increase safety.

Linguistic Manipulations

Numerous linguistic manipulations help dementia patients communicate by facilitating cognitive processing. They can be classi-

fied according to their impact on language comprehension and production.

Improving Language Comprehension

Language comprehension is a complex, multistage process (Rochon, Waters, & Caplan, 2000). Listeners must analyze the form, content, and context in which an utterance is spoken to derive the proposition(s) being expressed. Thus, techniques for facilitating comprehension can be subcategorized according to whether they involve primarily the form, content, or use of language.

Form

Use a Slower Than Normal Rate of Speech. As previously mentioned, the brain damage associated with dementing diseases results in slower information processing as does normal aging. By slowing the rate of speech, the load on memory is reduced because the more words spoken per minute, the more concepts the individual must process. The average rate of speech is 160 to170 words per minute but fast speakers produce 200 or more words per minute. Calculate your normal rate of speech and if you are a fast speaker, slow your rate to slightly less than average.

Provide Multimodal Input. For most individuals, learning and comprehension are better when information is experienced in more than one modality. Hearing information and being able to review it in written form is better than simply hearing it because of the rapid forgetting that characterizes many types of dementia. Providing information in one sensory modality and then another also capitalizes on the value of repetition for strengthening encoding. For example, to teach a name, it is better to explain the name, show the patient its written form, then have the patient read the name, write the name, and associate it with a face or picture that can be described.

Because Alzheimer's dementia patients retain the ability to read words far into the course of the disease, it is generally helpful to use the visual modality in addition to the auditory modality, for providing information. Similarly, because they have difficulty holding information in mind, it is better to provide the object being discussed (Hopper, Bayles, & Tomoeda, 1998).

Limit the Number of Conversational Partners. Keeping track of the topic, and who said what to whom, when several people are conversing, can overwhelm dementia patients because of deficits in attention and memory (Baddeley, Baddeley, Bucks, & Wilcock, 2001; Collette, Van der Linden, & Salmon, 1999). Many caregivers fail to appreciate this fact and are surprised when their dementia patient becomes agitated at large family gatherings. Dementia patients do best communicating one on one (Figure 13–1).

Use a Pleasant Accepting Vocal Tone. Everyone becomes uncomfortable when someone speaks in an unfriendly tone. Even dementia patients, who no longer have the capacity to process word meaning, respond to the prosodic and emotional characteristics of speech. Clinicians and caregivers who use an accepting vocal tone evoke a positive reaction from the patient. People who use a condescending or threatening tone create emotional distress that interferes with comprehension.

Content

Reduce the Number of Propositions in Sentences. The greater the number of propositions, the more cognitive resources listeners must garner to interpret and act on the message. Rochon, Waters, and Caplan (2000) administered a battery of working memory and sentence comprehension tests to AD patients and age- and education-matched elders. Individuals with AD were found to have reduced spans and impaired central

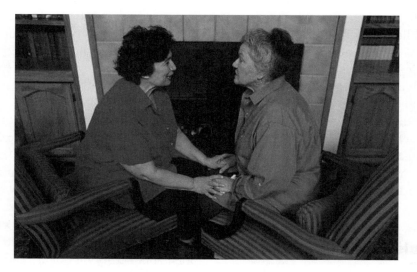

Figure 13–1. Limit the number of conversational partners. Individuals with dementia do best when communicating in a one-to-one situation.

executive processes. Rochon and colleagues observed that the number of propositions in stimulus sentences affected the performance of AD patients. When sentences contained a single proposition, AD patients performed like normal elders; when they contained two propositions, AD patient performance was significantly inferior to that of normal elders.

By simplifying syntax the number of propositions can be reduced. Consider the differences in cognitive demand of the following sentences.

1. **One proposition:** The airplane arrived late.
2. **Two propositions:** The airplane, that was coming from Seattle to Phoenix, arrived late. (*proposition 1: airplane was late; proposition 2: the airplane was coming from Seattle to Phoenix*)
3. **Three propositions:** He was traveling from Seattle to Phoenix on a recently refurbished airplane that took off late. (*proposition 1: he was traveling from Seattle to Phoenix ;proposition 2: the airplane was recently refurbished; proposition 3: the airplane took off late*)
4. **Four propositions:** The airplane, that was coming from Seattle, was late, but the airplane, that was coming from Phoenix, was early. (*proposition 1: the airplane was late; proposition 2: the airplane was coming from Seattle; proposition 3: the airplane was early; proposition 4: the airplane was coming from Phoenix*)

Simple subject-verb-object sentences, like sentence 1, require the fewest cognitive resources because they are the least demanding on memory. When embedded clauses are added, as in sentence 2, memory load is increased. Embedded clauses interrupt the main clause (airplane arrived late) and the listener must hold part of the main clause (airplane) in memory while processing the

embedded clause (that was coming from Seattle to Phoenix). Sentence 3 contains multiple propositions and embedding. In sentence 4, two main clauses are conjoined by a conjunction and both contain an embedded relative clause. Four propositions are expressed. Conjoining propositions increases memory load as does embedding.

Left-branching sentences with an initial dependent clause, such as "When he was traveling from Seattle to Phoenix, he developed air sickness," are harder to process than right-branching sentences, such as "He developed air sickness when he was traveling from Seattle to Phoenix." Dependent clauses occurring before the main clause must be held in mind until the listener/reader comes to the main clause.

Talk About the Here and Now. Because dementia patients have difficulty recalling episodic information, they do best when the conversation concerns something they can see and feel, in other words, something to which they can refer. Doing an activity with the patient provides something to talk about. Many clinicians have observed that patients talk more when doing an activity. Myriad activities like arranging flowers, building an object, sewing, and painting provide a topic for conversation about the here and now.

Simplify Vocabulary. All of us have stronger engrams for simple, high-frequency words than infrequently used words. The same is true for individuals with dementia. Thus, it is important to share information using common, high-frequency words. Although sentences A and B express the same meaning, sentence B is easier to comprehend.

A. The philatelist was a centenarian.
B. The stamp collector was a hundred years old.

Replace Pronouns with Proper Nouns. All pronouns have antecedents that must be remembered for pronoun and sentence comprehension. Dementia patients with episodic memory deficits have difficulty remembering antecedents. By repeating the proper noun, rather than using a pronoun, as in sentence 2, memory load is reduced and comprehension facilitated (Almor, Kempler, MacDonald, Andersen, & Tyler, 1999)

1. John and Mary went to see Bill before he left for college. They wanted to wish him well.
2. John and Mary went to see Bill before *Bill* left for college. *John and Mary* wanted to wish *Bill* well.

Revise and Restate That Which Was Not Understood. Occasionally, more than one explanation of a phenomenon or event is needed for us to comprehend. All of us know that some explanations are more comprehensible than others. When a dementia patient fails to comprehend, revising and restating the information may improve comprehension especially if done in a non-condescending way.

Use

Ask Multiple-Choice or Yes/No Questions. Some question forms are less cognitively demanding than others. Open-ended questions like "What did you do last night?" place your conversational partner in a free-recall situation. With a moment's reflection, healthy adults can mentally reconstruct the events of the previous night; however, individuals with AD and other dementias associated with episodic memory impairment cannot. Although questions like, "What do you want for dinner?" do not place individuals in a free-recall situation, they nonetheless pose difficulty because they require the generation of possibilities. Generating ideas is

another cognitive ability impaired early in dementia. Choice questions, like "Would you like chicken or steak for dinner?" do not place patients in a free recall situation or require them to generate possibilities, they simply make a choice. In Table 13–1 are examples of difficult and easier types of questions.

Use Direct Rather Than Indirect Speech Acts. Indirect speech acts are best explained by example. Frequently used ones are where person A says to person B, "Can you pass the sugar?" or "Why can't I ever find the TV guide?" In both of these examples, person A *is making a request* of the listener indirectly *by asking a question*. Being indirect is a way of being polite. When people are direct and say, "Pass the sugar" or "Find the TV guide," they can be perceived as demanding and rude. Nonetheless, direct statements, politely

Table 13–1. Difficult and Easy Types of Questions

Difficult types of questions:
Open-ended free recall:
Of the places you have visited, what are your favorites?
Open-ended generative:
What should we buy Susan for her birthday?
Easier types of questions:
Two-choice:
Did you like Hawaii or the Caribbean islands better?
Should we buy Susan a necklace or clock for her birthday?
Yes/No:
Do you like to travel?
Do you want to buy Susan a clock for her birthday?

worded, are often easier for dementia patients to understand, for example, "Please pass the sugar" or "Please help me find the TV guide."

Avoid Teasing and Sarcasm. In many forms of teasing and sarcasm, the speaker exaggerates or says something not meant literally. For example the nurse who said, "You look so good today that I'll bet all the girls will be asking you for a date" confused a nursing home patient who interpreted her literally. The interpretation of teasing and sarcasm frequently require sensitivity to context, an activity that is beyond the capacity of many demented individuals.

Avoid Talking to the Patient Like a Child. Talking to the patient like a child is demeaning and provides a poor model for other caregivers. Many patients will be offended even if they are unable to articulate their perceptions.

Try Amplifying the Voice of the Speaker. Many caregivers report the effectiveness of assistive listening devices (Figure 13–2) in communicating with AD patients. Assistive listening devices look similar to a conventional body-worn hearing aid and serve to provide general sound level gain. They improve the speech-to-noise ratio and can help patients focus their attention. This is especially true if the caregiver has a soft voice.

Improving Production of Language

Provide Something Tangible and/or Visible to Stimulate Conversation

This strategy is similar to talking about the here and now and helps both production and comprehension because it gives the patient and caregiver a point of reference. Furthermore, the apprehension by the patient of the tangible/visible object causes con-

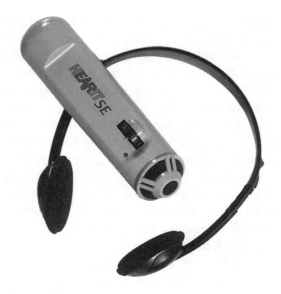

Figure 13–2. Example of an assistive listening device. Photo provided courtesy of Hearit LLC, a division of Speech Banana Therapies, http://www.hearitllc.com

cepts related to the object to be activated through the process of spreading activation. This often results in the patient being able to call to mind other information that can be shared in the conversation. Memory wallets and books containing information about the patient stimulate language production and are an excellent example of this technique. Bourgeois (1992) wrote a book about conversing with dementia patients through these memory assistive devices.

Bourgeois has shown that some dementia patients are more likely to make meaningful utterances when a memory wallet or book is the stimulus to conversation. The memory wallet is a compilation of pictures and sentences about the patient's life. The patient does not have to actively recall the pictured events, merely recognize them. Bourgeois observed that pictures and sentences enabled subjects in her studies to recall related information. The memory book is a larger version of the memory wallet. Memory books include biographical information and facts about people important to the patient that have been simply stated and paired with pictures and other memorabilia.

According to Bourgeois, mild dementia patients, those who score 19 to 24 on the MMSE, receive excellent benefit from the wallets and books. Then, too, mild patients are aware that they have the wallets and books and refer to them on their own. Moderately impaired patients, whose MMSE scores range between 12 and 18, typically require caregiver prompting to use the aids. Severely demented individuals, whose MMSE scores are lower than 12, may not benefit from the aids.

Hopper et al. (1998) used a single-subject experimental design with replications across subjects to investigate the efficacy of using dolls and stuffed animals to stimulate meaningful communication in four females with AD who were moderately demented. Study participants produced more relevant information units when the dolls and stuffed animals were used as conversational stimuli than when questions alone were used. Also, the AD patients clearly enjoyed the dolls and stuffed animals as evident by their increased animation when they were presented and their hugging and talking to them.

Avoid Placing Patients in a Free-Recall Situation. Recently we visited a patient and caregiver at home. Both greeted us at the door and the caregiver said, "You remember Cheryl and Kathryn, dear, they are here to test your memory." The patient responded, "Oh, yes, nice to see you again." Had the caregiver not provided our names and explained the purpose of our visit, the patient would have floundered and been embarrassed. The sensitivity of this caregiver to her spouse's inability to freely recall our names and appointment preserved his dignity. Clinicians should counsel caregivers to avoid placing the patient in a free-recall situation, especially in the presence of other people.

When the Patient Forgets the Topic, Summarize What Has Been Said. A classic problem for dementia patients is forgetting what they intended to say thereby causing the communicative interchange to fail. The thoughtful listener can summarize what has been said thereby allowing the patient to continue. This strategy helps the patient save face. The following is an example of the benefit of this strategy.

Context: An individual with dementia and her friend were talking during lunch that consisted of salad.

Patient: I used to have a garden and raised tomatoes. We would go out to the garden with a salt shaker you know and . . . (here the patient forgot what she was going to say), let me see, oh my, uh . . .

Caregiver: Going to the tomato garden with a salt shaker was a good way to get a snack.

Patient: Yes, we picked tomatoes and ate them right in the garden.

If the Patient Wishes to Write a Letter, Supply the Materials, a List of News Items, and a Picture of the Letter's Intended Recipient. This type of support makes it easier for the patient to be successful in producing a letter. Even healthy adults have trouble thinking of things to write. Having a few news items written down eliminates the need for the patient to remember and may stimulate related memories. Also, being able to see the person for whom the letter is intended helps the patient focus.

Have the Patient Read Aloud. Because the mechanics of reading remain intact for many patients late into the disease course, this is a language production activity they can do. One caregiver friend of ours had her husband read popular novels aloud while she worked in the kitchen preparing food. He felt useful and she enjoyed the story. We have heard many reports of elders with dementia who read story books to children in day care centers or their own grandchildren.

Do Not Repeatedly Correct the Patient. Dementia patients often make erroneous statements, and too often, caregivers embarrass them by correcting misinformation, particularly when other people are present. Once a patient has been put on the defensive, agitation and hostility may result, and he or she loses the desire to talk.

A strategy for indirectly correcting a patient who has an erroneous idea is to provide the correct information in the patient's memory wallet or scrapbook. Frequent use of the wallet or book may help the patient stay informed. One moderately demented AD patient repeatedly told caregivers that her son was coming home from school, and she needed to make supper. The caregiver put her son's picture in his Navy uniform on her nightstand and reviewed the fact of his being at sea daily. In a few days, the patient's confusion about her son's whereabouts

diminished, and she told people that her son was in the Navy.

Involve the Verbally Repetitious Patient in a Physical Activity to Reduce Perseveration. Admonishing repetitious patients to quit repeating is ineffective because their episodic memory problems cause them to forget admonitions. However, changing the activity, especially to one that is physical, may eliminate the cues that elicit the ideational repetition.

When moderate or late stage dementia patients produce disruptive vocalizations, it may be a sign they are experiencing physical discomfort, emotional distress, or have an unmet need (Sloane et al., 1997). Caregivers should be trained to consider these possibilities

Provide Food to Increase Sociability and Talking Among Patients. Refreshments create a social atmosphere and are a cultural trigger for conversation. Many long-term care facilities have programs in which residents gather daily to make breakfast and talk about world events (Figure 13–3). One program called, "The Breakfast Club," has

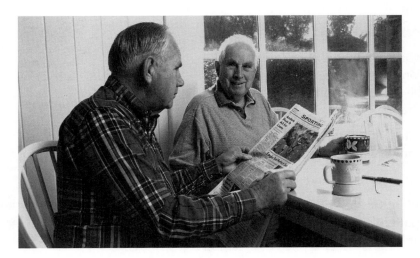

Figure 13–3. Providing refreshments or serving a meal creates a social context for communication.

been described by Boczko (1994) and Santo Pietro and Boczko (1998). Others have afternoon teatime. Many dementia patients enjoy preparing food and if done with supervision is a useful and pleasurable activity around which conversation can be built.

Environmental Manipulations

The goal of environmental manipulation is to create a safe, peaceful, and organized environment that evokes positive mood and behavior. The following suggestions will help achieve safety:

Remove guns or other weapons.

Lock up poisons, insecticides, solvents, paints, and medications.

Put a nightlight in the patient's bedroom and bathroom.

Install a safety gate at stairwells.

Fasten edges of rugs.

Secure sliding glass doors.

Place decals on glass doors.

Secure electric cords to prevent tripping.

Put on door locks that will prevent the patient from wandering away; however, be sure the patient has an exit in the event of fire.

Place a sturdy light by the patient's bed with a remote switch.

Put nonslip mats in tub and shower areas.

Have an identification bracelet made with the patient's name, address, and note about being memory impaired.

Give police a current photo or videotape of the patient.

Keep an article of worn clothing wrapped tightly in a plastic bag to be used to help track the lost patient.

Deter the patient from driving.

A safety issue for individuals with dementia and others is driving. Gilley and colleagues (1991) conducted a large study of driving and AD and discovered that the median duration of driving after disease onset was approximately 2½ years. Younger drivers and men were less likely to stop driving despite significant cognitive impairment. Twenty-two percent of the AD patients who were driving were involved in an accident in the previous 6 months. These investigators indicated that patients with MMSE scores of 18 or lower, who show evidence of visual spatial impairment, are unlikely to be safe drivers. Patients whose MMSE scores are 18 or higher and who have no visual spatial impairment or minimal impairment should be given an in-car driving evaluation to ensure that they can drive safely on familiar routes.

To create peaceful, organized environments that support basic ADLs, consider the following:

Keep the environment constant.

Minimize visual distractions.

Eliminate extraneous noise.

Remove clutter.

Keep needed objects visible (e.g., comb and brush).

Remove mirrors (patients may not recognize themselves and become alarmed at the presence of a "stranger").

Use orientation signs (e.g., bathroom, bedroom).

Display a calendar orienting the patient to the day's events, for example:

9:00	Get newspaper
10:00	Haircut at Sam's Barber Shop
11:00	Grocery store for milk
12:00	Lunch (egg salad sandwich and tomato soup)
1:00	Rest
3:00	Walk in the neighborhood
4:00	Visit from granddaughter Isabella
6:00	Dinner (chicken and rice)
Evening	Watch TV at home

The physical characteristics of an environment influence how people feel and respond. Each patient's environment should be analyzed in relation to what it evokes in terms of mood, language, and action. This analysis is particularly important for patients who are exhibiting negative behaviors and/ or are highly agitated. The following will help create a happy mood and positive behavior:

Accessible familiar objects

Pleasant aromas

Sufficient lighting

Culturally appropriate decor

Choice of well-liked foods

Pictures of past happy events

An energy outlet space where the patient can safely walk

Accessible craft materials and work tables

Music premorbidly preferred

Opportunities to do common procedures like folding laundry, raking leaves, setting the table

Regular touching through manicures, hair styling, massage

Dementia patients suffer confusion, and when left unoccupied, they often become agitated and afraid. Environments that provide stimulation, companionship, and opportunities for participating in activities combat the effects of confusion as well as improve the quality of life. The authors have an experience that demonstrates the truth of this statement. We went to a facility where dementia patients lived in an unstimulating environment to pilot-test the effect of various activities for engaging interest. The activities were singing, dancing, and bowling. The staff advised us that residents were unlikely to participate. But, in fact, the residents were very responsive to all three activities. We found that the musical activities stimulated singing, hand clapping, and smiles, and the majority of residents accepted our invitation to dance. Most of the ambulatory residents came outside with us for the bowling activity. Their attempts to throw the light-weight toy bowling ball were accompanied by laughter, and the activity of bowling brought to mind the language associated with bowling. Both the dancing and bowling provided needed exercise to residents. The personnel at the care facility were amazed at the responsiveness of the residents and what they could do when given an opportunity.

Music

Music is a potent tool for engaging patients and stimulating reminiscence. It has been shown to reduce agitation (Bright, 1986), loneliness, and depression (Summer, 1981), and stimulate participation in activities (Christie, 1992). Helmes and Wiancko (1997) reported that playing quiet baroque music significantly reduced noisemaking behavior in some dementia patients. Gerdner and Swanson (1993) observed that music preferred by dementia patients premorbidly produced a beneficial effect on behavior. Clinicians should obtain information about the music preferences of the patient and provide a means for turning off unwanted music.

Having Something to Nurture

A highly successful approach to designing nursing homes is to provide dementia patients something to nurture, for example, pets and plants (Figure 13–4). Thomas (1996) revolutionized the long-term care industry

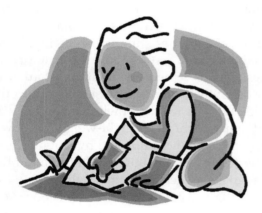

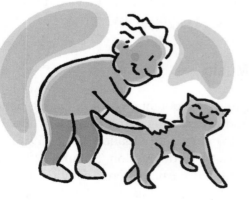

Figure 13–4. Individuals with dementia enjoy the opportunity to nurture plants and animals.

with his Eden Alternative™ system of care that he developed in response to the isolation and inactivity he observed in nursing home residents. Thomas advocated for nursing homes to be "human habitats" where residents live, feel useful and needed, and even thrive, as opposed to a place where they go to wait to die. A fundamental principle of the Eden Alternative model calls for residents to be given the opportunity to give as well as receive care. Using this approach, Thomas (1996) reported residents experienced fewer urinary tract infections, a decrease in upper respiratory infections, a decrease in medication use, and fewer deaths. Addditionally, use of the Eden Alternative resulted in decreased staff turnover. Resnick and Ransom (2001) documented fewer behavioral incidents and decreased restraint use in Eden nursing homes compared to traditional nursing homes, and Bergman-Evans (2004) reported lower levels of boredom and helplessness over a one-year period in residents of a certified Eden Alternative facility compared to residents of a non-Eden facility.

Facilitating Orientation

Many things can be done to facilitate orientation. Provide an easy to read calendar and digital clock to orient patients to day and time. If each weekday is associated with a unique activity, nursing home residents stay better oriented to the day of the week. Sterile, highly routinized environments with few activities make it difficult for dementia patients to distinguish one day of the week from another and can increase their helplessness and foster disorientation. Resident rooms with large windows that allow residents to see light changes in the day and seasonal changes facilitate orientation. Also, they combat sunlight deprivation. Being able to see the light change with the passage of the day is important because it enables our bodies to know when it is time for sleep. Finally, care facilities that make rooms look like what they are (kitchens like kitchens and bedrooms like bedrooms) foster orientation.

Many dementia patients forget the names of family members and caregivers. Name tags are helpful as is introducing yourself whenever you visit a patient.

Facilitating Prospective Memory

Prospective memory is remembering to remember, for example, remembering that you are supposed to take a pill at a certain time, or put the garbage out for pickup. Prospective memory failures are common in early stage dementia (Huppert, Johnson, & Nickson, 2000). Some investigators report that prospective memory deficit has a greater impact than retrospective memory deficit on the lives of caregivers of dementia patients (Smith, Della Sala, Logie, & Maylor, 2000). Many external memory aids (alarms, calendars, personal planners) can help mild dementia patients remember to do things.

Counseling Family About Choosing a Long-Term Care Facility

Many caregivers need to place loved ones in a nursing home or an assisted living facility to obtain the nursing and supervision the patient needs. Nursing homes vary greatly, and these variations affect the quality of the patient's life. The following is a list of questions that caregivers can ask themselves about potential placement sites:

What was my first impression?

Do I feel comfortable here?

Are residents smiling, agitated, staring into space?

Are residents well-groomed and clean?

Is the staff well-groomed and clean?

Is the facility clean?

Does the staff show respect to the patients?

Are many patients restrained?

What is the patient-to-staff ratio?

Is the staff well-trained?

What is the level of staff turnover?

Are staff members attentive to the patients?

What does the environment evoke in terms of emotion?

Does it smell like urine?

Are there places in which patients can move about?

Are patients confined to their rooms?

What does the environment evoke in terms of activity?

Is there an activity director?

Is the decor culturally appropriate for the patient?

Where are meals served?

Is the food appetizing?

Is help given to patients who are unable to feed themselves?

Are there handrails and support bars?

Is there unnecessary noise?

What is the level of medical support?

What is the policy on administration of drugs for behavioral management?

Is staff specially trained to care for dementia patients?

Is the home licensed?

Is the home approved to receive payments from Medicare?

What is the cost?

Counseling Professional Caregivers About Supporting Feeding

A common request for help from the speech-language pathologist is with feeding problems. Moderate and severely demented AD patients often require eating assistance. Environmental manipulations can improve functional feeding in many patients and the following suggestions are based on the observations of Van Ort and Phillips (1992):

a. Have the same individual feed the patient.
b. Feed the patient in the same place each time.
c. Have assistants feed one patient at a time.
d. Do not allow interruptions during the feeding.
e. Position the food so the patient can see it.
f. Use finger foods when possible.
g. Place a spoon in the patient's hand.
h. Provide a model of scooping food and taking it to the mouth.
i. Pace feeding so that the time between bites is about the same.
j. Avoid mixing and stirring foods.
k. Pair touch with the initiation of feeding and use it consistently as a cue.
l. Watch for cues from the patient that s/he wants another bite.
m. Offer drinks frequently during feeding.
n. Eliminate distractions such as a blaring television.
o. Provide social reinforcement for feeding such as hugs, touching, and compliments.

Summary of Important Points

- Indirect interventions involve modifying the linguistic and physical environments of individuals with dementia to improve cognitive-communicative functioning and quality of life.
- To improve linguistic comprehension, consider:
  - Using a slower than normal rate of speech.
  - Providing multimodal input.
  - Limiting the number of conversational partners.
  - Using a pleasant accepting vocal tone.
  - Reducing the number of propositions in sentences.
  - Talking about the here and now.
  - Using direct rather than indirect speech acts.
  - Avoiding teasing and sarcasm.
  - Avoiding talking to the patient like a child.
  - Amplifying the voice of the speaker.
- To improve the production of language, consider:
  - Providing something tangible and/or visible to stimulate conversation.
  - Avoiding placing patients in a free-recall situation.
  - When the patient forgets the topic, summarize what has been said.
  - If the patient wants to write a letter, supply materials, a list of news items, and a picture of the letter's intended recipient.
  - Respectfully supply the word the patient is struggling to remember.

- Have the patient read aloud to the caregiver or together with the caregiver.
- Do not repeatedly correct the patient.
- Engage patients in activities.
- Involve the verbally repetitious patient in a physical activity to reduce perseveration.
  - Provide food to increase sociability and talking among patients.
- The goal of environmental manipulation is to create an environment that is safe, peaceful, and organized and that evokes positive mood and behavior.
  - Left unoccupied, dementia patients become confused, agitated, and afraid. Thus, while they are awake, involve them in enjoyable activities and provide something for them to nurture.

References

Alm, N., Astell, A., Ellis, M., Dye, R., Gowans, G., & Campbell, J. (2004). A cognitive prosthesis and communication support for people with dementia. *Neuropsychological Rehabilitation, 14,* 117–134.

Almor, A., Kempler, D., MacDonald, M. C., Andersen, E. S., & Tyler, L. K. (1999). Why do Alzheimer patients have difficulty with pronouns? Working memory, semantics, and reference in comprehension and production in Alzheimer's disease. *Brain and Language, 67,* 202–227.

Baddeley, A. D., Baddeley, H. A., Bucks, R. S., & Wilcock, G. K. (2001). Attentional control in Alzheimer's disease. *Brain, 124,* 1492–1508.

Bergman-Evans, B. (2004). Beyond the basics: Effects of the Eden Alternative model on quality of life issues. *Journal of Gerontological Nursing, 30,* 27–34.

Boczko, F. (1994). The Breakfast Club: A multimodal language stimulation program for nursing home residents with Alzheimer's disease. *American Journal of Alzheimer's Disease and Other Dementias, 9,* 35–38.

Bourgeois, M. S. (1992). *Conversing with memory impaired individuals using memory aids.* Gaylord, MI: Northern Speech Services.

Bright, R. (1986). The use of music therapy and activities with dementia patients who are deemed "difficult to manage." *Clinical Gerontology, 6,* 131–144.

Christie, M. E. (1992). Music therapy applications in a skilled and intermediate care nursing home facility: A clinical study. *Activities, Adaptation and Aging, 16,* 69–87.

Cohen, G. (2000). Two new intergenerational interventions for Alzheimer's disease patients and families. *American Journal of Alzheimer's Disease and Other Dementias, 15,* 137–142.

Collette, F., Van der Linden, B. M., & Salmon, E. (1999). Phonological loop and central executive functioning in Alzheimer's disease. *Neuropsychologia, 37,* 905–918.

Gerner, L., & Swanson, E. (1993). Effects of individualized music on confused and agitated elderly patients. *Archives of Psychiatric Nursing, 7,* 284–291.

Gilley, D. W., Wilson, R. S., Bennett, D. A., Stebbins, G. T., Barnard, B. A., Whalen, M. E., et al. (1991). Cessation of driving and unsafe motor vehicle operation by dementia patients. *Archives of Internal Medicine, 151,* 941–946.

Helmes, E., & Wiancko, D. (1997). *Effects of music in reducing disruptive behavior in a general hospital.* Paper presented at the 16th Congress of the International Association of Gerontology, Adelaide, Australia.

Hopper, T., Bayles, K. A., & Tomoeda, C. K. (1998). Using toys to stimulate communicative function in individuals with Alzheimer's disease. *Journal of Medical Speech-Language Pathology, 6,* 73–80.

Huppert, F. A., Johnson, T., & Nickson, J. (2000). High prevalence of prospective memory impairment in the elderly and in early-stage dementia: Findings from a population-based study. *Applied Cognitive Psychology, 14,* S63–S81.

LoPresti, E. F., Mihailidis, A., & Kirsch, N. (2004). Assistive technology for cognitive rehabilitation: State of the art. *Neuropsychological Rehabilitation, 14,* 5–39.

Mihailidis, A., Fernie, G., & Barbenel, J. C. (2001). The use of artificial intelligence in the design of an intelligent cognitive orthotic for people with dementia. *Assistive Technology, 13,* 23–39.

Mynatt, E. D., Essa, I., & Rogers, W. (2000). *Increasing opportunities for aging in place.* ACM Conference on Universal Usability, Washington, DC (pp. 65–71). New York: ACM Press.

Ramakrishnan, S., & Pollack, M.E. (2000). Intelligent monitoring in a robotic assistant for the elderly. *Proceedings of the 16th National Conference on Artificial Intelligence,* Orlando, FL.

Resnick, O, & Ransom, S. (2001). The search for Eden: An alternative path for nursing homes. *Long-Term Care Interface, 2,* 45–48.

Rizzo, A. A., Schultheis, M., Kerns, K. A., & Mateer, C. (2004). Analysis of assets for virtual reality applications in neuropsychology. *Neuropsychological Rehabilitation, 14,* 207–239.

Rochon, E., Waters, G. S., & Caplan, D. (2000). The relationship between measures of working memory and sentence comprehension in patients with Alzheimer's disease. *Journal of Speech, Language, and Hearing Research, 43,* 395–413.

Santo Pietro M. J., & Boczko, F. (1998). Breakfast Club: Results of a study examining the effectiveness of a multi-modality group communication treatment. *American Journal of Alzheimer's Disease and Other Dementias, 13,* 146–158.

Sloane, P. D., Davidson, S., Buckwalter, K., Lindsey, B. A., Ayers, S., Lenker, V., et al. (1997). Management of the patient with disruptive vocalization. *Gerontologist, 37,* 675–682.

Smith, G., Della Sala, S., Logie, R. H., & Maylor, E. A. (2000). Prospective and retrospective memory in normal ageing and dementia: A questionnaire study. *Memory, 8,* 311–321.

Summer, L. (1981). Guided imagery and music with the elderly. *Music Therapy, 1,* 39–42.

Thomas, W. H. (1996). *Life worth living.* Acton, MA: VanderWyk & Burnham.

Van Ort, S., & Phillips, L. (1992). Feeding nursing home residents with Alzheimer's disease. *Geriatric Nursing, 13,* 249–253.

Zanetti, O., Zanieri, G., Vreese, L. P. D., Frisoni, G., & Binetti, G. (2000). *Utilizing an electronic memory aid with Alzheimer's disease patients. A study of feasibility.* Presentation at the Sixth International Stockholm/Springfield Symposium on Advances in Alzheimer Therapy. Stockholm, Sweden.

14

Care Planning

In previous chapters you read about dementia-producing diseases and their effect on cognition and communicative function and became familiar with standardized tests available for use in assessment. You also learned techniques for maximizing client function. However, before you can provide reimbursable services, you must understand the laws governing the provision of services and the rules for documenting what you do. This chapter begins with a discussion of the law and Medicare regulations and is followed by a discussion of how performance on the Arizona Battery for Communication Disorders of Dementia (ABCD) (Bayles & Tomoeda, 1993) or Functional Linguistic Communication Inventory (FLCI) (Bayles & Tomoeda, 1994) can be used to develop care plans and treatment goals. The chapter concludes with a discussion of caregiver education and training.

The Law and Medicare Regulations

With the "graying" of America, the demand for nursing home services dramatically increased as did scrutiny of the nursing home industry. Consumers became increasingly outraged by the prevalence of dirty, unsafe facilities that were negligent in their care of residents. When Congress became aware of the extent of the problem, legislation was passed that set new, higher standards for nursing homes. This legislation is known as the Omnibus Budget Reconciliation Act (OBRA, 1987). Its stated objective was the establishment of practices that maintain the *highest level of function* for long-term care residents and *promote quality of life*. To achieve this objective, OBRA mandated comprehensive assessment of all individuals admitted to long-term care facilities and the creation of care plans for sustaining them. A comprehensive assessment tool was created and is now used nationwide. This tool is called The Resident Assessment Instrument and is composed of the Minimum Data Set (MDS), which is a screening tool, and the Resident Assessment Protocols (RAPs) which specify "triggers" or issues to be addressed in care planning. These measures and further information about them can be found at: http://www.cms.hhs.gov.NursingHomeQualityInits/01_Overview.asp

Minimum Data Set (MDS)

The MDS is a tool for obtaining information about the status of an individual's history, physical and mental health, behavior, functional abilities, and special needs. Items of particular importance to SLPs include:

Section B. Cognitive Patterns

Memory (short-term and long-term)

Memory recall ability

Cognitive skills for daily decision-making

Indicators of delirium—periodic disordered thinking/awareness

Change in cognitive status

Section C. Communication/Hearing Patterns

Hearing

Communication devices/techniques

Modes of expression

Making oneself understood

Speech clarity

Ability to understand others

Change in communication/hearing

Section K. Oral/Nutritional Status

Oral problems

Height and weight

Weight change

Nutritional problems

Nutritional approaches

Parenteral or enteral intake

Section P. Special Treatment and Procedures Received in the Last 14 days

Medical treatments

Programs (including Alzheimer's/ dementia special care unit, training in skills required to return to the community)

Although a nurse generally oversees completion of the MDS, other health professionals may provide input related to their specialty and when they do, they sign the MDS form. Unfortunately someone other than an SLP generally completes the MDS sections related to cognitive-communicative functioning and swallowing. This is a concern because they generally lack the training necessary to make a valid judgment about the status of cognition, communicative function, and swallowing. Hopper, Bayles, Harris, and Holland (2001) reported that in a sample of 57 dementia patients, with deficits in communication and hearing as measured by objective testing, the majority were rated as having normal or adequate communication and hearing on the MDS when it was completed by a nurse. Furthermore, Hopper et al. (2001) reported that of those participants who had MDS-identified impairments in communication and hearing, *none* were referred for further evaluation.

Resident Assessment Protocols (RAPs)

The RAPS is used in partnership with the MDS. Each RAP identifies specific MDS responses that "trigger" the need for further evaluation of the resident to identify problems that can be remediated. Four of the 18 RAPS are of interest to SLPs:

- Cognitive Loss/Dementia
- Communication
- Nutritional Status
- Tube Feeding

A weakness that results in the RAP being triggered has to be addressed in the resident's plan of care unless justification to the contrary is entered in the medical record. For example, assume that the individual who completed the MDS checked that a resident "rarely/never understood." This would trigger the Communication RAP and require the facility to address the resident's comprehension problem unless a suitable explanation could be given as to why it should not be addressed. RAPs are used at the initial assessment and when there is a significant change in a resident's condition and annually. Unfortunately, when the individual who completes the MDS fails to recognize a problem with cognition, communication, hearing, and/or nutritional status, the patient receives no follow-up.

Centers for Medicare and Medicaid Services (CMS)

Under the executive branch of the federal government, the United States Department of Health and Human Services oversees the Medicare program. Within this agency are the Centers for Medicare and Medicaid Services that go by the acronym CMS. CMS has ten regional offices and is responsible for promulgating the regulations, guidelines, coverage rules, and medical review guidelines. The CMS established the following process that must be followed for individuals admitted to long-term care facilities:

- Residents must be *comprehensively evaluated* on admission to determine their level of functioning, needs, and patterns of activity.
- A *care plan* must be created based on results of comprehensive assessment. It must be designed to ensure the ability of the resident to attain/maintain his or her highest level of function and quality of life.
- Residents must be *reviewed and reassessed* by the MDS no less than every 3 months.
- A *comprehensive reassessment* (RAI) must be carried out after a significant change in

a resident's mental and/or physical health status but no less than every 12 months.

Basically, the passage of OBRA obligated care facilities to ensure that a resident's abilities in activities of daily living do not diminish unless the individual's clinical condition indicates that the loss of function was unavoidable. Inspectors visit nursing homes to ensure compliance with CMS regulations.

Role of the SLP

SLPs have a significant role in the care of dementia patients in long-term care (LTC) facilities because cognitive and communicative disorders significantly affect an individual's ability to function and quality of life. SLPs routinely evaluate residents, develop care plans, and periodically reassess residents. The care plans they develop may be restorative, that is, involve direct therapy with patients who have the potential to improve or be designed to maintain the individual at his or her current level of function. When a restorative plan is developed, the clinician must:

- provide objective evidence, or a clinically supportable statement of expectation, that the patient has the potential to improve
- demonstrate that the patient's maximum improvement is yet to be attained, and
- show that the anticipated improvement is attainable in a reasonable and predictable period of time.

The proposed therapy must require the special skills of the SLP, be necessary, and be physician approved. The provision of this documentation to claims reviewers makes obvious the need for information about the patient's deficits and any retained abilities that can be used to improve function. It also necessitates that the clinician be knowledgeable of best practice techniques that can improve function in a reasonable period of time.

When a patient lacks the potential to improve, a "Functional Maintenance Plan" (FMP) is developed by the SLP. FMPs are not carried out by the SLP but rather by support personnel and family caregivers. However, SLPs can receive reimbursement for writing the FMP, training support personal and caregivers in how to conduct it, and for supervising their efforts. The requirements of the FMP are that it be:

- Based on results of a comprehensive evaluation of the resident.
- Developed by the SLP.
- Explained to the resident and support personnel.
- Executed by support personnel or the resident.
- Signed by the referring physician.

A Relevant Question

Because individuals with dementia have progressive diseases and their dementia will inevitably worsen, one can reasonably ask whether they ever have the potential to improve. The answer is "yes," but with a qualification. Although behavioral therapy will not arrest the ultimate worsening of their dementia, it may enable individuals to use spared abilities to compensate for impaired abilities and therefore support them at the highest level of function of which they are capable, as the law requires.

Can SLPs Do Cognitive Therapy?

As you have learned, most techniques for improving the learning and retrieval of information are "cognitive," and historically

SLPs have had difficulty gaining approval from Medicare claims reviewers for providing cognitive therapy. Fortunately, that has changed as Medicare personnel and claims reviewers have come to understand that communication is a cognitive enterprise, and to improve it, one often has to work on those cognitive abilities that make communication possible. Today, Medicare policy statements clearly support coverage of cognitive therapy services provided by SLPs. Kander (2006) notes that the following excerpt can be cited when appealing denials of cognitive therapy coverage when rendered by an SLP:

Dementia is the general loss of cognitive abilities, including an impairment of memory and may include one or more of the following: aphasia, apraxia, agnosia, or disturbed planning, organizing, and abstract thinking abilities . . . Throughout the course of their disease, patients with dementia may benefit from pharmacologic, physical, occupational, speech-language pathology, and other therapies, according to CMS program memorandum AD-01-135, September 25, 2001 (p. 3).

Medicare Cap on Amount of Service Dollars

The Balanced Budget Act of 1997 required CMS to impose caps on outpatient physical, speech-language, and occupational therapy services. Occupational therapy was given its own cap, but a combined cap totaling 1,740 dollars was created for speech-language pathology and physical therapy. Thus, no more than this amount can be paid for speech-language pathology and physical therapy services combined. However, the Deficit Reduction Act of 2005, which became law in February 2006, directed CMS to create a process to permit exceptions to the therapy cap when additional services are medically necessary. The process that was created allows for automatic exceptions for certain diagnoses and manual exceptions (when the provider makes a formal request to the contractor who makes a determination based on evidence). The details regarding exceptions to the caps are detailed and can be found on the CMS Web site at: www.cms.hhs.gov/Manuals/IOM/list.asp#TopOfPage

The status of the therapy cap can change depending on future legislation. Consult the American Speech-Language-Hearing Association's Billing and Reimbursement Web page for updates on current reimbursement levels and rulings. Also, you can request specific information by sending an E-mail to reimbursement@asha.org

Using Test Performance to Develop Treatment Plans

CMS has standard forms for filing a treatment plan and reporting progress. Both require specification of the long-term goal and short-term treatment goals.

The long-term treatment goal is more general and specifies the *end state* to be achieved. For example:

■ The resident will be able to express needs with minimal cues 80% of the time.

Short-term treatment goals are the *means for achieving the end state* and may be numerous. For example:

■ The resident will learn to identify the features of a communication board to 100% accuracy through errorless learning techniques in daily 15-minute sessions for 2 weeks.
■ Thereafter, the resident will learn to utilize the communication board to make requests with 80% accuracy through spaced

retrieval training in daily 15-minute sessions for 2 weeks.

Proposed treatments must be related to the functional level of the patient, and it is important to realize that in the future, the clinician must compare treatment effects to the patient's functional level before therapy. The functional level of the patient is best discovered using standardized measures that have been demonstrated to yield reproducible results. Specify the standardized measure used in assessment on the treatment plan form. Finally, the clinician must provide evidence of the patient's potential to improve.

A Case Example: Restorative Care Plan

Mrs. Jane Doe is a resident of Country Acres Nursing Home who was admitted with a diagnosis of mild dementia. In the 6 months of her residency, staff has observed that Mrs. Doe rarely participates in activities, initiates conversation, or expresses her needs, and is hard to hear because of a barely audible voice. They are concerned because she is socially isolated. Her physician reports that she has no vocal pathology. The SLP administered the Arizona Battery for Communication Disorders to evaluate her cognitive-communicative functioning which also contains a speech discrimination hearing test (Figure 14–1). Additionally, they conducted a speech and voice evaluation. The SLP used Mrs. Doe's ABCD performance to complete the sections of the MDS related to cognitive-communicative functioning as can be seen in Table 14–1.

Mrs. Doe's performance on the ABCD, together with results of the hearing screening and speech and voice examinations, were used by the SLP to formulate the following long-term and short term goals for Mrs. Doe.

	CONSTRUCTS					Mrs. Doe's Score	Total Score Poss.
SUBTESTS	Mental Status	Episodic Memory	Linguistic Expression	Linguistic Comprehension	Visuospatial Construction		
Mental Status	3					9	13
Story Retelling - Immediate		3				4	17
Following Commands				4		8	9
Comparative Questions				3		5	6
Word Learning - Free Recall		3				2	16
Word Learning - Total Recall (free & cued)		3				8	16
Word Learning - Recognition		4				43	48
Repetition				3		45	75
Object Description			4			8	n/a
Reading Comprehension - Word				5		8	8
Reading Comprehension - Sentence				3		5	7
Generative Naming			4			8	n/a
Confrontation Naming			3			12	20
Concept Definition			2			24	60
Generative Drawing					5	13	14
Figure Copying					5	12	12
Story Retelling - Delayed		1				0	17
TOTAL of the scores for each Construct	3	14	13	18	10	**TOTAL OVERALL SCORE**	
Divide by this number	1	5	4	5	2		
AVERAGE Construct Summary Scores	3	2.8	3.2	3.6	5	17.6	

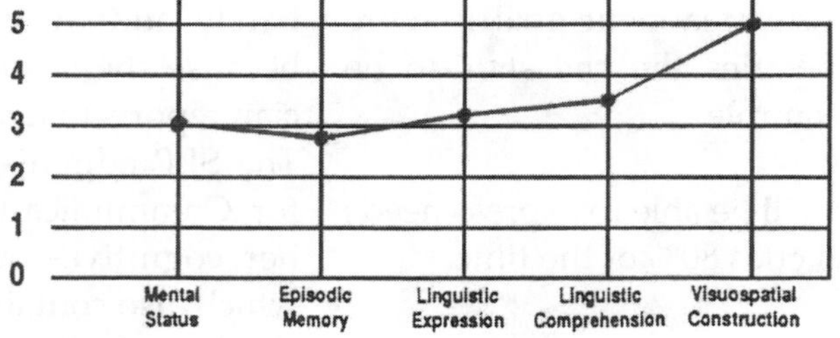

Figure 14–1. Mrs. Doe's performance on the ABCD.

Long-Term Goal

■ Resident will produce comprehensible language to express needs and participate in recognition-memory based activities through vocal loudness training to reduce social isolation.

Short-Term Goals

■ Spaced retrieval training to learn techniques for increasing vocal loudness by 50% daily for 3 weeks in 15-minute sessions.
■ Three times weekly participation in one 30-minute group reminiscence program

Table 14–1. Relating Mrs. Doe's ABCD Performance to MDS Items

Minimum Data Set (MDS) Functions	Information Provided by Analyzing ABCD Performance
Ability to Recall	• Disoriented for time but not for person. • Could recount only 24% of a short story immediately after hearing it; 20 minutes later, the story was forgotten. • Good recognition memory (83% accuracy). • Performance improves with cues.
Ability to Understand Communication/Hearing Patterns	• Read and comprehended single words with 88% accuracy. • Read and comprehended sentences with 71% accuracy. • Recognized and named objects with 60% accuracy. • Repeated with 60% accuracy. • Followed two-stage commands. • Answered comparative questions with 83% accuracy.
Making Self-Understood	• Generated items in a category. • Defined words with 40% accuracy. • Drew simple items with 50% accuracy.
Skills for Daily Decision-Making	• Patient was oriented for self. • Could answer simple questions. • Followed one- and two-step commands.
Indicators of Disoriented Thinking	• Disoriented for time.

that uses recognition paradigms and priming to stimulate participation.

Treatment Plan

The following information was provided on the CMS Treatment Plan Form. Note that the clinician included the reason for referral, Mrs. Doe's level of functioning, and data that suggest Mrs. Doe has the potential to improve.

Mrs. Jane Doe is a 77-year-old female who has resided in the care facility for 6 months.

REASON FOR REFERRAL: Staff report that patient has a hard to hear voice, rarely expresses needs or communicates with other residents and is socially isolated. Physician reports absence of vocal pathology.

LEVEL OF FUNCTION: The standardized Arizona Battery for Communication Disorders was administered as well as a speech and voice examination.

Cognition: Patient's test performance was typical of an individual with mild dementia. She was disoriented for time, could recount only 24% of a story immediately after hearing it and remembered nothing 15 minutes later.

Comprehension: Patient could read and comprehend sentences with 71% accuracy; name objects and repeat with 60% accuracy; follow two-stage commands; and answer questions with 83% accuracy.

Expression: Patient could generate items in a category and define words with 40% accuracy. She has good grammar and pragmatics.

Speech: Normal, no dysarthria.

Hearing: Able to discriminate speech with 90% accuracy.

Voice: Physician reports normal larynges and no pathology. Patient spoke in a barely audible voice 100% of the time but could increase loudness with cues.

OVERALL IMPRESSION: Mild cognitive-communicative deficit secondary to dementia. Voice is soft and hard to hear. Likely patient has withdrawn because others fail to hear her.

POTENTIAL: Excellent for stated goals because of good recognition memory, ability to follow two-stage commands, read with 71% accuracy, name with 60% accuracy, and answer questions with 83% accuracy. Patient could increase vocal loudness when stimulated to do so.

A Case Example: Functional Maintenance Plan (FMP)

As was the case with Mrs. Doe's restorative care plan, the FMP must be based on comprehensive evaluation of the patient. Whereas Mrs. Doe was a mild dementia patient for whom the ABCD was appropriate, Mr. John Doe's dementia is more severe. Both the Functional Linguistic Communication Inventory (Bayles & Tomoeda, 1994) and the Severe Impairment Battery (Saxton et al., 2005; Saxton & Swihart, 1989) were used to evaluate his mental status and level of communicative functioning. Mr. Doe's performance on the Functional Linguistic Communication Inventory is shown in Figure 14–2. Mr. Doe is both nonambulatory and incontinent; however, he is not bedridden. He is unable to control his wheelchair and therefore is often isolated from activities. Mr. Doe is docile and accepting of care and was an avid football fan before his illness.

When developing the FMP, the clinician noted Mr. Doe's strengths and weaknesses. His deficits are sufficiently severe that restorative therapy is not justifiable but he has many retained abilities that can be used to provide quality care; they are:

- Can give an appropriate verbal response
- Able to shake hands
- Can state own name
- Recognizes the written and spoken forms of his name
- Can answer some yes/no questions
- Able to write some words to dictation
- Recognizes some signs
- Can do some object to picture matching
- Can read single words
- Able to follow simple one-step commands
- Gave an appropriate response to a compliment
- Corrected misinformation given by the examiner
- Made an appropriate verbal response to examiner's closing remarks

Thus, the examiner formulated the following long-term goal and short-term steps for maintaining his function and quality of life:

Long-Term Goal

- Establish a routine of care that enables Mr. Doe to participate in activities daily that he enjoys through which he can have

Performance by severity level of standardization study subjects on FLCI subtests.

Plot performance of examinee on this graph to compare examinee to AD subjects in the standardization study.

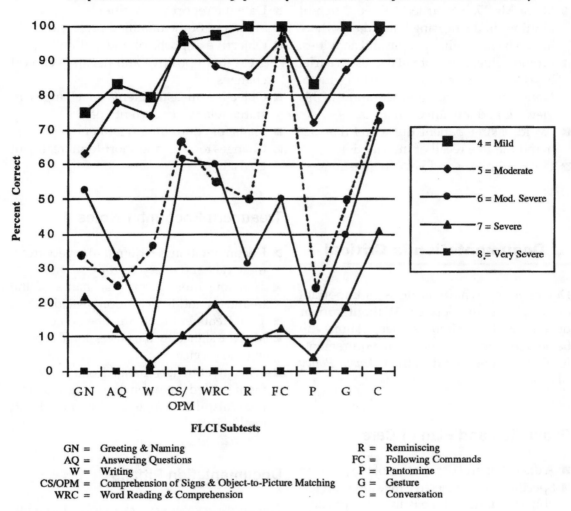

4 = Mild

5 = Moderate

6 = Mod. Severe

7 = Severe

8 = Very Severe

FLCI Subtests

GN =	Greeting & Naming	R =	Reminiscing
AQ =	Answering Questions	FC =	Following Commands
W =	Writing	P =	Pantomime
CS/OPM =	Comprehension of Signs & Object-to-Picture Matching	G =	Gesture
WRC =	Word Reading & Comprehension	C =	Conversation

Figure 14–2. Performance of Mr. John Doe on the FLCI.

social interchange with caregivers and other residents.

Care Program

- Address Mr. Doe by name when providing care.
- Shake hands when greeting Mr. Doe.
- Move from the handshake to a gentle massage of hands and arms.

- Talk to Mr. Doe in a nurturing voice about a tangible object (e.g., picture, ball) for at least 5 minutes daily.
- Encourage him to talk about the object.
- Place pictures related to patient's favorite football team in patient's immediate environment.
- Write single positive words on cards that relate to the pictures and place them where Mr. Doe can see them.

- Incorporate throwing and catching a small football in his daily activity schedule.
- Move Mr. Doe to at least three different locations in the nursing home daily where he can be near other people and activities.
- Provide videos of football games on a trial basis to see if he enjoys watching them. Note the frequency and duration of his viewing and any affect changes.
- Avoid asking patient questions that demand the free recall of information.
- Use recognition and yes/no questions.

Documentation Is Critical

Documenting what you do is as important as providing the service. Without proper documentation, reimbursement claims will be denied. The documentation requirements for CMS can be found in their *Benefit Policy Manual* and are outlined below.

Evaluation and Plan of Care

- A diagnosis and description of the problem
- Specification of objective measures, preferably standardized measures or functional outcomes measurement tools
- A clinical judgment of the patient's condition
- The need for treatment
- Certification that the client is under a physician's care.

Progress Notes

When treatment exceeds 10 treatment days or 30 calendar treatment days, whichever is less, progress notes must include:

- Date of the beginning of the treatment interval
- Date the report was written
- Signature of the qualified professional
- Objective reports of the patient's progress (both positive and negative clinical changes)
- Objective measurements of changes in status relative to current goals
- Plans for continuing treatment
- Changes to long- and short-term treatment goals.

Treatment Encounter Notes

- Documentation is required for every treatment day and every therapy service
- The note must record the name of the treatment and intervention provided
- Total treatment time must be noted
- Must be signed by the professional providing the service
- When treatment is changed, or a new treatment added between the progress note intervals, the change must be noted and justified.

Documentation Pitfalls

The necessary paperwork involved in gaining approval and reimbursement for services can be frustrating. Learn the rules early and adhere to them, it will reduce your frustration in the long run. The most common reason for denial of a claim is incomplete documentation, other reasons include:

- A skilled service is not being provided
- Therapy goals are not functional
- Requested services are not reasonable
- Requested services are not necessary
- The frequency and/or duration of therapy are inappropriate

- "Best practice" standards are not apparent in the treatment plan
- The therapy goal is to take the patient to a higher level than the patient was premorbidly.

Caregiving

The majority of Americans with dementia are cared for at home by family members. Because disease duration is generally long (exceeding 8 years on average for individuals with AD), the challenge caregivers face cannot be overstated. Mace and Rabins (1981, 1999) appropriately titled their book for caregivers "The 36-Hour Day." Schumock (1998) reported that caregivers of AD patients often spend 60 to 100 hours a week providing care.

Caregiving has been characterized as a role that is "devoid of formal training, choice, and compensation" (Pruchno, Kleban, Michaels, & Dempsey, 1990, p. 193). Schulz and Martire (2004) describe caregiving as

> . . . the provision of extraordinary care, exceeding the bounds of what is normative or usual in family relationships. Caregiving typically involves a significant expenditure of time, energy, and money over potentially long periods of time; it involves tasks that may be unpleasant and uncomfortable and are psychologically stressful and physically demanding (p. 240).

Dementia caregiving is recognized as the most stressful type of family caregiving (Ory, Hoffman, Yee, Tennstedt, & Schulz, 1999). Family caregivers have less time for themselves and other family members and have more work-related problems. Many caregivers of dementia patients are themselves elderly and coping with one or more chronic diseases. If a spouse is not available for care-

giving, the responsibility is often assumed by a middle-aged child of the patient and in many cases this means their leaving the work force (Biegel, Sales, & Schulz, 1991; Schulz, 2000).

Depression in Caregivers Is Common

Regardless of the age of the caregiver or their relation to the patient, they are likely to become depressed (Haley, 1997). Cohen and Eisdorfer (1988) reported that 55% of relatives who live with an AD patient met DSM-III criteria for clinical depression. Caregivers also are at increased risk for feeling anxious, hostile, and aggressive (Wiggins, Goldberg, & Appelbaum, 1971). Compared to people of the same age, who do not have the responsibilities of caregiving, caregivers use more psychotropic medications (George & Gwyther, 1986).

Health Risks of Caregiving

The chronic stress of caregiving takes a toll on physical and psychological health. Caregivers have more serious illnesses (Kiecolt-Glaser, Glaser, Gravenstein, Malarkey, & Sheridan, 1996; Shaw et al., 1997), higher prevalence and incidence of depressive and anxiety disorders (Kiecolt-Glaser, Dura, Speicher, Trask, & Glaser, 1991; Schulz et al., 1997; Schulz, O'Brien, Bookwala, & Fleissner, 1995; Teri, Logsdon, Uomoto, & McCurry, 1997), greater cardiovascular reactivity (King, Oka, & Young, 1994), slower wound healing (Kiecolt-Glaser, Marucha, Malarkey, Mercado, & Glaser, 1995), and an increased risk of mortality (Schulz & Beach, 1999). Schumock (1998) reported that caregivers use 71% more prescription drugs than age-mates and have 46% more visits to the doctor.

More alarming is the burgeoning literature on the alterations in the immune system that are suffered by caregivers (Kiecolt-Glaser et al., 1987; Mills, Yu, Ziegler, Patterson, & Grant, 1999; Vedhara et al., 1999). Kiecolt-Glaser and colleagues (1991) reported that compared to normal control subjects, caregivers had significantly more days of infectious illness and decrements on three measures of cellular immunity. Caregivers with the lowest levels of social support and the highest levels of distress had the most negative changes in immune system function.

Gender and Caregiving

The gender of the caregiver affects their vulnerability to caregiving stress, depression, and loneliness. Women are more stressed than men and report greater burden (Cantor, 1983; Sparks, Farran, Donner, & Keane-Hagerty, 1998; Zarit, Reever, & Bach-Peterson, 1980; Zarit, Todd, & Zarit, 1986), and female caregivers are more likely to experience depression than males (Beeson, 2004; Schulz et al., 1995; Stuckey, Neundorfer, & Smyth, 1996). Females also report significantly higher levels of loneliness (Beeson, 2004). Husbands are more likely to seek outside help and approach the problem of caregiving as they would a problem at work. Younger wives and older husbands report the greatest burden in caregiving (Fitting, Rabins, Lucas, & Eastham, 1986). The association between health variables and caregiving appears to be stronger among spousal caregivers than child caregivers (Baumgarten et al., 1992).

Family Strife and Violence

An infrequently recognized problem associated with caregiving is strife with other family members. The fact is that the existence of a dementia patient in a family often produces family conflict. In a study by Chenoweth and Spencer (1986), 60% of caregivers report that relations among family members deteriorated. Poulshock and Diemling (1984) and Cantor (1983) observed that increased burden is associated with adverse effects on caregiver-patient relations, and relations between the caregiver and other members of the family and friends.

Violence increases in families with dementia patients. Paveza et al. (1992) reported that violence is a "significant clinical challenge in families living with a relative diagnosed with Alzheimer's disease or a related dementia" (p. 493). More than half of all dementia patients exhibit aggressive behavior. Paveza and associates indicate that 15% of their sample of 184 families witnessed severe violence by the patient in the previous year and 5.4% of caregivers had been severely violent toward the patient. The overall prevalence of violence was 17.4%. According to Pillemer and Suitor (1992), the predictors of violence on the part of the caregiver include: physical aggression by the care recipient, disruptive behaviors, and a shared living situation. Spouses and older individuals appear more likely to become violent than other relatives.

Factors That Influence Caregiver Burden and Stress

Caregiver distress is highly related to the severity of the patient's behavioral problems. Teri (1997) found that patient depression, disruptive behaviors, and memory-related problems were associated with the highest levels of caregiver distress. Spouse caregivers of dementia patients in a study by Lieberman and Fisher (1995) reported greater somatic symptoms and anxiety/depression and lower levels of well being when patients had severe behavioral (not cognitive) problems. Similarly, Gallicchio, Siddiqi, Langenberg, and Baumgarten (2002), in their study of 327 caregiver-patient dyads, found a high association between behavioral disturbances and caregiver burden.

Family Counseling

Dementia is a family affair, and clinicians should consider the patient and caregiver as a unit because their health and well-being are highly interdependent. The American Medical Association (AMA), the American Psychiatric Association (APA), and the American Association for Geriatric Psychiatry (AAGP) all strongly recommend partnering with the patient and caregiver in managing dementia. The AMA has even developed an assessment tool for obtaining information about the caregiver called the Caregiver Self-Assessment Tool (American Medical Association, 2002). It comprises 18 questions about the caregiver's level of stress, health, and support. The AAGP views caregiver counseling as medically necessary.

When an individual is diagnosed with dementia, a family conference should be scheduled. This is especially true if the individual with dementia is living at home. When the diagnosis is recent, the caregiver may be in shock or denial. If so, much of what you say may not be comprehended or accepted in the initial conference, and a follow-up conference may be needed after the family has absorbed the diagnosis. Families caring for an individual with dementia benefit from periodic counseling. A good schedule is every six months or at least annually because new challenges arise as the disease progresses.

To appropriately counsel family, the clinician needs considerable information about the family including:

- Their understanding of the patient's disease
- Their methods of communication
- The degree of cooperation among members
- The existence and nature of major physical illness in other family members
- Their economic status
- And, very importantly, their cultural orientation.

Kleinman (1988), a Harvard psychiatrist and medical anthropologist, recommends that clinicians ask patients for an explanation of their illness or disability to uncover potential differences between the explanatory models of the patient and clinician. With this knowledge, the clinician can negotiate with the patient and caregiver about possible treatments and expected outcomes. Although these questions were developed for use by physicians (Kleinman, Eisenberg, & Good, 1978), they are of value to any health professional.

1. What do you think has caused your problem?
2. Why do you think it started when it did?
3. What do you think your sickness does to you? How does it work?
4. How severe is your sickness? Will it have a short or long course?
5. What kind of treatment do you think you should receive?
6. What are the most important results you hope to receive from this treatment?
7. What are the chief problems your sickness has caused for you?
8. What do you fear most about your sickness?

Culture Matters in Counseling

To counsel effectively, the clinician needs to understand and respect the culture of the client. What is culture? Culture is a shared way of perceiving the world. Lustig and

Koester (2006) define it as "... *a learned set of shared interpretations about beliefs, values, norms, and social practices, which affect the behaviors of a relatively large group of people*" (p. 25). How can a clinician become familiar with the culture of the client? The simple answer is by asking the right questions. Brislin (1994) identified critical features that distinguish the cultures of the world. These features are an excellent guide as to what questions to ask of clients or cultural informants.

- Importance of the group versus the individual in decision making
- Roles of men, women, and children
- Views of time and space
- Language
- Rituals and superstitions
- Significance of work
- Concepts about class and status
- Religion
- Values and beliefs about health

The Appendix at the end of the book contains a discussion of the major U.S. cultural groups and American culture. To provide culturally sensitive care, clinicians need to understand their own culture as well as that of clients. Questions are provided in Appendix A to help you discover your cultural orientation. Also included are resources for learning more about cultural diversity and developing intercultural skills.

Emphasize What the Patient Can Do

In counseling, regardless of the cultural orientation of the client, emphasize what the patient can do. Do not focus solely on the patient's deficits. Explain how the physical and linguistic environments and care regimen can be modified to provide safety and quality of life.

The following is a summary of problem areas and retained abilities by stage of dementia that can be used to counsel families. The information provided is based on the performance of individuals with Alzheimer's dementia (after Hopper, Bayles, & Kim, 2001).

Early Stage AD—Mild Dementia

This has been called the forgetful stage. The classic symptom is forgetting a recent experience. Patients often comment that they are having difficulty remembering and finding objects. They may accuse family members or housekeepers of taking the lost object. Affected individuals make more errors, often related to money. Then, too, individuals with mild AD frequently experience depression. Sometimes subtle personality changes are evident, such as apathy, increased irritability, and suspiciousness.

Retained Abilities

- Can sustain attention and selectively attend to stimuli
- Able to follow a three-stage command
- Good recognition memory
- Responsive to cuing
- Retain motor procedures and habits
- Semantic knowledge is generally intact
- Good grammar, syntax, and social language
- Able to read and comprehend at the sentence level
- Can write single words and comprehend gestures
- Independent in basic ADLs (toileting, bathing, feeding, and transferring)

Mid-Stage AD—Moderate Dementia

Mid-stage AD has been called the confused stage. Patients become disoriented, first for time and then place. Confusion results in poor job performance, money management difficulties, bad driving, and a deteriorating household. New environments are perplexing and travel becomes anxiety producing. Many mid-stage patients fatigue easily. Individuals with moderate dementia may withdraw from social gatherings especially with nonfamily members. Personality changes are common and can take many forms among them; paranoia, hostility, and aggressiveness. Well-practiced skills are usually maintained but caregivers observe the loss of functional activities of daily living particularly bathing and grooming. Also, during this stage patients become unaware of their deficits. Sleep-wake cycles may be disrupted. Some patients are awake at night and prone to restless wandering. It is not uncommon for them to become lost.

Retained Abilities

- Can sustain attention for limited amounts of time in a low distraction environment
- Can follow a two-step command
- Fair recognition memory
- Responsive to cuing
- Retain many motor procedures and habits
- Contents of semantic memory may be accessible with recognition strategies and cues
- Good grammar, syntax, and social language
- Can comprehend simple statements, yes/no questions, and most choice questions
- Can reminisce about tangible stimuli
- Generally able to perform basic ADLs with minimal assistance

Late Stage AD—Severe Dementia

In the advanced stages of dementia patients evolve to global intellectual deterioration. No longer do they have the capacity to reason, and they may fail to recognize family and even themselves. They require constant supervision and are unable to carry out the routines of life. They become totally dependent upon the caregiver. The images on television may confuse them as do new environments and unfamiliar persons. In the very late stage, patients typically are non-ambulatory, incontinent, unable to feed themselves, or chew, and they often have swallowing problems. Susceptibility to infection increases, and pneumonia is a common cause of death.

Retained Abilities

- May attend to positive stimuli for short periods
- Sometimes respond to cues
- Generally recognize own name
- Often can contribute to a conversation
- Retain some aspects of social language (greeting, leave taking, responding to a compliment)
- May read at the word level
- May answer simple yes/no and choice questions
- May feed self with minimal assistance

Caregiver Education and Training

The National Institute on Aging and the National Institute on Nursing Research have supported studies of the value of caregiver intervention. Results of studies to date indicate that interventions that target five types of risk to caregivers are best: safety, social support, health and self-care, emotional well-being, and care-recipient problem behaviors (Belle et al., 2003; Czaja, Schulz, Lee, & Belle, 2003).

Several investigators have studied the effect of formal caregiver education and training programs on patient care and caregiver burden (Bourgeois, Dijkstra, Burgio, & Allen, 2004; Dijkstra, Bourgeois, Burgio, & Allen, 2002; Irvine, Ary, & Bourgeois, 2003; McCallion, Toseland, & Freeman 1999; McCallion, Toseland, Lacey, & Banks, 1999; Orange & Colton-Hudson, 1998; Ripich, 1994; Ripich, Wykle, & Niles, 1995; Ripich & Ziol, 1999; Shulman & Mandel, 1988). Results of these studies were reviewed by the Academy of Neurologic Communication Disorders and Sciences and ASHA Committee to Establish Practice Guidelines for the Management of Dementia. The committee reported that educating caregivers on communication strategies may contribute to (a) more successful conversational exchanges, (b) reduced or increased caregiver burden, (c) improved quality of life for patients, (d) maintenance of patients' language skills, and (e) an increase in caregiver understanding of how and why communication breaks down (Zientz et al., in press). Based on their review of the methodological rigor of these studies, committee members recommended that an educational program have at least four sessions that include an opportunity for actual practice of strategies with individualized feedback.

Summary of Important Points

- The passage of OBRA mandated that long-term care facilities establish practices that maintain the highest level of function of long-term care residents and promote quality of life.
- All long-term care residents must be evaluated at admission and periodically thereafter using the MDS.
- Numerous MDS items are relevant to SLPs: cognitive patterns, communication and hearing patterns, oral/nutritional status, and special treatment and procedures.

- RAPs trigger the need for further evaluation of a long-term care resident to identify problems that can be remediated.
- The CMS oversees the Medicare program and has established a process that must be followed for individuals admitted to long-term care facilities.
- Speech-language pathology services are reimbursable by Medicare if the therapy requires the special skills of the SLP, is necessary and physician approved, and if the patient has the potential to improve in a reasonable amount of time.
- SLPs also can be reimbursed for creating functional maintenance plans and overseeing their implementation.
- Medicare will pay for cognitive therapy by an SLP when documentation supports the therapy plan.
- Medicare has a cap on the amount of dollars that can be spent per individual for SLP and occupational therapy services. However, CMS will make exceptions to the cap when additional services are medically necessary.
- CMS has standard forms for filing a treatment plan and reporting progress.
- Careful documentation and completion of forms according to CMS rules is necessary for Medicare approval of therapy and reimbursement.
- Personal caregivers of dementia patients are at risk for depression, diminished immune system function, and conflict with other family members.
- Clinicians should treat dementia as a family affair and consider the patient and caregiver as a unit because their health and well-being are interdependent.
- Knowledge of the culture of the patient and caregiver is critical to good counseling. Take time to gather information about the patient and caregiver's perception of the cause of the patient's problems.

■ When counseling family, emphasize what the patient can do and how the physical and linguistic environments and care regimen can be modified to provide safety and quality of life.

■ Families need counseling throughout the course of a dementing disease and may benefit from participation in a caregiver education and training program.

References

American Medical Association. (2002). *Caregiver Self-Assessment Tool.* Retrieved January 1, 2007 from http://www.ama-assn.org/ama/pub/category/5037.html

Baumgarten, M., Battista, R. N., Infant-Rivard, C., Hanley, J. A., Becker, R., & Gauthier, S. (1992). The psychological and physical health of family members caring for an elderly person with dementia. *Journal of Clinical Epidemiology, 45,* 61–70.

Bayles, K. A., & Tomoeda, C. K. (1993). *Arizona Battery for Communication Disorders of Dementia.* Austin, TX: Pro-Ed.

Bayles, K. A., & Tomoeda, C. K. (1994). *Functional Linguistic Communication Inventory.* Austin, TX: Pro-Ed.

Beeson, R. A. (2004). Loneliness and depression in caregivers. In R. W. Richter & B. Zoeller Richter (Eds.), *Alzheimer's disease: A physician's guide to practical management* (pp. 449–453). Totowa, NJ: Humana Press.

Belle, S. H., Czaja, S. J., Schulz, R., Zhang, S., Burgio, L. D., Gitlin, L. N., et al., REACH Investigators. (2003). Using a new taxonomy to combine the uncombinable: Integrating results across diverse caregiving interventions. *Psychology and Aging, 18,* 396–405.

Biegel, D., Sales, E., & Schulz, R. (1991). *Family caregiving in chronic illness: Heart disease, cancer, stroke, Alzheimer's disease, and chronic mental illness.* Newbury Park, CA: Sage.

Bourgeois, M. S., Dijkstra, K., Burgio, L. D., & Allen, R. S. (2004). Communication skills training for nursing aids of residents with dementia: The impact of measuring performance. *Clinical Gerontologist, 27*(1/2), 119–138.

Brislin, R. (1994). *Understanding cultural diversity: A model* [Videotape 1]. Tucson: University of Arizona National Center for Neurogenic Communication Disorders.

Cantor, M. H. (1983). Strain among caregivers: A study of experience in the United States. *Gerontologist, 23,* 597–604.

Chenoweth, B., & Spencer, B. (1986). Dementia: The experience of family caregivers. *Gerontologist, 26,* 267–272.

Cohen, D., & Eisdorfer, C. (1988). Depression in family members caring for a relative with Alzheimer's disease. *Journal of the American Geriatric Society, 36,* 885–889.

Czaja S. J., Schulz., R., Lee, C. C., & Belle, S. H. (2003). A methodology for describing and decomposing complex psychosocial and behavioral interventions. *Psychology and Aging, 18,* 385–395.

Dijkstra, K., Bourgeois, M., Burgio, L., & Allen, R. (2002). Effects of a communication intervention on the discourse of nursing home residents with dementia and their nursing assistants. *Journal of Medical Speech-Language Pathology, 10,* 143–157.

Fitting, M., Rabins, P., Lucas, M. J., & Eastham, J. (1986). Caregivers for dementia patients: A comparison of husbands and wives. *Gerontologist, 26,* 248–252.

Gallicchio, L., Siddiqi, N., Langenberg, P., & Baumgarten, M. (2002). Gender differences in burden and depression among informal caregivers of demented elders in the community. *International Journal of Geriatric Psychiatry, 17,* 154–163.

George, L. K., & Gwyther, L. P. (1986). Caregiver well-being: A multidimensional examination of family caregivers of demented adults. *Gerontologist, 26,* 253–259.

Haley, W. E. (1997). The family caregiver's role in Alzheimer's disease. *Neurology, 48*(Suppl.), 25–29.

Hopper, T., Bayles, K. A., Harris, F. P., & Holland, A. (2001). The relationship between Minimum Data Set ratings and scores on measures of communication and hearing among nursing home residents with dementia. *American Journal of Speech-Language Pathology, 10,* 370–381.

Hopper, T., Bayles, K. A., & Kim, E. (2001). Retained neuropsychological abilities of individuals with Alzheimer's disease. *Seminars in Speech and Language, 22,* 261–273.

Irvine, A. B., Ary, D. V., & Bourgeois, M. S. (2003). An interactive multimedia program to train professional caregivers. *Journal of Applied Gerontology, 22,* 269–288.

Kander, M. (2006, May 23). Medicare covers cognitive therapy. *The ASHA Leader, 11,* 3, 14.

Kiecolt-Glaser, J. K., Dura, J. R., Speicher, C. E., Trask, O. J., & Glaser, R. (1991). Spousal caregivers of dementia victims: Longitudinal changes in immunity and health. *Psychosomatic Medicine, 53,* 345–352.

Kiecolt-Glaser, J. K., Glaser, R., Gravenstein S., Malarkey, W. B., & Sheridan, J. (1996). Chronic stress alters the immune response to influenza virus vaccine in older adults. *Proceedings of the National Academy of Sciences of the USA, 94,* 3043–3047.

Kiecolt-Glaser J. K., Glaser, R., Shuttleworth, E. C., Dyer, C. S., Ogrocki, P., & Speicher, C. E. (1987). Chronic stress and immunity in family caregivers of Alzheimer's disease victims. *Psychosomatic Medicine, 49,* 523–535.

Kiecolt-Glaser, J. K., Marucha P. T., Malarkey W. B., Mercado, A. M., & Glaser, R. (1995). Slowing of wound healing by psychological stress. *Lancet, 346,* 1194–1196.

King A. C., Oka, R. K., & Young, D. R. (1994). Ambulatory blood pressure and heart rate responses to the stress of work and caregiving in older women. *Journal of Gerontology, 49,* 239–245.

Kleinman, A. (1988). *The illness narratives: Suffering, healing, and the human condition.* New York: Basic Books.

Kleinman, A., Eisenberg, L., & Good, B. (1978). Culture, illness and care: Clinical issues from anthropologic and cross-cultural research. *Annals of Internal Medicine, 88,* 251–258.

Lieberman, M. A., & Fisher, L. (1995). The impact of chronic illness of the health and well being of family members. *Gerontologist, 35,* 94–102.

Lustig, M. W., & Koester, J. (2006). *Intercultural competence.* Boston: Pearson, Allyn & Bacon.

Mace, N. L., & Rabins, P. V. (1981; 1999). *The 36-hour day: A family guide to caring for persons with Alzheimer's disease, related dementing illnesses, and memory loss in later life.* Baltimore: Johns Hopkins University Press.

McCallion, P., Toseland, R. W., & Freeman, K. (1999). An evaluation of a family visit education program. *Journal of the American Geriatrics Society, 47,* 203–214.

McCallion, P., Toseland, R.W., Lacey, D., & Banks, S. (1999). Educating nursing assistants to communicate more effectively with nursing home residents with dementia. *Gerontologist, 39,* 546–558.

Mills, P. J., Yu, H., Ziegler, M. G., Patterson, T., & Grant, I. (1999). Vulnerable caregivers of patients with Alzheimer's disease have a deficit in circulating CD62L-T lymphocytes. *Psychosomatic Medicine, 61,* 168–174.

Omnibus Budget Reconciliation Act of 1987. (1987). Publication No. 100–203, 483.15.

Orange, J. B., & Colton-Hudson, A. (1998). Enhancing communication in dementia of the Alzheimer's type. *Topics in Geriatric Rehabilitation, 14,* 56–75.

Ory, M. G., Hoffman, R. R., Yee, J. L., Tennstedt, S., & Schulz, R. (1999). Prevalence and impact of caregiving: A detailed comparison between dementia and nondementia caregivers. *Gerontologist, 39,* 177–185.

Paveza, G. J., Cohen, D., Eisdorfer, C., Freels, S., Semla, T., Ashford, J. W., et al. (1992). Severe family violence and Alzheimer's disease: Prevalence and risk factors. *Gerontologist, 32,* 493–497.

Pillemer, K., & Suitor, J. J. (1992). Violence and violent feelings: What causes them among family caregivers? *Journal of Gerontology, 47,* S165–S172.

Poulshock, S. W., & Deimling, G. T. (1984). Families caring for elders in residence: Issues in the measurement of burden. *Journal of Gerontology, 39,* 230–239.

Pruchno, R. A., Kleban, M. H., Michaels, J. E., & Dempsey, N. P. (1990). Mental and physical health of caregiving spouses: Development of a causal model. *Journal of Gerontology, 45,* 192–199.

Ripich, D. N. (1994). Functional communication with AD patients: A caregiver training program. *Alzheimer Disease and Associated Disorders, 8,* 95–109.

Ripich, D. N., Wycke, M., & Niles, S. (1995). Alzheimer's disease caregivers: The FOCUSED program. *Geriatric Nursing, 16,* 15–19.

Ripich, D. N., & Ziol, E. (1999). Training Alzheimer's disease caregivers for successful communication. *Clinical Gerontologist, 21,* 37–56.

Saxton, J., Kastango, K. B., Hugonot-Diener, L., Boller, F., Verny, M., Sarels, C. E., et al. (2005). Development of a short form of the Severe Impairment Battery. *American Journal of Geriatric Psychiatry, 13,* 999–1005.

Saxton, J., & Swihart, A. A. (1989). Neuropsychological assessment of the severely impaired elderly patient. *Clinics in Geriatric Medicine, 5,* 531–543.

Schumock, G. T. (1998). Economic considerations in the treatment and management of Alzheimer's disease. *American Journal Health-System Pharmacy, 55*(Suppl. 2), 17–21.

Schulz, R. (2000). *Handbook on dementia caregiving: Evidence-based interventions for family caregivers.* New York: Springer.

Schulz, R., & Beach, S. (1999). Caregiving as a risk factor for mortality: The caregiver health effects study. *Journal of the American Medical Association, 282,* 2215–2219.

Schulz, R., & Martire, L. M. (2004). Family caregiving of persons with dementia: Prevalence, health effects, and support strategies. *American Journal of Geriatric Psychiatry, 12,* 240–249.

Schulz, R., Newsom, J., Mittelmark, M., Burton, L., Hirsch, C., & Jackson S. (1997). Health effects of caregiving: the caregiver health effects study: An ancillary study of the Cardiovascular Health Study. *Annals of Behavioral Medicine, 19,* 110–116.

Schulz, R., O'Brien, A. T., Bookwala, J., & Fleissner, K. (1995). Psychiatric and physical morbidity effects of dementia caregiving: Prevalence, correlates, and causes. *Gerontologist, 35,* 771–791.

Shaw W. S., Patterson, T. L., Semple, S. J., Ho, S., Irwin, M. R., Hauger, R. L., et al. (1997). Lon-gitudinal analysis of multiple indicators of health decline among spousal caregivers. *Annals of Behavioral Medicine, 19,* 101–109.

Shulman, M. D., & Mandel, E. (1988). Communication training of relatives and friends of institutionalized elderly persons. *Gerontologist, 28,* 797–799.

Sparks, M. B., Farran, C. J., Donner, E., & Keane-Hagerty, E. (1998). Wives, husbands, and daughters of dementia patients: predictors of caregivers' mental and physical health. *Scholarly Inquiry for Nursing Practice, 12,* 221–234.

Stuckey, J. C., Neundorfer, M. M., & Smyth, K. A. (1996). Burden and well-being: the same coin or related currency. *Gerontologist, 36,* 686–693.

Teri, L. (1997). Behavior and caregiver burden: Behavioral problems in patients with Alzheimer's disease and its association with caregiver distress. *Alzheimer Disease and Associated Disorders, 11*(Suppl. 4), 35–38.

Teri, L., Logsdon, R. G., Uomoto, J., & McCurry, S. M.(1997). Behavioral treatment of depression in dementia patients: A controlled clinical trial. *Journals of Gerontology Series B-Psychological Sciences and Social Sciences, 52,* 159–166.

Vedhara, K., Cox, N. K., Wilcock, G. K., Perks, P., Hunt, M., Anderson, S., et al. (1999). Chronic stress in elderly carers of dementia patients and antibody response to influenza vaccination. *Lancet, 353,* 627–631.

Wiggins, J. S., Goldberg, L. R., & Appelbaum, M. (1971). MMPI content scale: Interpretive norms and correlations with other scales. *Journal of Consulting and Clinical Psychology, 37,* 403–410.

Zarit, S. H., Reever, K. E., & Bach-Peterson, J. (1980). Relatives of the impaired elderly: correlates of feelings of burden. *Gerontologist, 20,* 649–655.

Zarit, S. H., Todd, P. A., & Zarit, J. M. (1986). Subjective burden of husbands and wives as caregivers: A longitudinal study. *Gerontologist, 26,* 260–266.

Zientz, J., Rackley, A., Bond Chapman, S., Hopper, T., Mahendra, N., Kim, E., et al. (in press). Evidence-based practice recommendations for dementia: Educating caregivers on Alzheimer's disease and training communication strategies. *Journal of Medical Speech-Language Pathology.*

Providing Culturally Sensitive Care

Speech-language pathologists, who are certified by the American Speech-Language-Hearing Association (ASHA), have an ethical obligation to provide culturally appropriate services to their patients/clients. The following is a summary of the knowledge needed for achieving cultural competence (ASHA, 2004):

- Knowledge of the influence of one's own beliefs and biases in providing effective services.
- Respect for an individual's race, ethnic background, lifestyle, physical/mental ability, religious beliefs/practices, and heritage.
- Influence of the client's/patient's traditions, customs, values, and beliefs related to providing effective services.
- Impact of assimilation and/or acculturation processes on the identification, assessment, treatment, and management of communication disorders/differences.
- Recognition of the clinician's own limitations in education/training in providing services to a client/patient from a particular cultural and/or linguistic community.
- Appropriate intervention and assessment strategies and materials, such as food, objects, and/or activities that do not violate the patient's/client's values and/or that may form a constructive bridge between the client's/patient's home culture and community or communication environment.

- Appropriate communications with clients/patients, caregivers, and significant others, so that the values imparted in the counseling are consistent with those of the client/patient.
- The need to refer/consult with other service providers with appropriate cultural and linguistic proficiency, including a cultural informant/broker, as it pertains to a specific client/patient.
- Ethical responsibilities of the clinician concerning the provision of culturally and linguistically appropriate services.

ASHA (2004) specifies that it is the clinician's role to: "Advocate for and empower consumers, families, and communities at risk for or with communication/swallowing/balance disorders. This includes knowledge and skills related to:

- Community resources available for the dissemination of educational, health, and medical information pertinent to particular communities.
- High risk factors for communication/swallowing/balance disorders in particular communities.
- Prevention strategies for communication/cognition/swallowing/balance disorders in particular communities.
- The impact of regulatory processes on service delivery to communities.

- Incidence and prevalence of culturally-based risk factors (e.g., hypertension, heart disease, diabetes, fetal alcohol syndrome) resulting in greater likelihood for communication/cognition/swallowing/balance disorders.
- Appropriate consumer information and marketing materials/tools for outreach, service provision, and education" (p. 2).

Knowledge of One's Own Culture

The *first step* in achieving intercultural competence is to *become aware of one's own cultural orientation*. This knowledge is essential for understanding how others perceive and respond to you. To gain insight to your cultural identity, ask yourself the following questions.

1. What is the relative importance of the group/family compared to the individual?
2. What do you think are the roles of men, women, and children?
3. How important is your work in defining who you are?
4. How much do you value class distinctions and status markers?
5. What do you believe should be the relation of humans to the natural world?
6. How important is tradition?
7. What, if any, is your religion?
8. What is your style of communication—direct, indirect, assertive, nonassertive, fast or slow paced?
9. What language do you speak?
10. What is your orientation to activity? Do you focus on "being" or "becoming?

11. Are you relaxed about time or is keeping a schedule important to you?

Your answers to these questions, derived from the basic parameters that differentiate cultures (Brislin, 1994), should give you some insight to your cultural identity. Many readers will be Americans and have many, if not most of the values that characterize American culture. The following is a summary of values held by the majority of Americans (Kohls, 1984).

- Individualism and independence: Each individual is unique and has a right to make his or her decisions and a right to privacy.
- Time is valuable: Achievement of goals depends on productive use of time.
- Equality is a cherished value: Everyone should have the opportunity to succeed.
- Self-reliance: Respect is given for achievements not the accident of birth.
- Future-oriented.
- Work and action oriented: Wasting time is bad.
- Materialistic and acquisitive: Material goods are just rewards of hard work.
- Directness, openness, and honesty: Truth is more important than saving face.
- Change is linked to progress.
- Rank, status, and authority are not as highly valued as in many other cultures.
- Competition is good.
- Informality: Informality typifies American culture and influences behavior, dress, and language use.
- Personal control over the environment: People should control their environment.

Most human conflict stems from differences in values. By understanding a client's culture and how it differs from your own, you are better able to identify areas of possible conflict. You also are in a position to know how to modify your behavior to make your client feel comfortable. Thus, the *second step* in achieving intercultural competence is *developing an understanding of other cultures*. The following is an overview of the characteristics of the major cultural groups in the United States.

Characteristics of Major U.S. Cultural Groups

Four major cultural groups in the United States are: African American, American Indian, Asian, and Hispanic. Paniagua's (2005) book, *Assessing and Treating Culturally Diverse Clients*, contains a discussion of the characteristics of these groups. Paniagua emphasizes, and rightly so, that generalizations about a client's cultural group may not apply to the client. Members of a cultural group differ in myriad ways, among them: migration and relocation history, acculturation, facility with native and other languages, family composition, education, socioeconomic level, and degree of adherence to cultural beliefs (Cheng, 1993; Paniagua, 2005; Wong, 1985). Nonetheless, Paniagua's guide is a useful starting point for understanding these cultures.

African Americans

In the 2000 census, approximately 34.6 million Americans self-identified as "Black or African American" and another 1.8 million specified their race as Black or African American in combination with one or more other races (Grieco & Cassidy, 2001; U.S. Bureau of the Census, 2000). Although the census asked respondents for race designation and used these terms, clinicians should be aware that race designation and racial terminology can be offensive. Of the Census terminology, the term reputed to be most acceptable is African American because it lacks reference to color and emphasizes cultural heritage (Gibbs, Huang, & Associates, 2003; Ho, 1992; Paniagua, 2005; Sue & Sue, 2003).

Cultural Characteristics

- Family (nuclear and extended, biologic, and nonbiologic) may be important.
- Roles of men, women, and children are flexible. The family head may not be the father.
- For many, religion and its celebration are integral to daily life.
- Some members have folk beliefs.
- Black or African-American English is widely spoken.
- Some individuals have a "healthy paranoia" about members of other cultural groups because of past experiences.
- Celebrations, such as Kwanza, help establish African-American identity.

Considerations in Providing Culturally Sensitive Care

- Develop trust and establish expectations.
- Do not focus on problems but rather solutions.
- Show flexibility.
- Be supportive rather than authoritative and judgmental.
- Acknowledge the role of family.
- Emphasize empowerment.
- Remember that Black or African-American English are not substandard forms of English, merely different forms.

American Indians

More than 4 million people reported being American Indian or Alaskan Native in the 2000 census (U.S. Bureau of the Census, 2000). This group comprises 556 federally recognized tribes that speak more than 200 different languages making it a very heterogeneous group. Consequently, it is extremely hard to generalize about American Indian culture. Cognizant of this fact, Paniagua (2005) and Jervis, Cullum, and Manson (2006) offer the following considerations in treating American Indians.

Cultural Characteristics

- Clan and tribal relationships are important.
- The family unit may have primacy over the individual.
- Clients often bring family members with them for medical care.
- Sharing (of material goods, time, and solutions to problems) is valued.
- Less emphasis on clock time and more on the time it takes to complete an event.
- Many American Indians place emphasis on nonverbal forms of communication and listening may be more important than talking.
- Working together as a group is generally important.
- Many American Indians seek treatment from traditional healers and prefer to keep the procedures used by traditional healers to themselves.
- Individuals who reside on reservations, or live in rural areas, may be more traditional than those residing in urban areas.
- Much cultural life and many traditions revolve around nature.
- Children are encouraged to make their own decisions.

Considerations in Providing Culturally Sensitive Care

- Take time to gain the individual's trust.
- Be aware that, for many tribes, looking directly into the client's eyes is offensive.
- Many American Indians shake hands with a light grip.
- Avoid being too formal in demeanor, dress, and testing environment.
- Many American Indians may be reluctant to divulge personal information, especially if they are not assured of confidentiality.
- Avoid taking too many notes, it can be seen as disrespectful.
- Avoid technical jargon.
- Pay attention to nonverbal behavior.
- Don't ask too many questions early in the relationship. Use an indirect approach to discover issues.
- Recognize that the client may be reluctant to ask questions because of a belief that to do so would be disrespectful.
- Avoid rushing the client.
- Be flexible about time.
- Respect the role of traditional healers.

Hispanic-Americans

In 2000, approximately 35.3 million Hispanics resided in the United States (U.S. Bureau of the Census, 2000). The majority were Mexican Americans (58.5%). Puerto Ricans were the second largest group (3.4 million) followed by Cubans (1.2 million). Approximately 1.7 million reported Central American heritage and 1.4 million reported South American heritage. By the year 2020, the Hispanic population will approximate 54.3 million (Dana, 1993). California has the largest Hispanic population followed by Texas and New York. The term Hispanic is generally used to refer to individuals who label themselves as such or are descended from people who were from Spain, Mexico, South America, Central America, or the Caribbean.

Cultural Characteristics

- For men, the personal quality of machismo is important. It connotes physical strength, masculinity, and respect from others.
- For women, the personal quality of marianismo is valued. Marianismo connotes submissiveness, obedience, dependence, gentleness, and virginity before marriage.
- For most Hispanic-Americans, family relationships are paramount and the father is the head of the family.
- Warmth in interpersonal relationships is valued.
- Fatalism, or belief in divine providence, is a common characteristic.
- Some members of Hispanic culture hold folk beliefs.

Considerations Important in Providing Culturally Appropriate Care

- Take time to determine the degree of the client's acculturation early in your relationship.
- Explore the individual's belief about the cause of mental health problems and be prepared to function in both the client's belief system and the scientific system.
- Display respect for the client's culture.
- Avoid being "distant" and too formal when working with Hispanic individuals. Take time to acknowledge the person and family before proceeding with testing and counseling.
- Acknowledge the importance of family in solving problems.
- Avoid interrupting and rushing the client.

Asian-Americans

The generic term, "Asian," is widely used to refer to three major subgroups of the U.S. population: Asian American, Asian Pacific Islanders, and Southeast Asian refugees (Chung, Kim, & Abreu; 2004; Iwamasa, 2003). Asian-American includes Japanese, Chinese, Filipino, Asian Indians, and Koreans. Asian Pacific Islanders includes Hawaiians, Samoans, and Guamanians. Southeast Asian refugees include Vietnamese, Cambodians, and Laotians. In the 2000 census, 10.3 million individuals self-identified as Asian only and 398,835 self-identified as Native Hawaiian or Pacific Islander. Approximately 1.6 million individuals reported being Asian in combination with one or more other races (Grieco & Cassidy, 2001).

Cultural Characteristics

- Collectivistic: The needs of the family take precedence over the needs/desires of the individual.
- Family relationships are strong.
- The role of many Asian women is obedience to their husbands and fathers.
- Children are expected to respect their parents and follow their parent's desires.
- Many Asians avoid expressing family problems to nonfamily members.
- Saving face is extremely important.
- Ancestry is very meaningful and ancestor worship is prevalent.
- Sharing success is expected.
- Shame may be used to enforce family values.
- Silence (a sign of respect) and lack of eye contact are widely used forms of indirect communication.
- Mental problems may be expressed in somatic terms (e.g., stomach problem, rash).

- Many women do not shake hands with men. Bowing may be more appropriate than hand-shaking.
- Expertise is valued.

Considerations in Providing Culturally Appropriate Care

- Use your professional title.
- Exhibit your expertise (display credentials).
- Mention prior experience.
- Establish expectations
- Emphasize family needs.
- Avoid actions and words that produce loss of face or shame.
- Respect the authority of men.
- Focus on practical solutions.
- Avoid being too informal.

Using Interpreters

Clinicians who treat a diverse clientele often need an interpreter. The following are guidelines for using interpreters.

- Whenever possible, use a trained interpreter with knowledge of clinical methods.
- Speak in easily translatable language.
- Avoid jargon and technical words.
- Talk directly to the patient and not the interpreter.
- Avoid nonverbal behaviors that may be misinterpreted.
- Periodically check that the client and family understand you.
- Reinforce verbal information with written materials.
- Be cautious about using a family member or friend to translate, especially a very young individual. Lack of objectivity can be an issue.
- Meet with the interpreter prior to the session.

- Explain your purpose.
- Decide on forms of address.
- Explain the topic areas to be covered.
- Estimate session length.
- Emphasize the importance of translating exactly what the client says.
- If the interpreter is bicultural, ask if there are any culturally sensitive factors you should be aware of.
- Stress the confidentiality of information shared in the session.
- Advise the interpreter that the patient's responses may not make sense.

References

American Speech-Language-Hearing Association. (2004). Knowledge and skills needed by speech-language pathologists and audiologists to provide culturally and linguistically appropriate services. *ASHA Supplement, 24,* 1–7. Available online at: http://www.asha.org/members/deskref-journals/deskref/DRVol4.htm#ks

Brislin, R. (1994). *Understanding cultural diversity: A model* [Videotape 1]. Tucson: University of Arizona National Center for Neurogenic Communication Disorders.

Cheng, L. L. (1993). Asian-American cultures. In D. E. Battle (Ed.), *Communication disorders in multicultural populations* (pp. 38–77). Stoneham, MA: Butterworth-Heinemann.

Chung, R. H., Kim, B. S. K., & Abreu, J. M. (2004). Asian American Multidimensional Acculturation Scale: Development, factor analysis, reliability, and validity. *Cultural Diversity and Ethnic Minority Psychology, 10,* 66–80.

Dana, R. H. (1993). *Multicultural assessment perspectives for professional psychology.* Boston: Allyn & Bacon.

Gibbs, J. T., Huang, L. N., & Associates. (2003). *Children of color: Psychological interventions with culturally diverse youth* (2nd ed). San Francisco: Jossey-Bass.

Grieco, E. M., & Cassidy, R. C. (2001). *Overview of race and Hispanic origin: 2000 (Census 2000 Brief C2KBR/01-1)*. Washington, DC: U.S. Department of Commerce, Economics and Statistics Administration, Bureau of the Census.

Ho, M. K. (1992). *Minority children and adolescents in therapy*. Newbury Park, CA: Sage.

Iwamasa, G. Y. (2003). Recommendations for the treatment of Asian American/Pacific Islander populations. In Council of National Psychological Associations for the Advancement of Ethnic Minority Interests (Ed.), *Psychological treatment of ethnic minority populations* (pp. 8–12). Washington, DC: Association of Black Psychologists.

Jervis, L. L., Cullum, C. M., & Manson, S. M. (2006). American Indians, Cognitive Assessment, and Dementia. In G. Yeo & D. Gallagher-Thompson (Eds.), *Ethnicity and the dementias* (pp. 87–101). New York: Routledge, Taylor & Francis Group.

Kohls, L. R. (1984). *The values Americans live by* [pamphlet]. Washington, DC: Meridan House International.

Paniagua, F. A. (2005). *Assessing and treating culturally diverse clients* (3rd ed.). Thousand Oaks, CA: Sage Publications.

Sue, D. W., & Sue, D. (2003). *Counseling the culturally diverse*. New York: John Wiley & Sons.

U.S. Bureau of the Census (2000). *Statistical abstract of the United States* (119th ed.). Washington, DC: U.S. Department of Commerce.

Wong, H. Z. (1985). Training for mental health service providers to Southeast Asian refugees: Models, strategies and curricula. In T. C. Owan (Ed.), *Southeast Asian mental health treatment, prevention services, training and research* (pp. 345–390). Washington, DC: National Institute of Mental Health.

Resources on Cultural Diversity

Books

Battle, D. E. (2001). *Communication disorders in multicultural populations* (3rd ed.). Stoneham, MA: Butterworth-Heinemann.

Brislin, R. (1981). *Cross-cultural encounters: Face-to-face interaction*. Elmsford, NY: Pergamon.

Lustig, M. W., & Koester, J. (2006). *Intercultural competence* (5th ed.). Boston: Pearson, Allyn & Bacon.

Paniagua, F. A. (2005). *Assessing and treating culturally diverse clients*. Thousand Oaks, CA: Sage Publications.

Yeo, G., & Gallagher-Thompson, D. (Eds.). (2006). *Ethnicity and the dementias* (2nd ed.). New York: Routledge, Taylor & Francis Group.

Other

American Speech-Language-Hearing Association. (2002). Communication development and disorders in multicultural populations: Readings and related materials. Available online at: http://www.asha.org/about/Leadership-projects/multicultural/readings/

American Speech-Language-Hearing Association. (2007). Self-assessment for cultural competence. Available online at: http://asha.org/about/leadership-projects/multicultural/Gotit.htm

U.S. Department of Health and Human Services, OPHS Office of Minority Health (2001, March). *National Standards for Culturally and Linguistically Appropriate Services in Health Care*. Washington, DC: Author.

Index

A